Chronic Illness
Research and Theory for Nursing Practice

Ruth Bernstein Hyman, PhD, is a founding editor of *Scholarly Inquiry for Nursing Practice* and has been a consulting reviewer to numerous other journals. She has been a member of the graduate faculty of Adelphi University and the faculty of the department of Epidemiology and Social Medicine at the Albert Einstein College of Medicine. She has consulted and authored books, reports, and articles in the fields of Nursing, Mental Health, Evaluation, Instrument Development, and Epidemiology. She holds a PhD in Educational Research. Her specialties are measurement, statistics, adult developmental psychology, and mammography utilization.

Juliet M. Corbin, DNSc, RN, FNPC, is currently a lecturer in the School of Nursing at San Jose State University, where she has taught clinical and lecture courses to undergraduate and graduate students for over 20 years. In addition, she teaches clinical students in a Nurse Managed Center run under the auspices of San Jose State School of Nursing, where, with her group of undergraduate students, she is able to implement a program of chronic illness care based upon the trajectory model. She has also more recently become affiliated with the International Qualitative Research Institute in Alberta Canada, where she teaches workshops in qualitative analysis as an adjunct professor. Her clinical specialty is community gerontology and her focus is on chronic illness management. She has written articles, books, and made presentations worldwide about chronic illness and qualitative methodology. Her latest research concerns the impact of life-threatening, early-onset cardiac disease on people's lives.

Editors of *Scholarly Inquiry for Nursing Practice*

Ruth Bernstein Hyman, PhD, Independent Scholar
Elizabeth R. Lenz, PhD, FAAN, Columbia University School of Nursing
Kathleen Southerton, RNC, PhD, SUNY University Hospital and Medical Center
Janice L. Thompson, RN, PhD, University of Southern Maine
Pierre Woog, PhD, Adelphi University

Chronic Illness
Research and Theory for Nursing Practice

Ruth Bernstein Hyman, PhD
Juliet M. Corbin, DNSc, RN, FNPC
Editors

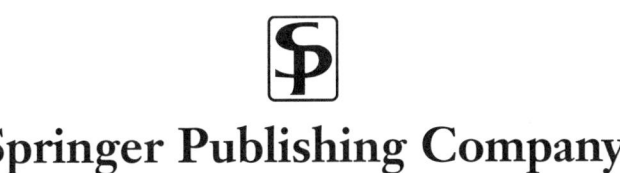

Springer Publishing Company

Copyright © 2001 by Springer Publishing Company, Inc.

All rights reserved

No part of this publication may be reproduced, stored in a retrieval system, or transmitted in any form or by any means, electronic, mechanical, photocopying, recording, or otherwise, without the prior permission of Springer Publishing Company, Inc.

Springer Publishing Company, Inc.
536 Broadway
New York, NY 10012-3955

Acquisitions Editor: Ruth Chasek
Production Editor: Helen Song
Cover design by Susan Hauley

00 01 02 03 04 / 5 4 3 2 1

Library of Congress Cataloging-in-Publication Data

Chronic illness: research and theory for nursing practice / Ruth Bernstein Hyman and Juliet M. Corbin, editors.
    p. ; cm.
  A compilation of articles from the journal Scholarly inquiry for nursing practice.
  Includes bibliographical references and index.
  ISBN 0-8261-1353-2 (hardcover)
    1. Chronic diseases—Nursing. 2. Chronic diseases—Social aspects.
3. Nurse and patient. I. Hyman, Ruth Bernstein. II. Corbin, Juliet M., 1942– III. Scholarly inquiry for nursing practice.
  [DNLM: 1. Chronic Disease—nursing—Collected Works.
2. Chronic Disease—psychology—Collected Works. 3. Clinical Nursing Research—methods—Collected Works. 4. Nurse-Patient Relations—Collected Works. WY 152 C55758 2000]
  RT120.C45 C495 2000
  616'.044—dc21   00-022099

Printed in the United States of America

Contents

Contributors		*vii*
Prologue by Ruth Bernstein Hyman		*ix*
1	Introduction and Overview: Chronic Illness and Nursing *Juliet M. Corbin*	1
2	A Description of the Nature and Dynamics of Coping Following Coronary Bypass Surgery *Nancy S. Redeker* *Response by Susan R. Gortner*	16
3	Women Recovering from Coronary Artery Bypass Surgery *Mary H. Hawthorne* *Response by Sally H. Rankin* *Response by Jonathan N. Tobin*	36
4	Health-Promoting Behaviors and Quality of Life Among Individuals With Multiple Sclerosis *Alexa K. Stuifbergen* *Response by N. Margaret Wineman and Kathleen M. Schwetz*	75
5	Families and Children's Chronic Conditions: Knowledge Development and Methodological Considerations *Virginia E. Hayes* *Response by Bonnie Holaday* *Response by Janet A. Deatrick*	106

6 Toward a Practice Theory of Caring for
   Patients with Chronic Skin Disease   152
   Marit Kirkevold
   Response by Nancy E. White and Judith R. Richter

7 Coping Amid Uncertainty:
   An Illness Trajectory Perspective   180
   Carolyn L. Wiener and Marylin J. Dodd
   Response by Marilyn T. Oberst

8 Chronic Sorrow: A Lifespan Concept   202
   Carolyn L. Lindgren, Mary L. Burke,
   Margaret A. Hainsworth, and Georgene G. Eakes
   Response by Ida M. Martinson

9 Operationalizing the Corbin and Strauss Trajectory
   Model for Elderly Clients with Chronic Illness   223
   Linda A. Robinson, Catherine Bevil, Virginia Arcangelo,
   JoAnne Reifsnyder, Nancy Rothman, and Suzanne Smeltzer
   Response by Juliet M. Corbin

10 End-of-Life Family Decision-Making From
   Disclosure of HIV Through Bereavement   245
   Barbara M. Stewart
   Response by Kathleen M. Nokes
   Response by Anselm L. Strauss

11 Epilogue: A Proactive Model of Health Care   294
   Juliet M. Corbin and Julie Cheitlin Cherry

Index   *301*

Contributors

Virginia Arcangelo, PhD, NPC
Cherry Hill Family Medical Associates
Cherry Hill, New Jersey

Catherine A. Bevil, RN, EdD,
College of Nursing,
University of Nebraska Medical Center, Omaha

Mary L. Burke, DNSc, RN
Department of Nursing
Rhode Island College
Providence, Rhode Island

Julie Cheitlin Cherry, RN, MSN
Health Hero Network, Inc.
Mountain View, California

Janet A. Deatrick, PhD, RN, FAAN
University of Pennsylvania School of Nursing
Philadelphia, Pennsylvania

Marylin J. Dodd, PhD, MSN, RN, FAAN
University of California San Francisco

Georgene G. Eakes, RN, EdD
East Carolina University School of Nursing
Greenville, North Carolina

Susan R. Gortner, PhD, RN, FAAN
University of California San Francisco (Emeritus)

Margaret A. Hainsworth, PhD, RNC, CS
Rhode Island College (Emeritus)
Providence, Rhode Island

Mary H. Hawthorne, PhD, RN
Duke University School of Nursing
Durham, North Carolina

Virginia E. Hayes, RN, PhD
School of Nursing
University of Victoria
Vancouver, British Columbia

Bonnie Holaday, DNS, RN, FAAN
Clemson University School of Nursing
Clemson, South Carolina

Marit Kirkevold
Institute of Nursing Science
University of Oslo, Norway

Carolyn L. Lindgren
Wayne State University College of Nursing
Detroit, Michigan

Ida M. Martinson, PhD, RN, FAAN
University of California San Francisco

Kathleen M. Nokes, PhD, RN
Hunter-Bellevue School of Nursing
New York, New York

Marilyn T. Oberst, PhD, RN, FAAN
Wayne State University College of Nursing
Detroit, Michigan

Sally H. Rankin, RN-C, PhD, FAAN
University of California San Francisco

Nancy S. Redeker, PhD, RN
Rutgers, the State University of New Jersey
Newark, New Jersey

JoAnne Reifsnyder, PhD, RN, AOCN
Ethos Consulting Group LLC
Merchantville, New Jersey

Judith R. Richter, RN, PhD
University of Northern Colorado School of Nursing
Greeley, Colorado

Linda Robinson, PhD, RNCS
Hahn School of Nursing and Health Science
University of San Diego

Nancy Rothman, EdD, RN
Temple University
Philadelphia, Pennsylvania

Kathleen M. Schwetz, RN, MS
Mellen Center for Multiple Sclerosis Treatment and Research
Cleveland Clinic Foundation
Cleveland, Ohio

Suzanne Smeltzer, RN, EdD, FAAN
Villanova University College of Nursing
Villanova, Pennsylvania

Barbara M. Stewart, PhD, RN
Pace University
Pleasantville, New York

Anselm Strauss, PhD
Deceased

Alexa K. Stuifbergen, PhD, RN, FAAN
University of Texas School of Nursing
Austin, Texas

Jonathan N. Tobin, PhD
Clinical Directors Network
New York, New York

Nancy E. White, RN, PhD
University of Northern Colorado School of Nursing
Greeley, Colorado

Carolyn L. Wiener, PhD
School of Nursing
University of California San Francisco

N. Margaret Wineman, RN, PhD
University of Akron College of Nursing
Akron, Ohio

Prologue

The Editors of *Scholarly Inquiry for Nursing Practice* (SINP) are very pleased to present *Chronic Illness: Research and Theory for Nursing Practice*. This volume is a compilation of the best articles on the topic of chronic illness that have previously appeared in the journal. To assure quality, coherence, and currency of the compilation we invited Juliet Corbin, R.N., D.N.Sc., a recognized expert in the field, to join in producing this volume.

This book represents a continuation for us of a long history with Juliet Corbin and Anselm Strauss. In 1992, Springer Publishing Company published a special issue of SINP edited by Pierre Woog on "The Chronic Illness Trajectory Framework" in book format. The book won book of the year awards from both *The American Journal of Nursing* and *Nurse Practitioner* and was also translated into both German and Japanese.

Since then, both Corbin and Strauss have responded to many of our articles related to chronic illness and to their trajectory framework. We sorely miss the possibility of Anselm Strauss's contribution to the current project due to his death in 1996, but are very pleased that Juliet Corbin consented to take on the task, and that she invited Julie Cheitlin Cherry to coauthor the Epilogue.

Corbin became interested in the area of chronic illness while working on her doctoral dissertation in 1979 and has been doing research, teaching, and practice in the area ever since. Her publications in the area of chronic illness include two books coauthored with Anselm Strauss, *Unending Work and Care* (1988) and *Shaping a New Health Care System* (1988), as well as numerous articles. Over the years her emphasis on chronic illness has broadened to include not only its management but the potential role of nursing in its prevention, primary through tertiary.

For this volume, Corbin has assembled a group of articles and interpreted them in light of the phases of the chronic illness trajectory framework that she formulated with Anselm Strauss and with a keen eye toward the special, often invisible, contribution of nursing to the treatment of chronic illness. In the epilogue, she and Cherry build on the actual and potential contributions of nursing to present their vision for a proactive model of health care.

I have been responsible for working with Juliet Corbin to produce this volume. Since it is compiled from many years (primarily the first 10) of *Scholarly Inquiry for Nursing Practice*, however, it results not only from the work of Corbin, Cherry, and the authors whose articles are included. It is a product of all editors of *Scholarly Inquiry for Nursing Practice*, current and past, who are listed below.

Ruth Bernstein Hyman, Ph.D.

Current SINP Editors

Ruth Bernstein Hyman, Ph.D.
Elizabeth R. Lenz, Ph.D., F.A.A.N.
Kathleen Southerton, R.N.C., Ph.D.
Janice L. Thompson, R.N., Ph.D.
Pierre Woog, Ph.D.

Editors Emeritae

Harriet R. Feldman, Ph.D., R.N., F.A.A.N.
Audrey G. Gift, R.N., Ph.D., F.A.A.N.
Ruth Beall Harris, Ph.D., R.N., C.C.R.N.
Dorothea R. Hays, Ed.D., R.N., C.S.
Barbara Kos-Munson, Ph.D., R.N., C.S.
Carol Ann Mitchell, Ed.D., R.N.

Chapter 1

Introduction and Overview: Chronic Illness and Nursing

Juliet M. Corbin

In these times of rapid change one thing remains the same: The existence of chronic illness. A chronic illness is defined as any physical or mental condition that requires long-term (over 6 months) monitoring and/or management to control symptoms and to shape the course of the disease. Although the incidence tends to increase with age, chronic conditions can be found among all age groups, socioeconomic levels, and genders. Despite the emphasis on genetic research and the promise of new cures, it is highly unlikely that chronic conditions will disappear soon. In fact, their rate is expected to increase during the next decades. By the year 2030 it is projected that 150 million Americans will have one or more chronic conditions. Of that number, 42 million will have activity limitations restricting their ability to work and live independently (Institute for Health & Aging University of California San Francisco, 1996, p. 8). The conditions on the rise are those associated with the stresses and strains of modern living, which over time take their toll on the human body, such as mental illness, lung, and cardiac disease ("Chronic Illnesses," September, 16, 1996). At the same time, because of advances in modern medicine, persons with chronic conditions are living longer and more productive lives. Addressing their varied health care needs is one of *the major challenges* facing the present health care delivery system.

This volume on chronic illness has been assembled to illustrate the complexity and range of problems that result from living with chronic illness. *More important* these chapters demonstrate that nurses do more than carry out technical tasks. They do highly sophisticated problem solving, teaching, counseling, monitoring, advocating, early intervention, and referral making, all with the aim of helping patients and their families to gain and maintain control over their illness conditions, and in doing so, their lives.

Unfortunately, much of what nurses do as part of chronic illness care is either invisible to or undervalued by society, because outcomes are difficult to sort out and measure. With medical interventions, such as the use of antihypertensive drugs to control elevations in blood pressure, it is relatively easy to demonstrate a cause and effect relationship. The blood pressure either goes down or it doesn't. Nursing interventions, however, are only one part of the total care provided to chronic patients. They are often integrated into a range of services provided by a team of health care workers consisting of physicians, social workers, and a variety of therapists. What is special and different about nursing is that nurses teach patients how to integrate their regimens into their lives and how to recognize signs of complications. Nurses pick up on the subtle signs that indicate changes in the status of an illness and advise patients when to seek medical assistance. These are *indirect and intangible actions.* Yet, when it comes to chronic illness management, these indirect actions are just as vital as medical regimens. Regimens are useless unless persons carry them out and doing so is dependent upon patients' understanding and acceptance of their disease and the regimens. It is in providing the knowledge and support *that lead to patient understanding and acceptance* that nurses have the potential to make one of their greatest contributions to health care management.

Another reason why chronic illness care is undervalued and unrecognized by society is that the work is not very dramatic. The adrenaline rush that comes from saving a patient's life in the Emergency Room or in the Intensive Care Unit is lacking when it comes to patient teaching or case managing. Yet, nurses who work with the physically and mentally chronically ill realize that the care they provide is anything but dull and routine. The problems that persons with chronic conditions face each day are so varied and complex that in order to manage them nurses must draw upon their entire repertoire of skills and knowledge. They must push the boundaries of their practice to the limits, challenging the very health care delivery system that they work in. Anyone can apply an antibiotic to the skin or insert a Foley catheter. Patients and their families perform these tasks and many more difficult ones every day. Nurses, on the other hand, incorporate assessing, teaching, counseling, comforting, advocating for, advising, and case managing into the performance of these hands-on skills. They provide a total package of care that only professional nurses can provide.

The strength of the following chapters is in their cumulative impact. Reading them one after the other makes one realize the actual and potential contributions professional nurses do and can make to patients' management of chronic conditions. This recognition is especially important considering what one young man with early onset cardiac disease recently related in an interview, "They thought that when they stabilized me and sent me home that it was all over, but that [coming home] was just the beginning." (Personal communication, March 12, 1999.) As he dramatically conveys, surviving a crisis is just the entry into a longer trajectory. Afterwards comes living with a chronic condition, including all its ups and downs, and that is where nursing comes in.

To capture the complexity of living with a chronic condition the term trajectory was borrowed from the physical sciences (Corbin & Strauss 1988, 1992; Glaser & Strauss, 1965). A trajectory is defined as a course of illness over time, *plus the actions* taken by patients, families, and health professionals to manage or shape that course. Interestingly enough, in this day of medical specialization and compartmentalization, nursing is the one profession that stretches across the entire trajectory. Nurses can be found in all settings: hospitals, homes, rehabilitation units, hospices, doctor's offices and clinics, and a variety of other agencies. It was to nurses that the young man quoted above turned when he began to rebuild his life. Uncertain about what activities he could and could not resume and to what degree, he turned to nurses for guidance. Why nurses? He replied, "because they were always there for him." They were there around the clock when he was hospitalized and it was they who checked in on him when he returned home.

Over time, the course of chronic conditions tends to vary, unless the condition is very mild and invariable. Symptoms increase and decrease; physiological status changes. To capture the dynamic and changing character of chronic conditions, the concept of phasing has been added to trajectory. Nine different trajectory phases have been identified. See Table 1.1 for a list of these phases.

The chapters in this book are arranged to highlight some of these different phases. Not all phases of chronic illness are represented, as the chapters (which originated as articles in the journal *Scholarly Inquiry for Nursing Practice*) were not written with the Corbin and Strauss Chronic Illness Trajectory Framework in mind. Rather, while reading the chapters, this author was struck by how they speak to different phases of chronic illness. In addition, the interventions suggested by the

TABLE 1.1 Trajectory Phases

Phase	Definition	Goal of Management
Pretrajectory	Genetic factors or lifestyle behaviors that place an individual or community at risk for the development of a chronic condition.	Prevent onset of chronic illness.
Trajectory onset	Appearance of noticeable symptoms, includes period of diagnostic workup and announcement by biographical limbo as person begins to discover and cope with implications of diagnosis.	Form appropriate trajectory projection and scheme.
Stable	Illness course and symptoms are under control. Biography and everyday life activities are being managed within limitations of illness. Illness management centers in the home.	Maintain stability of illness, biography, and everyday life activities.
Unstable	Period of inability to keep symptoms under control or reactiviation of illness. Biographical disruption and difficulty in carrying out everyday life activities. Adjustments being made in regimen with care usually taking place at home.	Return to stable.
Acute	Severe and unrelieved symptoms or the development of illness complications necessitating hospitalization or bed rest to bring illness course under control. Biography and everyday life activities temporarily placed on hold or drastically cut back.	Bring illness under control and resume normal biography and everyday life activites.

TABLE 1.1 *(continued)*

Phase	Definition	Goal of Management
Crisis	Critical or life-threatening situation requiring emergency treatment or care. Biography and everyday life activities suspended until crisis passes.	Remove life threat.
Comeback	A gradual return to an acceptable way of life within limits imposed by disability or illness. Involves physical healing, limitations stretching through rehabilitative procedures, psychosocial coming to terms, and biographical reengagement with adjustments in everyday life activities.	Set in motion and keep going the trajectory projection and scheme.
Downward	Illness course characterized by rapid or gradual physical decline accompanied by increasing disability or difficulty in controlling symptoms. Requires biographical adjustment and alterations in everyday life activity with each major downward step.	To adapt to increasing disability with each major downward turn.
Dying	Final days or weeks before death. Characterized by gradual or rapid shutting down of body processes, biographical disengagement and closure, and relinquishment of everyday life interests and activities.	To bring closure, let go, and die peacefully.

authors are very specific to problems by phase. The phases represented in this book are comeback, acute, stable, unstable, downward, and dying phases of illness.

Comeback Phase

The first two chapters pertain to the comeback phase of chronic illness. These are the chapters by Redeker (1992) and Hawthorne (1993). Comeback refers to a process of returning to a satisfactory way of life following an acute or crisis phase of a chronic condition within any residual physical or psychosocial limits imposed by the condition. The work of comeback is threefold. It involves physical recovery, limitations stretching, and psychosocial reintegration (Corbin & Strauss, 1991). "Physical recovery" refers to the healing process that occurs after major body trauma. "Limitations stretching" refers to the formal rehabilitation process, and, just as important, to the discoveries made about the body once persons are at home and on their own. Often, they discover that they can stretch their limitations through repeated attempts and reach levels of activity higher than originally expected. But there are limits to how far one can stretch and the disabilities that remain must be lived with. "Psychosocial reintegration" refers to the psychological and social aspects of learning to live with those remaining limitations, plus the identity reconstitution that occurs as the illness and its ramifications are incorporated into the larger framework of persons' lives. Comeback is a gradual process and it is difficult to say whether or not it is ever fully achieved.

Though nurses are an important part of the rehabilitation team, their part in the comeback process is often obscured, occurring mainly behind the scenes. Their efforts are directed more at promoting patient rehabilitative efforts, teaching families, and coordinating the work of other professionals, rather than doing the actual rehabilitation work per se. Promoting comeback, however, is a complicated process that requires locating individuals and their families within the total framework of their lives, including the physical condition and psychological and social contexts, and then using that information to help patients embark and remain upon the comeback trail until they reach their potential. Nurses by virtue of "being there" are the ones to guide this process.

The chapter by Redeker (1992) with a response by Gortner (1992) brings out the salience of this last point. Redeker's research examined the dynamics of coping during the first 6 weeks after coronary artery bypass surgery. The sample consisted of 129 persons, including both men and women; however, the majority of the study participants were White, married males with a high school education or higher, and a mean age of 62. The findings revealed that persons use a variety of coping strategies following bypass surgery, the most frequently cited strategy being "seeks social support." The predominant coping style demonstrated was "problem-focused coping," indicating that persons attempt to take an *active* role in their recovery. It follows that the most appropriate nursing interventions during comeback are those that encourage social support seeking and self-care behaviors. These include: allowing more flexible visiting hours, making follow-up phone calls after discharge, monitoring and coaching the recovery process, exploring persons'- plans for recovery prior to surgery, and assessing individuals' coping styles and their appropriateness for the stage of recovery.

Cardiac disease has traditionally been viewed as a man's disease. As a consequence, early diagnosis of cardiac disease and the specialized problems of women after bypass surgery are often overlooked. Hawthorn's chapter and the accompanying responses by Rankin (1993) and Tobin (1993) bring out some of these issues. The findings are just as relevant today as they were at the time the research was conducted. Hawthorn utilized a qualitative approach in her research. The sample consisted of 10 women recovering from bypass surgery. The relevance of this study lies in the gender differences discovered by Hawthorn when she compared the findings from the study of women with those derived from her previous study of men. Perhaps the most troublesome finding was "delayed access to care." Neither the research participants nor their health care providers recognized the seriousness of early cardiac symptoms. As a consequence, surgery often was performed under emergency conditions. Other gender differences also emerged. Women were found to be more passive and deferent in their communication with caregivers. They were less concerned than men about the surgery itself, but more disturbed by the surgical incision. Since women are the primary caregivers in families, their surgery caused considerable family disruption, creating the need to revamp family relationships. Also, in contrast to men, women gauged resumption of activity based more on level of fatigue and perceived role responsibilities than on medical guidelines. Though women made successful recoveries, both Hawthorne and Rankin emphasize that gender and family roles can significantly facilitate or hinder the recovery process. The research suggests a wide range of nursing interventions. These include teaching women about the early signs and symptoms of heart disease and how to be more assertive with their practitioners—plus helping them learn to read their body cues during the recovery period so that they may gauge their level of activity appropriately.

Stable Phase

The next two chapters, one by Stuifbergen (1995) and the other by Hayes (1998), relate to the stable phase of chronic illness. A stable phase denotes a period within the illness course during which symptoms, with small variations, are under control. For some conditions, stability indicates that the illness condition is in remission. When an illness is stable, most chronically ill persons do not consider themselves to be ill. They lead fairly normal lives within the limitations imposed by any disabilities. Reaching and maintaining stability, however, requires adhering to regimens and adopting lifestyles that promote health and well-being. In addition to being costly and time consuming, regimens can be tiresome and demanding. They often conflict with activities of daily living. The realities of life have a way of subverting even the best intentions to carry out regimens, increasing the possibility of complications and destabilization.

The chapter by Stuifbergen (1995), with a response by Wineman and Schwetz (1995), examines the relationship between health promotion behaviors and quality of life in persons diagnosed with multiple sclerosis. The sample consisted of 61, mostly White, well-educated, and married females. This study reinforces just how difficult it is to carry out health-promoting activities on a daily basis when one has a chronic condition. Fatigue, inconvenience, disabilities, lack of time and money, and conflicting role responsibilities were the reasons given for not exercising on a routine basis. For this reason contact by nurses with chronically ill persons to provide ongoing monitoring and reinforcement of healthy lifestyles is essential, even during stable periods, to minimize the incidence of relapses and complications.

Illness management is not only the work of ill persons, as the chapters in this book indicate. Families share in the constant work associated with carrying out regimens and handling disabilities. Even when they take no part in regimen management, chronic conditions in one partner can bring about role reversals and new tasks to contend with. Often, persons are unprepared and resentful of having to carry these additional burdens. When the ill person is a child, developmental and sibling issues may also compound the problems. Despite the heavy workloads, during stable phases of illness families receive little support from the health care system precisely because everything is supposedly "under control." Though some families are able to manage quite well without assistance, others are overwhelmed by the unending work and care involved and family life is severely compromised. A greater safety net of resources and nursing support is needed during periods of stability to help families avert crises both of the illness and in family life.

Hayes (1997), with responses by Holaday (1997) and Deatrick (1997), explores the many gaps and contradictions in the literature on chronic illness and children. Studies tend to focus on specific family members and not on the interaction between them as a whole. She attributes this incomplete state of knowledge, in part, to the inability of present research methods to capture the dynamics of family interaction. Hayes challenges readers to develop methods that are sensitive enough to elicit interactional data, so that nurses can intervene more appropriately.

Acute Phase

The chapter by Kirkevold (1993) addresses the acute phases of chronic illness. An acute phase denotes an exacerbation of symptoms or the development of illness complications requiring major medical intervention, even hospitalization, to stabilize the condition. Sometimes it is an acute episode, such as a myocardial infarction, that signals the presence of a chronic condition. During an acute phase, a person is "sick" and, more than in any other period in the overall trajectory, requires the comprehensive care of nurses. Reading the chapter by Kirkevold makes one realize how shortsighted our present health care system is. In order to contain costs, it takes professional nurses away from the patient's beside and replaces them with less expensive workers. The latter may be able to do the technical tasks but are not educated to handle the underlying issues that interfere with regimen management and that bring persons with chronic conditions back into the hospital for repeated admissions. The chapter by Kirkevold reveals just how necessary is the presence of professional nurses.

Kirkevold (1993) examined the implicit practice theory of 13 experienced Norwegian registered nurses working on a unit that specializes in the care of patients with skin conditions. What emerged from her study was that many patients stopped caring for their skin conditions during the months prior to hospitalization because they "couldn't take" the continued stress and strain of repeatedly carrying out what they considered time-consuming and uncomfortable regimens. Nor could they handle the stigma associated with outbreaks of their skin disease. The practice theory that nurses developed to handle the situation consisted of two main strategies. First, they nurtured the patients, "alleviating" them of all illness management tasks. During this initial period, nurses addressed patients' identity issues as well as their medical problems. Then, when the patients were emotionally and physically able, the nurses taught patients the self-care skills they would need to prevent future skin outbreaks. When viewed from this perspective, the long-term cost to benefit ratio of nurses working at the bedside is shifted in favor of nursing, making it a good financial investment.

Unstable Phase

The chapter by Weiner and Dodd (1993) relates to the concept of uncertainty, a problem of particular significance during unstable phases of chronic illness. An unstable trajectory denotes a period in the chronic illness when a person is not considered "acutely ill," yet symptoms are not under control and direct medical intervention is needed to stabilize the condition. It may be that environmental factors such as allergens render a regimen for asthma ineffective. Or an exacerbation of an illness such as multiple sclerosis necessitates adjustments in lifestyle. The uncertainty associated with unstable phases comes from not knowing whether the condition will continue to worsen and whether or not a regimen can be found to control symptoms and stabilize the course. Patients question: What will the future be like? Is it possible to bring the symptoms under control? Will the disabilities increase? Was the disease discovered early enough? With conditions such as cancer, the uncertainty is even greater, because one never knows what the outcome will be. Often it is not until treatment has been completed that it is known whether or not the condition has been "cured." During periods of instability carrying out the activities of daily living can be problematic and individuals and their families are suspended in a state of biographical limbo. Since medical management of unstable conditions is often done on an outpatient basis, persons and their families often have to cope with the side effects of treatment and the uncertainties about the future on their own.

Weiner and Dodd (1993), with a response by Oberst (1993), report the results of a qualitative research project examining the impact of chemotherapy on cancer patients. The qualitative data were collected as part of a larger quantitative study. Analysis of the qualitative data indicated that the major problem facing patients during the time of chemotherapy is "tolerating the uncertainty that permeates the disease of cancer." Uncertainty has three dimensions: temporality, body, and identity, each with its own unique facets. To gain some control over their lives during periods of uncertainty persons engage in what the authors termed "Uncertainty Abatement Work." The process includes strategies aimed at reducing anxiety, such as: "pacing of activities," "becoming professional patients," "engaging in reviews," "choosing a support network," "setting goals," "finding a safe place to let down," "seeking reinforcing comparisons," and "taking charge." By reaching out into the community and maintaining contact with persons during unstable periods, nurses can help persons to develop strategies for managing the uncertainties that illness brings into their lives.

Downward Phase

The sixth chapter in this series is one by Lindgren, Burke, Hainsworth, and Eakes (1992). Though the authors do not talk specifically about downward phases of illness, their concept of chronic sorrow is one that is especially pertinent to this phase. A downward phase is a period in the chronic illness course characterized by progressive bodily deterioration during which symptoms and disabilities intensify despite efforts to contain them. Deterioration may progress until death. It also can be arrested at any point along the trajectory and interspersed between long periods of stability. With each major downward phase, persons are asked to come to terms with new losses increasing their sorrow. Though some persons are able to endure symptoms and disability and remain engaged despite progressive debilitation, others go on until one day there is just one loss too many and they reach a breaking point. They question the meaning of life under these difficult conditions, pull inward, and withdraw from life.

Lindgren, Burke, Hainsworth, and Eakes (1992), with a response by Martinson (1992), explore the concept of Chronic Sorrow as applied to persons with chronic conditions and to their caregivers. They differentiate chronic sorrow from prolonged grief and depression by defining chronic sorrow as a normal reaction to chronic illness, a difficult situation in life, which has no predictable end. Chronic sorrow can be triggered by internal or external events, is cyclic or recurrent, and may or may not be progressive. It may intensify even years after the initial body and identity insults. Nurses can greatly influence how persons and their families experience deteriorating conditions. According to the authors, nurses working with the chronically ill and their families should inform persons who are suffering that their sorrow is not pathological, but a normal reaction to repeated loss. Their support and advice may be all that are needed to keep a person and family functioning despite increasing symptoms and the overwhelming sense of loss.

A second chapter in this section on downward phases is one by Robinson, Bevil, Arcangelo, Reifsnyder, Rothman, and Smeltzer (1993). Though chronic conditions may be found among all age groups, the incidence of chronic deteriorating conditions increases in elderly persons, who often have more than one chronic condition. In addition to their chronic illnesses, elderly persons must contend with the physical changes that accompany aging, compounding their losses. Since lifespans are extending, the challenge to health care professionals is how to help persons retain their independence and sense of well-being by slowing down the rate of deterioration. This can be done through proper regimen management, ongoing monitoring, and early intervention.

Staying on top of chronic conditions and slowing down the rate of decline is the goal of the research reported by Robinson, Bevil, Arcangelo, Reifsnyder, Rothman, and Smeltzer (1993). Their project examined delivery of care to chronically ill elderly persons living in the community. The Corbin and Strauss Chronic Illness Trajectory Model (1991) provided the theoretical framework for their research. Since the major concepts of the framework had not been operationalized, this became the researchers' first task. From the newly operationalized concepts, the authors developed assessment guides for each illness phase. The findings from the study indicate that the management of chronic conditions in the elderly is a very complicated process. They have multiple chronic conditions and, despite efforts to control the conditions, the tendency is for complications to develop, necessitating frequent hospitalizations. More important, the authors found that there was very little coordination of care between hospital and home. The authors suggest that the assessment protocols developed as part of this research project could be used to coordinate care, easing transitions between settings. They would also enable multidisciplinary practitioners to develop integrated plans of care specific to the patients who may be in different phases of each chronic condition.

Dying Phase

The final chapter is by Stewart (1994). It addresses some of the problems associated with dying trajectories. Modern medicine is making some conditions that were once fatal "chronic," while "curing" some that once were thought to be incurable. In doing so it is redefining the meaning of "chronic illness." Despite the advances in medicine, people are still dying. The dying period is characterized by profound physiologic and pyschosocial changes. Because of the finality of this stage of life and the difficulties persons have coping with it, dying and death are almost always stressful for families. The stress may be even greater when the condition leading to death is a stigmatizing one such as AIDS. In this situation persons must come to terms with the overlying (and sometimes covert) biographical issues as well as the dying ones.

Stewart's (1994) research, with responses by Nokes (1994) and Strauss (1994), investigated end-of-life decision-making in families from the time that a person disclosed testing positive for the AIDS virus to the period of bereavement following death. The sample for this qualitative study consisted of 59 families in which 1 family member had AIDS. The findings indicate that patients with aids (PWA) and their families undergo a very complex adjustment process over the illness trajectory. Individuals with HIV disclose their state to their families because they need their support during the illness and at the time of dying. Yet, all of the families experienced some degree of hopelessness and ineffective coping. Some families never moved beyond using what Stewart called an "emotional decision-making" model. They did not seek outside support or assistance, choosing instead to handle the problems on their own. Though mourning rituals provided some relief from the travail that families had endured, there remained in many a "shadow of grief that never left them." Again the need for nursing presence during the difficult months and weeks of dying cannot be overemphasized.

Summary

The management of chronic conditions and the "human aspects" of that management present a tremendous challenge to the American health care system. Of all the health care professionals, nurses, by virtue of their educational preparation and the scope of their professional practice, are the group most prepared to meet that challenge. When reading this book keep in mind that it is *nursing* and not the illnesses themselves that you should focus upon. Nurses can no longer remain in the shadows of health care delivery. The rise in the incidence of chronic conditions and the increasing demands for health care services call for a shift in how the nation thinks about health care and the role that nursing has in its future. This topic will be elaborated in the epilogue that follows at the end of the book.

REFERENCES

Chronic illnesses expected to rise. (Monday, September 16, 1996). San Jose, CA: San Jose Mercury News.

Corbin, J. M. (1993). Response to "Operationalizing the Corbin & Strauss Trajectory Model for elderly clients with chronic illness." *Scholarly Inquiry for Nursing Practice, 7*, 265–268.

Corbin, J., & Cherry, J. (1997). Caring for the chronically ill elderly in the community. In L. Swanson & T. Tripp-Reimer, (Eds.), *Advances in Gerontological Nursing* Vol. 2, (pp. 62–81). New York: Springer.

Corbin, J., & Strauss, A. (1988). *Unending work and care: Management of chronic illness at home.* San Francisco: Jossey Bass.

Corbin, J., & Strauss, A. (1991). Comeback: Overcoming disability. In G. Albretch & J. Levy (Eds.), *Advances in medical sociology, II* (pp. 137–159). Greenwich, CT: JAI Press.

Corbin, J., & Strauss, A. (1992). A nursing model for chronic illness management based upon the trajectory framework. In P. Woog, (Ed.), *The Chronic Illness Trajectory Framework: The Corbin and Strauss nursing model.* (pp. 9–28). New York: Springer.

Deatrick, J. A. (1997). Response to "Families and Children's chronic conditions: Knowledge development and methodological considerations." *Scholarly Inquiry for Nursing Practice, 11*, 295–298.

Glaser, B., & Strauss, A. (1965). *Awareness of dying.* Chicago, IL: Aldine.

Gortner, S. R. (1992). Response to "A description of the nature and dynamics of coping following coronary artery bypass surgery." *Scholarly Inquiry for Nursing Practice, 6*, 77–79.

Hawthorne, M. H. (1993). Women recovering from coronary artery bypass surgery. *Scholarly Inquiry for Nursing Practice, 7*, 223–248.

Hayes, V. E. (1997). Families and Children's chronic conditions: Knowledge development and methodological considerations. *Scholarly Inquiry for Nursing Practice, 11*, 259–290.

Holaday, B. A. (1997). Response to "Families and Children's chronic conditions: Knowledge development and methodological considerations." *Scholarly Inquiry*

for Nursing Practice, 11, 291–293.
The Institute for Health & Aging University of California, San Francisco. (1996). *Chronic Care in America: A 21st century challenge.* Princeton, NJ: A Robert Wood Johnson Foundation Publication.
Kirkevold, M. (1993). Toward a practice theory of caring for patients with chronic skin disease. *Scholarly Inquiry for Nursing Practice, 7*, 37–52.
Lindgren, C. L., Burke, M. L., Hainsworth, M. A., & Eakes, G. G. (1992). Chronic sorrow: A lifespan concept. *Scholarly Inquiry for Nursing Practice, 6*, 27–40.
Martinson, I. M. (1992). Response to "Chronic sorrow: A lifespan concept." *Scholarly Inquiry for Nursing Practice, 6*, 41–42.
Nokes, K. M. (1994). Response to "End-of-life family decision-making from disclosure of HIV through bereavement." *Scholarly Inquiry for Nursing Practice, 8*, 357–359.
Oberst, M. T. Response to "Coping amid uncertainty: An illness trajectory perspective." *Scholarly Inquiry for Nursing Practice, 7*, 33–35.
Rankin, S. H. (1993). Response to "Women recovering from coronary artery bypass surgery." *Scholarly Inquiry for Nursing Practice, 7*, 245–248.
Redeker, N. S. (1992). A description of the nature and dynamics of coping following coronary artery bypass surgery. *Scholarly Inquiry for Nursing Practice, 6*, 63–75.
Robinson, L. A., Bevil, C., Arcangelo, V., Reifsnyder, J., Rothman, N., & Smeltzer, S. (1993). Operationalizing the Corbin & Strauss Trajectory Model for elderly clients with chronic illness. *Scholarly Inquiry for Nursing Practice, 7*, 253–264.
Stewart, B. M. (1994). End-of-life family decision-making from disclosure of HIV through bereavement. *Scholarly Inquiry for Nursing Practice, 8*, 321–352.
Strauss, A. (1994). Response to "End-of-life family decision-making from disclosure of HIV through bereavement." *Scholarly Inquiry for Nursing Practice, 8*, 353–355.
Stuifbergen, A. K. (1995). Health behaviors and quality of life among individuals with multiple sclerosis. *Scholarly Inquiry for Nursing Practice, 9*, 31–50.
Tobin, J. N. (1993). Response to "Women recovering from coronary artery bypass surgery." *Scholarly Inquiry for Nursing Practice, 7*, 249–252.
White, N. E., & Richter, J. R. (1993). Response to "Toward a practice theory of caring for patients with chronic skin disease." *Scholarly Inquiry for Nursing Practice, 7*, 53–57.
Wiener, C. L., & Dodd, M. J. (1993). Coping amid uncertainty: An illness trajectory perspective. *Scholarly Inquiry for Nursing Practice, 7*, 17–31.
Wineman, N. M., & Schwetz, K. M. (1995). Response to "Health behaviors and quality of life among individuals with multiple sclerosis." *Scholarly Inquiry for Nursing Practice, 9*, 51–55.

Chapter 2

A Description of the Nature and Dynamics of Coping Following Coronary Artery Bypass Surgery

Nancy S. Redeker

OVERVIEW

The purpose of this study was to explore the nature and dynamics of coping following coronary artery bypass surgery (CABS). The coping strategies of 129 subjects recovering from (CABS) were assessed at 1 and 6 weeks following surgery using the Revised Ways of Coping Checklist. The most frequently used coping strategy was "seeks social support," followed, in descending order of frequency, by problem-focused coping and the emotion-focused coping strategies of "blamed self," wishful thinking, and avoidance. There was an overall decrease in coping between 1 and 6 weeks following CABS. "Seeks social support," "blamed self," and wishful thinking coping were used significantly less frequently at 6 weeks than at 1 week following CABS. The decreases in problem-focused and avoidance coping, however, were not statistically significant. This study provides insight into the process of coping following CABS and supports the need for development of nursing strategies to promote coping in this population.

Note: Originally published in *Scholarly Inquiry for Nursing Practice: An International Journal*, Vol. 6, No.1, 1992. New York: Springer Publishing Company.

INTRODUCTION

Researchers have focused increasing attention on the experience of recovery from coronary artery bypass surgery (CABS). Despite relief of angina, improved exercise tolerance, decreased need for anti-anginal medications, and the potential for extended life expectancy in persons with stenosis of the left main coronary artery or triple vessel disease (CASS Principal Investigators and Their Associates, 1983; European Coronary Surgery Study Group, 1982; Read, Murphy, Hultgren, & Takaro, 1978), many persons who have undergone CABS experience psychosocial problems (Allen, 1990; Mayou, 1986; Stanford, 1982). Expected beneficial outcomes of CABS, such as return to work, resumption of social and leisure activities, and sexual activity, have not been consistently found (Allen, 1990), and a significant incidence of emotional distress has been reported (Mayou, 1986). Although the stressful nature of CABS has been the focus of nursing research (Carr & Powers, 1988; Flynn & Frantz, 1987; Gortner et al., 1989; King, 1985; Kos-Munson, Alexander, Hinthorn, Gallagher, & Goetze, 1988; O'Connor, 1983; Penckover & Holm, 1984), the discrepancy between the physiologic and psychosocial outcomes of CABS has been poorly understood.

The cognitive appraisal model of coping suggests that persons who cope successfully are able to function effectively in work or social living, and attain positive morale or life satisfaction, and somatic health (Lazarus & Folkman, 1984). Coping appears to be the mechanism used to deal with the stress of recovery from CABS and achieve adaptation. Differences in coping may explain the discrepancy between positive physiologic outcomes and poor psychosocial adaptation in certain individuals. Knowledge of the process of coping supports development of nursing strategies to promote adaptation. The purposes of this study, part of a broader investigation which also examined the relationship between uncertainty and coping (Redeker, 1990), were (a) to identify coping strategies used following CABS and (b) to examine the nature of the change in coping between 1 and 6 weeks following CABS.

RELATED LITERATURE

Coping is defined as constantly changing cognitive and behavioral efforts to manage specific internal and/or external demands that are appraised as taxing or exceeding the resources of the person (Lazarus

& Folkman, 1984). Two broad types of coping are emotion-focused coping (strategies used to manage the emotions arising from a stressful situation including wishful thinking, avoidance, and blamed self and problem focused coping (strategies directed toward changing a stressful situation). A third type of coping, seeks social support, describes problem focused and emotion-focused coping strategies that deal with receiving emotional, informational, and tangible aid from another person (Lazarus & Folkman, 1984).

According to Lazarus and Folkman (1984), coping is neither a personality style nor a defense mechanism, but a dynamic process influenced by the interaction between the person and the environment. Although there is variability in individual coping responses, similarity between different individuals' coping responses in particular contexts has been found. For example, in a study of community-residing adults, problem-focused coping was used more in work contexts than in health or family contexts, while emotion-focused coping was used more in health contexts than family contexts (Folkman & Lazarus, 1980). Emotion-focused and seeks social support coping have been found to predominate in conditions involving personal physical health threats (Folkman, Lazarus, Dunkel-Schetter, DeLongis, & Gruen, 1986). In contrast, Vitaliano and others (1990) found that seeks social support, followed (in descending frequency of use) by problem-focused, wishful thinking, avoidance, and blamed self coping were used by persons with physical health problems. This coping profile was different from the coping profile used by psychiatric patients, medical students, and spouse caregivers of Alzheimer Disease patients.

Christman and others (1988) found that myocardial infarction patients used confrontive (problem-focused) coping more frequently than emotion-focused coping and that the level of confrontive coping did not change between hospitalization and 4 weeks following discharge. Emotion-focused coping decreased between hospitalization and 1 and 4 weeks following discharge. King (1985) described the dynamics of coping in 50 patients undergoing CABS. Participants reported using direct action (problem-focused coping) more frequently following surgery than preoperatively and turned to family and friends more often three weeks following surgery than preoperatively or in the early postoperative period. The level of avoidance coping did not change postoperatively.

Personal characteristics of age, education, and gender have been suggested as correlates of coping. Consistent relationships, however, have not been found (Christman, McConnell, Pfeiffer, Webster, Schmitt, &

Ries, 1988; Folkman & Lazarus, 1980, 1985; McCrae, 1982, 1985; Pearlin & Schooler, 1978; Vitaliano, Russo, Carr, Mauiro, & Becker, 1985; Webster & Christman, 1988).

Although the cognitive appraisal model of coping supported by theoretical and clinical research suggests the dynamic and multidimensional nature of coping, the direction and timing of the change in the context of recovery from CABS remain unclear. Better understanding of the coping strategies employed and the nature of the changes in coping is necessary to enhance understanding of the CABS experience. The following exploratory research questions were posed:

1. Which coping strategies are used most frequently at 1 and 6 weeks following CABS?
2. Does problem-focused, seeks social support, and emotion-focused (avoidance, blamed self, wishful thinking) coping change between 1 and 6 weeks following CABS?
3. What are the relationships between age, education, gender, and coping strategies used at 1 and 6 weeks following CABS?

METHODS

Sample

A purposive sample of 129 adults recovering from a first coronary artery bypass surgery in a 550-bed open-heart surgery center was selected. A computer-generated daily list of all patients hospitalized for cardiac surgery was obtained from the cardiothoracic surgery office in the hospital, and medical records were reviewed to identify all persons meeting the delimitations of the study. Eligibility criteria included ability to read and write English and absence of acute physical or emotional distress at the time of completing the instruments. To control for severity of illness, persons were not included in the study if they had been transferred from the surgical intensive care unit less than 24 hours prior to participation in the study, required the use of the intra-aortic balloon pump or mechanical ventilation for more than 48 hours following CABS, or had undergone concurrent surgical procedures. Persons with histories of chronic physical or mental disease, other than diabetes mellitus or hypertension, which are risk factors for coronary artery disease (American Heart Association, 1989), were also excluded.

As presented in Table 2.1, the participants were predominantly white, male, and married. The mean age was 62 ± 9.7 years (range = 38–78 years). Thirty-six percent were retired, and 40% were employed fulltime and planning to return to work. The mean highest educational level was 13 ± –2.4 years. Twenty-five percent reported highest educational levels less than high school, 33% had graduated from high school, and 41% had completed at least 1 year of college.

Approval was obtained from the IRB of the medical center, and consent was obtained from all participants. A repeated measures design was used. The investigator obtained pertinent historical and clinical data from medical records. Participants completed a demographic data form and the Revised Ways of Coping Checklist (WCCL) (Vitaliano, 1987) 1 week following CABS in the hospital. This time period was chosen because it corresponds to the "resolution phase" in which persons begin to prepare for discharge to home (Jillings, 1978).

At 6 weeks following surgery, participants completed the WCCL at home. The WCCL was mailed to the participants and returned to the investigator by mail. The 6 week time period was selected because persons begin to return to normal activities of daily living at about this time.

The sample of 129 represents those participants who responded at both 1 and 6 weeks. At one week, the WCCL was completed by 167 persons. At 6 weeks, one person was deceased, one had not provided an address, and a third requested that a second survey not be sent. Of 164 potential responses, 134 were received. Four of these were not usable due to missing data, and one was returned too late to be included. The 129 usable questionnaires represent a response rate of 79% between 1 and 6 weeks.

Instrument

The 42-item Revised WCCL (Vitaliano, 1987), which was developed from the Ways of Coping Scale (Folkman & Lazarus, 1980) was used. This scale was chosen because it measures three major coping domains: emotion-focused, problem-focused, and seeks social support coping.

Emotion-focused coping describes efforts to manage the emotions arising from a stressful situation (Lazarus & Folknan, 1984), as measured by subscale scores on *avoidance* strategies (10 items) to psychologically distance oneself from the situation, *blamed self* strategies (3 items) to hold oneself culpable for a situation, and *wishful thinking* strategies (8

TABLE 2.1 Demographic Characteristics of the Sample *(N = 129)*

Variable	Category	n	Percent
Sex			
	Female	27	21
	Male	102	79
Race			
	Black	9	7
	Hispanic	1	<1
	Oriental	2	2
	White	116	90
	Other	1	<1
Marital Status			
	Never married	9	7
	Married	92	71
	Divorced	8	6
	Separated	3	2
	Widowed	15	12
	Missing	2	2
Employment Status			
	Not Employed	2	2
	Employed Full Time	40	31
	Employed Part Time	5	4
	Medical Disability (present illness)	17	13
	Medical Disability (other illness)	4	3
	Retired	47	36
	Homemaker	7	5
	Missing	7	5
Highest Educational Level			
	Some High School	32	25
	Completed High School	43	33
	Some College	20	15
	Completed College	17	13
	Graduate Work	17	13

items) to escape by using fantasy (Lazarus, Averill, & Opton, 1974, p. 261). *Problem-focused coping* describes strategies directed toward changing a stressful situation, as measured by the problem-focused subscale (15 items). *Seeks social support coping*, measured by the seeks social support subscale (6 items), describes both problem-focused and emotion-focused coping strategies used to receive emotional, informational, and tangible aid from another person (Lazarus & Folkman, 1984, p. 245).

Vitaliano, Russo, Carr, Mauiro, and Becker (1985) reported construct validity, concurrent validity, and internal consistency for the WCCL, which has been used to study coping in medical students, spouses of persons with Alzheimer's disease, persons with chronic low back pain, and persons with chest pain (Turner, Clancy & Vitaliano, 1987; Vitaliano, Katon, Maiuro, & Russo, 1989; Vitaliano et al. 1987; Vitaliano et al., 1985). See Table 2.2 for the internal consistencies of the coping subscales for the present study which are comparable to those reported by Vitaliano et al. (1985).

The WCCL is completed in a 5 point Likert format. Responses range from 0, "not appropriate" to 4, "regularly used." For the present study, the tense of the WCCL items was changed from the past to the present, and directions were changed to elicit the participant's response to the specific stressor of CABS, rather than a stressor of choice.

Data Analysis

Raw scores were obtained by summing the ratings for items on each of 5 subscales. Raw scores were divided by the number of items on respective scales to allow comparability of subscale scores. The resulting coping scores range from 0 to 4. High scores indicate more frequent use of coping strategies. Relative coping scores were obtained by dividing the coping score for the particular scale by the sum of the coping scores for all of the subscales (total coping effort) and multiplying by 100. For example, the relative coping score for problem-focused coping was obtained as follows (Vitaliano et al., 1987):

The use of relative coping scores allows assessment of the magnitude of each coping strategy relative to the individual's total coping effort (Vitaliano et al., 1987). It allows meaningful comparison between persons reporting high levels of all forms of coping and persons reporting high levels of selected coping strategies.

Means, standard deviations, and ranges of coping scores and relative scores were used to examine levels of coping. Multivariate analysis of

$$\text{PF Relative} = \frac{\text{PF} \times 100}{\text{PF}+\text{WT}+\text{SS}+\text{BS}+\text{AV}}$$

variance for repeated measures (MANOVA) and posthoc dependent *t*-tests were used to examine changes in coping strategies between one and six weeks. All hypotheses and research questions were tested at the .05 level of significance.

RESULTS

As presented in Table 2.3, all measured coping strategies were used. Seeks social support was used most frequently, followed by problem-focused coping and the emotion-focused coping strategies of blamed self, wishful thinking, and avoidance. The greatest variability was found in seeks social support coping at 6 weeks following CABS and wishful thinking and blamed self coping at 1 and 6 weeks. Use of these strategies ranged from never used to regularly used.

Examination of the mean relative coping scores for survey 1 reveals that seeks social support accounted for 27% of the total coping effort, and problem-focused coping accounted for 24%, followed by blamed self (16.7%), wishful thinking, (16.5%), and avoidance coping (15.6%). Forty-eight percent of the total coping effort at 1 week and 46% of the total coping effort at 6 weeks was attributed to emotion-focused coping (the sum of the mean relative scores for avoidance, blamed self, and wishful thinking). The mean relative coping scores for survey 2 are of similar magnitude to those for survey 1, suggesting that the relative

TABLE 2.2 Internal Consistence of WCCL ($N = 129$)

	Cronbach's Alpha	
Subscale	One Week	Six Weeks
Avoidance	.88	.79
Blamed Self	.86	.90
Problem-Focused	.69	.91
Seeks Social Support	.72	.87
Wishful Thinking	.88	.86

TABLE 2.3 Means, Standard Deviations, and Ranges of Coping Scores and Relative Scores at One and Six Weeks following CABS ($N = 129$)

Subscale	One Week		Six Weeks	
	Mean SD	Range* Min.–Max.	Mean SD	Range* Min.–Max.
Avoidance				
Coping Score	1.78 ± .61	.10 – 3.60	1.69 ± .67	.2 – 3.10
Relative Score	15.63 ± 3.59	1.55 – 24.87	16.49 ± 4.81	5.16 – 34.68
Blamed Self				
Coping Score	1.96 ± .99	0 – 4.00	1.72 ± 1.06	0 – 4.00
Relative Score	16.66 ± 6.36	0 – 29.87	15.36 ± 7.91	0 – 35.01
Seeks Social Support				
Coping Score	2.93 ± .66	.50 – 4.00	2.67 ± .75	0 – 4.00
Relative Score	26.77 ± 7.04	8.20 – 62.18	26.89 ± 8.53	0 – 58.14
Problem-Focused				
Coping Score	2.68 ± .52	.87 – 3.67	2.58 ± .66	.20 – 3.73
Relative Score	24.40 ± 4.72	13.86 – 35.33	26.16 ± 7.29	10.61 – 70.00
Wishful Thinking				
Coping Score	1.91 ± .87	0 – 4.00	1.68 ± .95	0 – 4.00
Relative Score	16.54 ± 5.72	0 – 32.77	15.10 ± 6.55	0 – 35.48

*Potential range = 0–4.00

importance of particular coping strategies did not change substantially between 1 and 6 weeks following CABS. Scrutiny of the maximum and minimum values and standard deviations, however, reveals great intraindividual variation in the percentage of total coping effort attributed to the 5 coping strategies.

Coping scores were positively correlated with one another (see Table 2.4), with the exception of seeks social support, which was not significantly correlated with avoidance or wishful thinking coping at 1 week. In particular, the emotion-focused coping strategies avoidance, blamed self, and wishful thinking were more highly correlated with one another than with problem-focused or seeks social support coping at 1 and 6 weeks. Problem-focused and seeks social support coping were more highly correlated with one another than with the emotion-focused coping variables.

Multivariate analysis of variance (MANOVA) for repeated measures was used to measure the change in the entire set of coping scores (avoidance, blamed self, problem-focused, seeks social support, and wishful thinking) over time. Use of this statistical procedure to assess overall change in correlated variables, prior to measuring univariate changes in the coping scores, reduces the likelihood of inflating Type I error. There was an overall decrease in coping between 1 and 6 weeks ($F(5, 124) = 4.21$, $p = .001$). Post hoc dependent groups t-tests were performed to assess changes in individual coping strategies. There were no significant changes in the levels of problem-focused or avoidance coping. Seeks social support ($t(128) = 3.42$, $p = .001$), blamed self ($t(128) = 2.84$, $p < .01$), and wishful thinking coping ($t(128) = 3.40$, $p < .01$) decreased significantly.

DEMOGRAPHIC CORRELATES OF COPING

Age was significantly negatively related to blamed self and to seeks social support at 1 week, but was not related to use of the other coping strategies. Highest level of education was significantly, negatively related to avoidance and wishful thinking and positively related to seeks social support coping. At 6 weeks, education was negatively related to wishful thinking and blamed self (see Table 2.5).

Men sought social support significantly more often than women ($t(127) = 2.28$, $p < .05$). There were no significant differences in use of

TABLE 2.4 Correlations between Coping Variables at One and Six Weeks Following CABS ($N = 129$)

	1	2	3	4	5
Survey 1 (one week following CABS)					
1. Avoidance	1.00	.55***	.40***	.08	.72***
2. Blamed Self		1.00	.33***	.19**	.47***
3. Problem-Focused			1.00	.46***	.24**
4. Seeks Social Support				1.00	.08
5. Wishful Thinking					1.00
Survey 2 (Six weeks following CABS)					
1. Avoidance	1.00	.58***	.48***	.28**	.66***
2. Blamed Self		1.00	.39***	.27**	.55***
3. Problem-Focused			1.00	.53***	.15*
4. Seeks Social Support				1.00	.16*
5. Wishful Thinking					1.00

*$p < .05$ **$p < .01$ ***$p < .001$

TABLE 2.5 Correlations between Age, Education, and Coping ($N = 129$)

Variables	Age	Education
Avoidance		
Survey 1	.03	–.23***
Survey 2	–.02	–.14
Blamed Self		
Survey 1	–.14*	–.05
Survey 2	–.13	–.18*
Problem-Focused		
Survey 1	.02	.04
Survey 2	–.06	.08
Seeks Social Support		
Survey 1	–.25***	.18*
Survey 2	.06	.08
Wishful Thinking		
Survey 1	.00	–.22**
Survey 2	–.04	–.22**

* $p < .05$
** $p < .01$
*** $p < .001$

avoidance, blamed self, wishful thinking or problem-focused coping between men and women.

DISCUSSION

The high proportion of the total coping effort attributed to seeks social support coping indicates that it was used most frequently following CABS. Social support can be provided by family, friends, and health professionals by expressing positive affect between persons, affirming or endorsing another's behavior or perceptions, and giving symbolic or material aid (Norbeck, Lindsey, & Carrieri, 1981). Nurses can assist this process in several ways, e.g., by providing flexible visiting hours and support groups for patients and families to enhance social support for hospitalized persons. Telephone call-back systems, which provide contact between patients and nurses following hospital discharge, have also been found to provide support, reduce anxiety, and increase information following CABS (Beckie, 1988).

The decrease in use of seeks social support at 6 weeks following CABS contrasts with King's (1985) finding that persons turned to others most often 3 weeks after CABS. This apparent contradiction suggests that the relevance of different sources and functions of social support may change between 1 and 6 weeks. King (1985) suggested that sources of social support may change throughout the experience of CABS. Persons may turn to health professionals or others who have undergone CABS for "expert" advice early in the experience and turn to family and friends to a greater extent following discharge from the hospital. Further study, using an instrument that discriminates sources and functions of social support, is needed to elaborate on these findings.

The high relative frequency of problem-focused coping at 1 and 6 weeks suggests that persons attempt to take an active role in recovery in the weeks following CABS. Providing cognitive and psychomotor information to promote self-care during and following hospitalization are nursing strategies that may support problem-focused coping in this population.

Similar levels of problem-focused coping appear to be used at 1 and 6 weeks following CABS. The behaviors which comprise problem-focused coping, however, may change in relevance according to changes in the person and environment. No attempt was made to differentiate among particular problem-focused behaviors in this study. Closer scrutiny of different forms of problem-focused coping such as confrontive, self-controlling, and planful problem-solving (Lazarus & Folkman, 1984; Moos & Billings, 1982) over a longer time frame may reveal core specific changes over time.

The individual emotion-focused coping strategies avoidance, blamed self, and wishful thinking were used less frequently than problem-focused and seeks social support coping. The sum of the relative frequencies of the emotion-focused coping strategies, however, accounted for almost 50% of the total coping effort, implying the general importance of emotional distress at both 1 and 6 weeks. The variability in wishful thinking and blamed self coping indicates that while some persons used a great deal of emotion-focused coping, others used none at all.

Nurses play a significant role in identifying emotional distress and should intervene to support emotion-focused coping where it may be an effective means of stress reduction. Nurses may support avoidance or wishful thinking when they serve a protective function by allowing emotional "escape" for persons who are not yet ready to confront the outcomes of CABS or the details associated with post-CABS care. On the other hand, nurses may need to intervene to reduce avoidance and wishful thinking when they impede recovery by preventing persons from taking action on their own behalf. Further research is needed to identify persons who are likely to use more emotion-focused coping, examine the effectiveness of the various coping strategies, and test supportive nursing interventions.

Blaming oneself, the most frequently used emotion-focused coping strategy in this sample, may be a normal response to CABS, when persons perceive their own behaviors, such as diet, smoking, and lack of exercise to have led to coronary artery disease and subsequent CABS. Active listening, realistic reassurance, and focusing on positive aspects of the situation, combined with concrete strategies for changing problematic health behavior, may be useful strategies for assisting these individuals.

The overall decrease in coping between 1 and 6 weeks suggests a general decline in the stressful nature of recovery. The continued use of all measured coping strategies at 6 weeks, the approximate time at which persons begin to resume normal roles and activities, however, supports the need for development of nursing strategies to support coping throughout recovery.

The "profile" of coping found in this study, consisting of seeks social support, problem-focused, blamed self, wishful thinking, and avoidance coping (in descending order of magnitude) is similar to the coping profile described by Vitaliano et al. (1990) in persons with physical health problems. This suggests that persons with a variety of health problems may cope in similar ways. The positive correlations among the coping scores suggest that coping strategies tend to be used together. These correlations also suggest that some persons may consistently report high levels of use of all forms of coping, while others may consistently report lower levels.

There was no consistent relationship between age and coping. The negative relationships between educational level and emotion-focused coping strategies, however, indicate that educational level should be considered in future research. Because of the small number of women in this sample, gender differences in seeks social support coping and the absence of gender differences in the other measured forms of coping warrant further investigation.

This study has contributed to knowledge of the nature and dynamics of coping, within the cognitive appraisal model of stress and adaptation. Investigations of individual patterns of coping, the relationships between coping and emotional distress, the effectiveness of coping in reducing stress, and the nature and dynamics of coping in samples, including more women and minority group members, are recommended. Longitudinal studies are essential because of the lengthy and dynamic nature of recovery. These efforts have the potential to lead to long-term improvement of psychosocial adaptation following coronary artery bypass surgery.

REFERENCES

Allen, J. K. (1990). Physical and psychosocial outcomes after coronary artery bypass graft surgery: Review of the literature. *Heart and Lung, 19*, 49–54.

American Heart Association. (1989). *Heart facts.* Dallas, TX: Author.

Beckie, T. (1989). A supportive-educative telephone program: Impact on knowledge and anxiety after coronary artery bypass graft surgery. *Heart and Lung, 18*, 46–55.

Carr, J. A., & Powers, M. J. (1986). Stressors associated with coronary bypass surgery. *Nursing Research, 35*, 243–246.

CASS Principal Investigators and Their Associates. (1983). Coronary artery surgery study (CASS): A randomized trial of coronary bypass surgery. Survival Data. *Circulation, 68,* 939–950.

Christman, N. J., McConnell, E. A., Pfeiffer, C., Webster, K. K., Schmitt, M., & Ries, J. (1988). Uncertainty, coping, and distress following myocardial infarction: Transition from hospital to home. *Research in Nursing and Health, 11,* 71–82.

European Coronary Surgery Study Group. (1982). Long-term results of prospective randomized study of coronary artery bypass surgery in stable angina pectoris. *Lancet, 2,* 1173–1180.

Flynn, M. K., & Frantz, R. (1987). Quality of life after coronary artery bypass. *Heart and Lung, 16(2),* 159–166.

Folkman, S., & Lazarus, R. S. (1980). An analysis of coping in a middle-aged community sample. *Journal of Health and Social Behavior, 21,* 219–239.

Folkman, S., & Lazarus, R. S. (1985). If it changes it must be a process: Study of emotion and coping during three stages of a college examination. *Journal of Personality and Social Psychology, 48,* 150–170.

Folkman, S., Lazarus, R. S, Dunkel-Schetter, C., DeLongis, A., & Gruen, R. J. (1986). Dynamics of a stressful encounter: Cognitive appraisal, coping and encounter outcomes. *Journal of Personality and Social Psychology, 50,* 992–1003.

Folkman, S., Lazarus, R. S., Gruen, R. J., & De Longis, A. (1986). Appraisal, coping, health status, and psychological symptoms. *Journal of Personality and Social Psychology, 50,* 571–579.

Folkman, S., Schaefer, C., & Lazarus, R. S. (1979). Cognitive processes as mediators of stress and coping. In V. Hamilton & D. M. Warburton (Eds.), *Human stress and cognition: An information processing approach* (pp. 265–298). London: Wiley.

Gortner, S. R., Gilliss, Moran, J. A., Sparacino, P, & Kenneth, H. (1985). Expected and realized benefits from coronary bypass surgery in relation to severity of illness. *Cardiovascular Nursing, 21(3),* 13–18.

Gortner, S. R., Gilliss, C. L., Paul, S. M., Leavitt, M. B., Rankin, S., Sparacino, P. A., & Shinn, J. A. (1989). Expected and realized benefits from cardiac surgery: An update. *Cardiovascular Nursing, 25(4),* 19–24.

Jillings, C. R. (1978). Phases of recovery from open-heart surgery. *Heart and Lung, 7,* 987–994.

King, K. B. (1985). Measurement of coping strategies, concerns, and emotional response in patients undergoing coronary artery bypass grafting. *Heart and Lung, 14,* 579–586.

Kos-Munson, Z. A., Alexander, L. D., Hinthorn, P.A.C., Gallagher, E. L., & Goetze, C. M. (1988). Psychosocial predictors of optimal rehabilitation postcoronary artery bypass surgery. *Scholarly Inquiry for Nursing Practice, 2,* 171–193.

Lazarus, R. S., Averill, J. R., & Opton, E. M. (1974). The psychology of coping: Issues of research and assessment. In G. V. Coelho, D. A. Hamburg, & J. E. Adams (Eds.), *Coping and adaptation* (pp. 249–315). New York: Basic Books.

Lazarus, R. S. & Folkman, S. (1984). *Stress, appraisal and coping.* New York: Springer Publishing Co.
Lazarus, R. S., & Launier, R. (1978). Stress-related transactions between person and environment. In L. A. Pervin & M. Lewis (Eds.), *Perspectives in interactional psychology* (pp. 287–327). New York: Academic Press.
Mayou, R. (1986). Invited review: The psychiatric and social consequences of coronary artery surgery. *Journal of Psychosomatic Research, 30,* 255–271.
McCrae, R. R. (1984). Situational determinants of coping responses: Loss, threat, and challenge. *Journal of Personality and Social Psychology, 46,* 919–928.
McCrae, R. R. (1982). Age difference in the use of coping mechanisms. *Journal of Gerontology, 37,* 454–460.
Mishel, M. H., & Braden, C. J. (1987). Uncertainty, a mediator between support and adjustment. *Western Journal of Nursing Research, 9,* 43–57.
Moos, R. J., & Billings, A. J. (1982). Conceptualizing and measuring coping resources and processes. In L. Goldberger & S. Breznitz (Eds.), *Handbook of stress: Theoretical and clinical aspects* (pp. 212–230). New York: Free Press.
Norbeck, J. S., Lindsey, A. M., & Carrieri, V. L. (1981). The development of an instrument to measure social support. *Nursing Research, 30,* 264–269.
O'Connor, A. M. (1983). Factors related to the early phase of rehabilitation following aortocoronary bypass surgery. *Research in Nursing and Health, 6,* 107–116.
Pearlin, L. & Schooler, C. (1978). The structure of coping. *Journal of Health and Social Behavior, 19,* 2–21.
Penckofer, S. H., & Holm, K. (1984). Early appraisal of coronary revascularization on quality of life. *Heart and Lung, 33*(2), 60–63.
Read, R., Murphy, M., Hultgren, H., Takaro, T. (1978). Survival of men treated for chronic stable angina pectoris, a cooperative randomized study. *Journal of Thoracic and Cardiovascular Surgery, 75,* 1–16.
Redeker, N. S. (1990). *Uncertainty and coping following coronary artery bypass surgery.* Ann Arbor, MI: University Microfilms International.
Stanford, J. L. (1982). Who profits from coronary artery bypass surgery? *American Journal of Nursing, 82,* 1068–1072.
Stanton, B. A., Jenkins, C. D., Savageau, J. A., Harkin, D. E., & Aucoin, R. (1984). Perceived adequacy of patient education and fears and adjustments after cardiac surgery. *Heart and Lung, 13,* 525–531.
Turner, J., Clancy, S., & Vitaliano, P. P. (1987). Relationships of stress, appraisal and coping to chronic low back pain. *Behavioral Research and Therapy, 25,* 281–288.
Vitaliano, P. P. (1987). *Manual for Revised Ways of Coping Checklist (WCCL).* Seattle, WA: The Stress and Coping Project.
Vitaliano, P. P, Katon, W., Maiuro, R. D., & Russo, J. (1989). Coping in chest pain patients with and without psychiatric disorder. *Journal of Consulting and Clinical Psychology, 57,* 338–343.
Vitaliano, P. P., Maiuro, R. D., Russo, J., Katon, W., DeWolfe, D., & Hall, G. (1990). Coping profiles associated with psychiatric, physical health, work, and family problems. *Health Psychology, 9*(3), 348–376.

Vitaliano, P. P., Maiuro, R. D., Russo, J., & Becker, J. (1987). Raw versus relative scores in the assessment of coping strategies. *Journal of Behavioral Medicine, 10*(1), 1–18.

Vitaliano, P. P., Russo, J., Carr, J. E., Mauiro, R. D., & Becker, J. (1985). The ways of coping checklist: Revision and psychometric properties. *Multivariate Behavioral Research, 20,* 3–26.

Acknowledgment. This study was partially supported by a grant from the Gamma Nu Chapter of Sigma Theta Tau, Seton Hall University College of Nursing, South Orange, New Jersey.

Response
Susan R. Gortner

This study of recovery from coronary artery bypass surgery concentrates on the early recovery period and describes the nature of coping used by the respondents. This period generally is difficult for patients and families, even with professional and family support and an absence of complications. As noted by Redeker, several studies have documented the value of telephone contact to monitor recovery and coach in the recovery process. With this large male and well-educated sample, it might be expected that patients and their caretakers would take an active role in recovery and use problem-focused recovery strategies as well as social support. These expectations are borne out by study data and suggest that continued support by clinicians, particularly nurses, would be helpful in the recovery process. At one week post-discharge, the need for a professional or skilled tutor seems apparent, at six weeks, there is less need because: (a) recovery tends to be well advanced at this time; (b) persons are resuming presurgery social roles, including return to work; and, (c) the predominantly male CABS population tends to approach the process of recovery in an instrumental or work-oriented pattern.

Keeping these features in mind, clinicians might explore with patients and spouses during hospitalization (and even as early as the day of admission presurgery) expectations for recovery and plans for the recovery process. We have found that expected goals or benefits from surgery differ for elders in comparison with younger patients (Gortner et al. 1990). An interesting finding of the Redeker study at the one week testing period was the negative relation between age and the use of blamed self and seeking-social support strategies. Elders appear to be more realistic in their expectations of surgery and have reported a high proportion of realized benefits following surgery; even when expectations for resumption of activity were not met, elders indicated that they would consider surgery again (Gortner et al., 1990). Further, they enter surgery with the support of family and friends. These findings suggest that elders represent a group that clinicians might "target" for special attention following bypass surgery, maximizing the life experience that the elder patient brings to the surgery and the ways in which elders and their families have in the past coped with stressors.

The design and two-time assessment schedule used in the Redeker study did not allow for examination of the dynamics of recovery. Yet clinical follow-up can provide just that "window" into the recovery process, allowing clinicians to assess the progress of physical and emotional recovery and determine appropriate interventions.

Another group that clinicians may wish to target is persons under the age of 50 and all women undergoing surgery. Lifespan development theory suggests that the need for bypass surgery can interrupt professional careers and personal relations. Doordan (1991) found higher measured anxiety before CABS surgery and at six weeks after surgery in 65 men as compared with 16 women also assessed at these same times. Gilliss (1984) found 20% of families still not recovered at 6 months post-CABS surgery. We found in our first trial that those under 50 years of age reported more disturbed mood state and fewer realized benefits than those over 70 (Gortner, Gilliss, Shinn, Sparacino, Rankin, Leavitt, Price, & Hudes, 1988). Most of these persons were men. Yet women of all ages appear to have difficulty following cardiac surgery (Rankin, 1990). Why this is the case for women is not clear, but the Redeker study does show differences between genders in the seeking of social support, as was demonstrated also by Rankin (1990). In a study of 81 cardiac surgery patients, Doordan (1991) found lack of support and recovery information to be related to higher levels of psychological distress on the Brief Symptom Index (BSI) for both men and women.

Exploration of patient and family plans for rehabilitation needs to occur early in the hospitalization period and be followed by at least one post discharge telephone call within a day or two of discharge for all patients. Based on the information obtained, certain groups of patients, e.g., those reporting unusually difficult recovery, should be considered for special follow-up intervention. What might these interventions be? As noted by Redeker, they should include support of patient and family actions and decisions to hasten recovery, dealing with symptomatology, and maintenance of risk factor reduction behaviors. As noted by Tack and Gilliss (1990), ineffective coping was the most frequent nursing diagnosis in the sample of cardiac surgery patients coached by telephone. Telephone coaching was individualized and continuous over time, i.e., patient and family decisions were supported, ventilation of feelings and emotions were allowed for, maintenance of heart healthy behaviors was encouraged, and anticipatory guidance was provided for the next week of recovery. While the investigators did not carry out home visits, these would be an excellent adjunct from the practice site.

It is too soon to suggest interventions specific to coping styles based on data from the Redeker study, intriguing as this idea may be. Emotion-focused coping may be specific to the initial time period studied, i.e., one week after surgery and to the sample studied, but not to the general population. In the study by Doordan (1991) it was found that confrontive coping was the most frequently used strategy, followed by emotion-focused coping, which decreased significantly from discharge to six weeks. A preferred alternative in the absence of supporting evidence regarding one or more coping strategies at particular time points in the recovery trajectory would be to query patients on their preferred coping strategy, and to adapt professional advice accordingly. As Redeker states, more needs to be known about coping preferences in the management of recovery from cardiac events. To this, I would add that further study is needed in the immediate recovery period to explore age and gender differences (if real) and in the later period (past the usual six month end point). In this way, middle-range theory regarding immediate and long-term recovery from cardiac events might be built that would be of interest both to clinicians and scientists.

REFERENCES

Doordan, A. (1991). Psychosocial correlates of cardiac recovery. Unpublished doctoral dissertation, University of California San Francisco.

Gilliss, C. (1984). Reducing family stress during and after bypass surgery. *Nursing Clinics of North America*, 19, 103–112.

Gortner, S.R., Gilless, C. L., Shinn, J.A., Sparacino, P.A., Rankin, S., Leavitt, M., Price, M., & Hudes, M. (1988). Improving recovery following cardiac surgery: A randomized clinical trial. *Journal of Advanced Nursing, 13,* 649–661.

Gortner, S. R., Miller, R., Doordan, A., Paul, S., Wolfe, M. M., & Gaudiani, V. M. (1990). "Would you do it again?" Indicators of treatment satisfaction in cardiac elders. (Abstract). *Circulation Supplement, 82(4),* III–706.

Rankin, S.H. (1990). Differences in recovery from cardiac surgery: A profile of male and female patients. *Heart and Lung, 19(5),* 481–485.

Tack, B., & Gilliss, C.L. Nurse-monitored cardiac recovery: A description of the first eight weeks. *Heart and Lung, 19(5),* 491–499.

Chapter 3

Women Recovering from Coronary Artery Bypass Surgery

Mary H. Hawthorne

OVERVIEW

Coronary heart disease is the leading cause of death among American women over 50, and women are undergoing surgical revascularization procedures in ever increasing numbers. There are, however, few research-based data upon which to guide the nursing care of these patients. This study explored the nature of the recovery process for women following coronary bypass surgery in order to extend our understanding of the posthospitalization phase of the recovery trajectory. Ten patients participated in semi-structured interviews that were analyzed using thematic analysis. Data revealed significant problems with caregiver recognition and access to care. Barriers to care may also exist due to women's traditional subordinate role in American society and their use of gender specific interactive skills. Recovery for women was found to differ significantly from that of men due to the later developmental stage when women are more likely to experience cardiac illness.

INTRODUCTION

Coronary heart disease is the leading cause of death among American women over 50 and the second leading cause of death in women between 35 and 39. An estimated 250, 000 women die each year from this disease (American Heart Association, 1989; Thom, 1987). Despite these

Note: Originally published in *Scholarly Inquiry for Nursing Practice: An International Journal,* Vol. 7, No. 4, 1993. New York: Springer Publishing Company.

impressive statistics, coronary heart disease is generally thought of as a disease primarily of men in their middle years (Hawthorne, 1991; Wingate, 1991). This view is reflected in both the clinical diagnosis and management of women with coronary heart disease and the research underpinning the decision tree for treatment. For example, several recent studies of gender bias in physicians' use of diagnosis and treatment options indicate that women in several major cardiac centers have not been undergoing procedures such as coronary angioplasty and artery bypass procedures as frequently as men (Ayanian & Epstein, 1991; Kahn et al., 1990; Tobin et al., 1987; Wenger, 1990).

The apparent gender bias operating in diagnosis and treatment and also in clinical trials involving patients with coronary heart disease has special significance for nursing. A consequence is that the assumptions and knowledge base that guide nursing management of these patients may be based upon incomplete or even inaccurate information. The lack of research-based data to guide nursing care for women with cardiac disease is particularly worrisome in the case of women recovering from infarction or cardiac surgery, where recovery outcomes have been linked to patients' perceptions of illness events (Evart et al., 1986; Mishel, 1980; Peel, Semple, Wang, Lancaster, & Dall, 1962). A major aspect of the nursing care of these patients is enhancement of the patient's understanding of illness events through providing appropriate information and correcting misconceptions.

Patients recovering from coronary artery surgery may be viewed as facing a novel phase within a chronic illness trajectory (Corbin & Strauss, 1988; Hawthorne, 1990). This illness phase is characterized by ambiguity and uncertainty as symptoms that have guided illness management are significantly altered or even eradicated. Nurses can help patients foresee the recovery phase of the illness trajectory and also help them to understand the new demands of illness. Patients are assisted to construct plans to meet regimen demands and renegotiate relationships (Corbin & Strauss, 1988). Patient and family expectations can then approach alignment with clinical realities, enabling the patient to manage the work of recovery.

A necessary antecedent to this kind of nursing care is an understanding of the patient's interpretation of clinical events (Paterson & Zderad, 1976). This understanding requires acknowledging the individual's own interpretive framework, which operates from within to assign meaning to lived events (Shutz, 1967). Unfortunately, for women recovering from cardiac surgery, patients' views of the surgical experience and recovery trajectory have not yet been described.

BACKGROUND OF THE STUDY

Coronary artery bypass surgery is, and is anticipated to remain, one of the most frequently performed surgical procedures in the United States (Becker, Corrao, & Alpert, 1988; Kinney & Craft, 1992). In recent years there has been a small but significant increase in the referral of women for this procedure, perhaps reflecting the beginning of resolution of the gender bias in patient referrals for surgery (Eaker, Packard, & Thom, 1989; Gillum, 1987; Tobin et al., 1987; Wenger, 1990). Women, however, have less favorable outcomes from coronary surgery than men, with higher reported rates of operative mortality, perioperative infarction, early and late graft reocclusion, and incomplete revascularization. Women also report less symptomatic relief and lower activity levels than men (Khan et al., 1990; Penckofer & Holm, 1990; Richardson & Cyrus, 1986).

These less favorable surgical outcomes reflect important preexisting differences between gender groups. First, coronary artery disease occurs 10 to 20 years later in the lifespan of women; hence when women undergo surgery, outcomes may reflect the not unexpected comorbidity of older patients (Eaker et al., 1989). Also, since there is an inverse relationship between body size and graft patency rates, it is not surprising that women have higher reocclusion rates (Tobin et al., 1987). The diagnosis of coronary artery disease is also more complex in women than in men because the extent of occlusive disease and angina are not correlated in women (Glazer & Hurst, 1986). Diagnosis is further complicated by the higher association of vascular spasm with angina in women than in men. These differences probably operate to delay diagnosis and surgical referral. Thus, women are likely to reach surgery later in their illness course and as older patients who are more likely to experience comorbidity. In fact, female gender is fifth among the five most important predictors of mortality following coronary bypass surgery (Christakis et al., 1989).

The literature suggests that the recovery trajectory following major cardiac events such as myocardial infarction and cardiac surgery may differ significantly for women and men (Boogaard, 1984; Gilliss, 1984; Murdaugh, 1986; Parchert & Creason, 1989; Vavaro, 1991; Wenger, 1990).

Boogaard (1984), for example, found that women and men resumed different types of activities during recovery after myocardial infarction. Men allowed themselves a period of "passivity" or no activity after hospital discharge; women began household work soon after they returned home. These findings suggest that women and men use different cues and parameters to guide activity resumption, which is consistent with what is currently known about gender and role differences in response to illness and surgery in general (Baker, 1989; Hibbard & Pope, 1983; Nathanson, 1975; Verbrugge, 1979). The multiple roles that women assume can significantly influence self-care and the resumption of activities; indeed, role demands may supersede physiologic cues as parameters that shape activity progression. There is also evidence that these demands add significant stress during recovery from cardiac illness (Rankin, 1989a).

Women may also have special difficulties during the recovery phase that are related to family structure and demographics. For example, women are more likely to outlive their spouses; thus, women bypass patients frequently live alone, and may have limited resources for caregiving. In contrast, male patients, typically younger, usually have their spouse available to care for them during a major illness (Rankin, 1989a). Their differing clinical responses and a higher incidence of comorbity, along with the influences of age and society, make it probable that the process of recovery and the experience of women during this phase of illness differ significantly from the experience of men.

PURPOSE OF THE STUDY

The major purposes of this qualitative study were to explore the nature of the recovery process for women following coronary artery surgery and to interpret these findings from within the context of the abundance of available literature about male patients who undergo this procedure. The overall intent of this research was to extend our understanding of the recovery trajectory for women. By choosing to examine a particular phase within a chronic illness trajectory, when major changes in illness management would be necessary, the author hoped to discover important characteristics about how women perceive and manage cardiac illness.

The study focused on the period of convalescence, defined as the phase of an illness trajectory when treatment ends or becomes predictable and the patient begins to reestablish patterns of daily living (Corbin & Strauss, 1988; Davis, 1987; Miller, 1983). Convalescence is characterized by uncertainty and unpredictability; it is usually experienced at home, and may be complicated by significant changes in symptom management due to the surgical intervention. Physical limitations and activity tolerance are also tested during this phase of recovery. Patients resume activities according to physiologic cues and role responsibilities (Baker, 1989; Gilliss, 1984; Hawthorne, 1990). All patients were asked to describe the story of their cardiac illness, surgery, and recovery, focusing upon the recovery phase of illness experienced at home. All patients recruited into the study, regardless of how long ago they had experienced surgery, had experienced the first 3 months of recovery at home. Although the author was aware that patient perspectives might vary with time from surgery, she chose not to control for this variation, believing that reflective time on behalf of the subjects would only contribute to the insight they might have into the process of recovery and thus enhance the researcher's opportunity for discovery.

The following four questions were used to guide this research on women's recovery process:

1. What is the nature of the recovery process for women convalescing from coronary artery surgery? What themes emerge that describe the recovery process?
2. What are the cues and parameters that women use to assess progress in recovery?
3. How important are social factors in shaping the recovery and illness management within the illness trajectory?
4. What are the key variables that influence recovery outcomes?

METHODS

From the population of female postoperative coronary artery surgery patients at Duke University Medical Center, subjects meeting the following inclusion criteria were selected: 1) having had surgery for the first time and being at least 3 months into recovery, 2) able to participate in the interview, 3) being between the ages of 45 and 75, and 4) giving informed consent to participate. In an effort to ensure diversity and increase the opportunity for discovery, purposive sampling was used to obtain the initial list of patients (Sandelowski, Davis, & Harris, 1989). The final sample size was determined by the rule of redundancy, or the point at which the interviewer reaches data saturation and hears no new information (Bogdan & Bilken, 1992).

Potential subjects were contacted by the researcher by telephone. Those who gave informed consent to participate were interviewed in their own homes, using prepared or "grand tour" questions to focus the interview (Spradley, 1979). Interviews averaged 2 1/2 hours in length. As points of interest emerged, the interviewer asked the participant to elaborate; also, using the techniques of "restatement" and "incorporation," described by Spradley (1979, p.63), the researcher returned to these points in a later phase of the interview, to obtain validation of the information. The researcher used some of the themes from her previous study of men after coronary artery surgery (Hawthorne, 1990) to generate discussion with participants regarding gender differences in illness. These techniques were only employed in the latter part of the interviews to avoid biasing subject responses. Finally, as the study progressed, the researcher also validated themes that emerged from preliminary analysis of prior interviews.

DATA ANALYSIS

Using the technique for thematic analysis outlined by Bogdan and Bilken (1992), fieldnotes of the researcher and the verbatim interview transcripts were coded and analyzed for the themes best articulating the essence of the recovery process for women recovering from coronary artery surgery. An initial coding scheme of 60 categories was developed; these were collapsed into groups that composed the final themes. An expert in qualitative methodology and women's health reviewed samples of the data and coding schema to support the validity of the analysis process.

THE SAMPLE

All potential subjects contacted agreed to participate in the study. Ten women, nine Caucasian and one Afro-American, participated; all were treated at one major cardiac referral center where the majority needed emergency surgical intervention. All participants had been born and raised in the South, although one had worked for 20 years as a nurse in Manhattan. The ages of subjects ranged from 42 to 72 years; nine were between 62 and 72. The average time since surgery was 21 months, with a range of 6 to 30 months. Six of the subjects had experienced recurrence of angina; a crucial time for this was the 1-year mark from surgery. Subjects reported that their symptoms (NYHA Angina Class II) were stable at the time of the interviews. Only one subject reported being unable to care for herself; this individual was not limited by her cardiac disease, however, but by peripheral vascular occlusive disease and diabetes.

Six participants reported living alone; two of these, however, lived adjacent to their daughters' homes. Four subjects were married and living with their spouses; four were divorced, and the remaining participants were widows. Of the four married participants, three had spouses who were chronically ill. Seven participants reported spending a significant amount of time caring for either unwell parents, chronically ill spouses, or grandchildren. Two of the four divorced women had even cared for sick spouses through major illness, such as cardiac surgery, after their divorces. Three of the participants were employed full time outside the home at the time of the study. Sample characteristics are also presented in Tables 1 and 2.

FINDINGS

Analysis of the transcripts and field notes yielded seven major themes describing key elements or characteristics of the recovery trajectory for women after coronary artery surgery. An important characteristic of these themes is that they contain comparative information from the experience of men from both the available literature and the author's previous study of men. Although these comparisons may suggest at first blush that the author failed to examine the experiences of women as unique, they reflect, instead, the research process necessary to enable full interpretation of the data. Interpretive research such as this study relies upon new understandings emerging from interpretation of data from within the context of an existing body of knowledge. Therefore, the references to men that are contained in both the themes from this study and their discussion, reflect the mass of information available about men and coronary artery surgery. The themes are presented below, and their implications for practice and research are briefly discussed.

Theme #1

Women understate and minimize the impact of the cardiac surgical experience. Cardiac surgery is assigned neither the power nor the significance assigned to it by men.

TABLE 3.1 Demographic Characteristics

Women: Subject	Age	Marital Status	Caregiving Responsibility	Living Arrangement	Employment Status
#1	67	widowed	no	alone	disabled
#2	65	divorced	yes	alone	yes(FT)
#3	71	married	yes	with spouse	no
#4	71	divorced & widowed	yes	alone	no
#5	68	married	no	with spouse	no
#6	62	divorced	yes	alone	yes(FT)
#7	42	divorced	yes	alone	yes(FT)
#8	65	married	yes	with spouse	no
#9	70	married	yes	with spouse	no
#10	72	widowed	no	alone	no

TABLE 3.2 Illness Characteristics

Women: Subject	Emergency Surgery	Time lapsed since surgery	Recurrence of angina	Attended formal rehab
#1	yes	24 months	yes	no
#2	yes	9 months	no	yes
#3	yes	24 months	no	no
#4	yes	24 months	no	no
#5	yes	15 months	no	yes*
#6	yes	18 months	yes	yes*
#7	yes	23 months	yes	yes
#8	yes	18 months	yes	no
#9	yes	24 months	yes	no
#10	yes	30 months	yes	no

*Left program early due to home or work responsibilities

One of the most fascinating and revealing discoveries of this study was the revelation that while all subjects were receptive to participation, all expressed doubt about the importance of their stories of illness and surgery. Interviews with these women were correspondingly more difficult in terms of flow of information and significantly shorter than the interviews with men in the author's previous study. The interviews also lacked the intense, almost cathartic emotionality that characterized the interviews in the previous study. Women became emotional only when they discussed the loss of a dear one, not when they discussed the experience of surgery. They attributed no extraordinary meaning to this experience, unlike the men who described it as a "near death" experience, often with the quality of epiphany.

These variations in interview tone and style reflect major gender differences in the meanings assigned to the surgical experience. These differences, however, may be in large part age related. The cardiac surgical experience is assigned meaning from within the context of the patient's developmental trajectory. As noted earlier, women develop coronary occlusive disease 10 to 20 years later in their life course than their male counterparts. Clearly, for the patient who views herself as being in a later stage of life, the discovery of cardiac illness may not be a shock. Indeed, the older patient may view cardiac illness as a "to be expected" event within the life cycle. This is consistent with Neugarten's concept of the "internal clocks" that determine our expectations for various stages in the life cycle (Neugarten, 1979): events consistent with perceived "timeliness" do not bring the distress that "untimely" or unexpected events bring.

Men typically encounter cardiac illness during midlife when the developmental crisis of these years may be underscored or even confounded by cardiac illness and surgery. In the author's previous study, interview data indicated that the surgical experience simulated a midlife crisis for men, serving to increase their awareness of emotions and the importance of their relationships with significant others (Hawthorne, 1990). In contrast, from early childhood women have an awareness of the importance of "connectedness" to others. According to contemporary feminist psychology, this awareness reflects an inherent difference in gender development. Early male gender development is centered upon individuation and separation from the mother; in contrast, the female child does not have to separate from the mother to achieve gender identity (Chodorow, 1978; Gilligan, 1982; Miller, 1986).

This developmental difference is thought to account for the relationship orientation of women and their greater capacity for empathy.

Major cardiac illness and cardiac surgery, then, in terms of meaning assigned from the framework of psychological and emotional development, may be potentially less disruptive for women than for men. There is some research that supports this view. In a study of matched cardiac surgery patients, examined preoperatively and followed for 6 weeks, Rankin (1990) found that the Profile of Mood States reflected significantly less emotional distress for female patients than for male patients at all data collection points.

The unique life experiences of women are key influences in the interpretation of the cardiac surgical experience. The women in the current study, not unlike many women in American society, were no strangers to illness; subjects came to the experience as veterans of major life and death events, who had served primarily as caregivers. All of these women had borne children and many had cared for elderly parents and/or spouses and had helped friends and family through illness, death, and loss. Other research also indicates that women have greater exposure to death than men (Russo, 1991). When cardiac surgery is considered within the context of such life experiences, it is not surprising that women perceive it as less significant than men, for whom illness is a novel experience. One participant in the study expressed it this way:

> I don't feel like I've been very helpful to you because I don't I dwelt more on other things than the heart because it has seemed more insignificant than other problems.

This study suggests that the life experiences of women may be helpful preparation for cardiac surgery. The experience of having cared for others during illness may reduce the fears that often accompany major surgery and the uncertainty and unpredictability that characterize the period of recovery. Perceiving cardiac surgery as a not-unexpected event in the life of an older adult, women may find integrating the experience and getting back to the business of everyday living easier than their male counterparts find it:

> ... and that [cardiac surgery] is not a focal point for me, really ... I don't even like to look back on it because I feel like we've come through it and life is going on ... and I feel like you do from day to day what you have to do.

Theme #2

Gender bias was strikingly apparent in the evidence of delayed recognition of symptoms of coronary disease in these women; diagnosis was postponed and as a consequence surgical intervention was done almost universally under emergency conditions. The data suggest that neither caregivers nor patients are "tuned-in" to the possibility of coronary artery disease in women. This affects all phases of the illness trajectory from prevention to rehabilitation.

As noted earlier, the literature points to significant gender differences in the use of available diagnostic and treatment procedures for the management of coronary heart disease (Ayanian & Epstein, 1991; Kahn et al., 1990; Tobin et al., 1987; Wenger, 1990). Although this group of female patients did not suffer gender bias in the hospital where they received surgical care, several subjects related poignant stories of delayed recognition of symptoms and extreme difficulty in receiving needed care from providers in outlying communities.

One woman, a 65-year-old Afro-American mother of 11 who had worked many years alongside her husband in the tobacco fields, complained to her physician for 2 years about classic angina. She received no treatment and experienced no improvement; finally she sought the opinion of another physician, a younger female, who sent her for exercise testing and referred her for needed angiography and subsequent surgical intervention. The subject described the experience this way:

> . . . I would just have, you know, sharp pains, and when it would come, it would go through this left breast, and down into my arm . . . And he [her physician] thought it was coming from a gas pocket that had developed in my gallbladder. He kept tending me and I didn't get no better and still I kept having those pains and all that, so I changed doctors and went to Dr. J . . . And when she examined me, she told me that this was no gas bubble, this was my heart.

The youngest subject in the study, who had undergone surgical menopause 17 years earlier and had a family history of premature coronary heart disease, told of extreme difficulty in getting care recognition of her cardiac illness. She had accompanied her brother to the coronary care unit when he experienced an infarction; sitting at his bedside, she recognized that she was experiencing the very same symptoms. In her, however, the symptoms had been diagnosed and treated as indigestion. The researcher asked the subject why she thought that physicians, and sometimes patients themselves, were reluctant to acknowledge cardiac disease in women. This was her response:

> ... I think we're brainwashed ... [we think] it's going to happen to the men, but it's not going to happen to women ... and if it does happen to women, how can we make the doctors understand that it's happening? They don't hear you. They didn't hear me. I mean, I didn't know what was wrong with me prior to that [her brother's infarction]. You know, I was being treated with Tagament, I was stressed out, and like I said, he was asking me if I was having, my menstrual cycle. I hadn't had one since I was 25 years old.

These two stories illustrate extreme difficulties in gaining access to care. Some of the difficulties may in part be related to the myth that coronary artery disease is a male illness. Or it may be that care providers are slower to refer or treat women because they believe that the disease is not as amenable to the available treatment options with the same success as with men. They may consider it not economically worthwhile to use expensive technology for women when the outcomes appear not as successful. These possibilities need explanation. Fortunately, they appear to be receiving increased attention, as indicated by national research guidelines and initiatives (Office of Women's Health, U.S. Public Health Service, 1991).

One way to improve patient access to care is to increase caregiver awareness of and sensitivity to these issues and enhance incentives for research efforts on them. It is equally important to explore problems from the patient's perspective. Delayed entry into the health care system is a long-standing problem in the treatment of coronary heart disease, for patients of both genders; this is especially troublesome in the current time of anticoagulant therapy, when the mantra is "time is muscle." Timely entry may be especially difficult for women, who may themselves buy into the myth that coronary heart disease is an illness of men.

Women may delay treatment because they lack awareness of their vulnerability to cardiac illness or believe that cardiac illness is an inevitable consequence of aging. Such belief in the inevitability of illness has indeed been documented as a significant barrier to effective treatment for elderly patients (Rodin, 1980). The data from this study indicate that women may not be as aware of symptoms and may not as readily attend to symptoms of cardiac illness as men. This lack of awareness is underscored by women's lack of attention to risk factor monitoring and modification in the postoperative period and their strikingly low participation in formal rehabilitation programs.

The lack of self monitoring as a self-caring behavior is worrisome. Again, it can be explained in part by gender differences. Women are known to be more "other" than self focused, and to take major responsibility for providing care to others (Miller, 1986). As caregivers, women may find it difficult to focus on their own needs, especially in the face of multiple role demands.

Multiple role responsibilities were a major obstacle to the participation of these subjects in a formal postoperative rehabilitation program. Several patients found the program too demanding; one said she had no energy left to meet home responsibilities after rehabilitation activities were accomplished. This subject reported that the men in the program had nothing to do but the rehab program and she had a house to run when she came home. Another subject stopped participating because her work hours conflicted with the program schedule.

In summary, the problems of illness recognition and access are multifaceted, as these patient stories clearly indicate. Their stories also point to a mammoth deficit in our knowledge of whether and how cardiac illness presents differently in women and men. Research is needed to explore the language of cardiac illness so that patterns of illness development can be mapped and women's medical histories can be attended to as "reliable." Such research will contribute significantly to eliminating the diagnostic problem noted by Glazer and Hurst (1987) in their article on gender differences and coronary heart disease:

> The history, then, has considerable diagnostic value in men with significant coronary atherosclerotic heart disease, but its value is limited in women except in the subgroup over 70 with definite angina pectoris. In the majority of women, the history establishes an intermediate level of disease likelihood and further diagnostic testing is in order (p. 63)

Theme #3

Women's interactions with caregivers reflect traditional sex-role and status differences. Such patterns of communication as deference to individuals holding higher status and/or males hinder the therapeutic exchange. This phenomenon has the potential to significantly compromise the quality of care as well as health outcomes.

The characteristics of the interviews in this study suggest major differences in the communication style of women and men recovering from coronary artery surgery. For instance, the general communication style of these women was noted to be passive, with the participants relying upon the investigator to actively guide the semi-structured interviews. The investigator needed to employ many more direct open ended questions and "probes" to elicit information and elaboration of key points from women than were needed in the study of men. Despite repeated efforts to get participants to elaborate freely upon issues important to them, control of the interviews remained in the hands of the researcher (in terms of turn-taking in dialogue, as the researcher made a concentrated effort not to direct the content of the discussion). The interviews were also significantly shorter than the interviews with men.

These participants' passivity and deference in communication are consistent with the traits thought to be dominant in women's personality development within Western cultures. Such personality traits (e.g., being less independent, less adventurous, less competitive, more suggestible, more excitable in crises, more emotional, less effective, and more illogical than men) reflect women's inferior status in societies founded upon the presumption of male dominance (Carmen, Russo, & Miller, 1981; Miller, 1986; Scully & Bart, 1973). In such societies, passivity in women's communication reflects both their heritage of inferior societal status and power base, and the cultural norms that serve to maintain male dominance (Goody, 1978; Shurpin, 1989).

Research in the area of mental health indicates that passive personality characteristics can adversely affect women's psychological development and are linked with unfavorable health outcomes:

> ... girls and women have been encouraged to develop passive and indirect psychological strategies—a more complex task [than that of men who must develop active mechanisms for coping and resolving conflicts]. Behaviors such as inhibition, passivity, and

submissiveness do not lead to favorable outcomes and play a role in the development of psychological problems (Carmen, Russo, & Miller, 1981, p. 1321).

Indeed, researchers have hypothesized that the higher rates of mental illness found among women (Gove & Tudor, 1972) result from female sex-role "learned helplessness," that is, the expectation of powerlessness and inability to control one's destiny, whether real or perceived, prevents effective action on one's behalf (Carmen, Russo, & Miller, 1981).

How such passive behaviors influence therapeutic interactions and subsequent health outcomes in female cardiac patients has yet to be described; however, the potential consequences of inability to take effective action on one's own behalf are not difficult to imagine. For example, even in the process of obtaining the patient's history, there is great potential for the female patient to be passive and only respond to direct questions from the caregiver, given the presumed superior social status and power of the caregiver. Deference and passivity may inhibit the patient from offering critical information, seriously diminishing the validity of clinical assessments and undermining treatment plans. Further, given that the stresses associated with the ineffectiveness of women's communication patterns are believed to contribute to mental illness, these same communication patterns may also be an important factor in cardiac illness, in which emotional stresses are known to be a contributing factor (Lown, 1984; Perlman, Ferguson, Bergeum, Isemberg, & Hammerstein, 1971).

Brown's (1976) research provides further insight into the compromised interactions between female patients and their caregivers. He contends that power gradients between communicants can also inhibit the skills of the individual with greater power in the interaction; status differences and efforts to ensure socially polite communication preclude the formulation and asking of appropriate questions. Thus, clinical interactions with female patients may be significantly disadvantaged both from the inadequate communication skills of the caregiver and the passive and deferential communication style of the patient.

There are other important gender-related phenomena that may serve, in combination with passivity and deference, to underline communications with female patients. Primary among these is the view that the long-standing inferior status of women has resulted in the development of separate spheres of communication; women, long banished from the public sphere, actually have a separate language (Shurpin,

1989). That language not only reflects the passivity related to inferior social status, but also contains gender specific content and form consistent with the home orientation of the woman's world. Thus, an innate language barrier is believed to exist between genders. This barrier is likely to be magnified in the clinical setting when combined with the obvious differences between the language of medical science and the vernacular. The effects of such barriers are worsened by the continued romance of American medicine with scientism, where only objective clinical data are "believed" by clinicians (Cassell, 1986; Oakley, 1976). Women's symptoms are often reported in terms of feelings and ability to care for others rather than in terms of objective facts and figures. As a result, their reports of symptoms are frequently not taken seriously in the paternalistic world of medicine (Ehrenreich & English, 1979; Pollack, 1985).

Theme #4

> A major task during the period of recovery is the remapping of relationships so that patient needs are met and family functions continue. This process is influenced by the "otherness" orientation of the subject.

The stories of these women recovering from coronary artery surgery confirm the intense family disruption that has been reported to accompany major cardiac illnesses and surgery (Gilliss, 1984; Rankin, 1989b; Vavaro, 1991) and provide additional insights into family functioning in illness. Several subjects' experiences illustrate the complex family situations that nurses will inevitably confront with the "graying of America."

One subject related an amazing story of her difficulties during the first month following surgery. This 72-year-old former nurse reported that everything went very well for the first 2 weeks at home. She had planned well for basic needs to be met for both herself and her husband, who had healing leg ulcers secondary to peripheral vascular disease. In Week 3, however, her husband required hyperbaric treatment for his ulcers, which meant relocation of the couple to a hotel adjacent to the medical center where he was receiving daily treatments. Meeting physical needs during the 2 weeks of his treatment was something this very intelligent woman negotiated well, but coping with her husband's despondency about his own illness was almost more than she could bear.

The situation led to a serious confrontation between the couple; the subject was then able to redirect some attention to her own needs. Her situation illustrates the difficulty that older couples may have when the synergy of chronic illness in both parties exhausts their resources. This experience also suggests that when the woman has assumed a primary role in meeting family needs, couples are at risk for significant disruption in functioning during the period of the wife's recovery. Interestingly, however, research indicates that in such families, if the wife has experienced illness prior to the major cardiac event, the family disruption is less than in families where the wife has never experienced illness (Vavaro, 1991).

Women in this culture have traditionally focused upon meeting the needs of the others; thus, meeting their own needs during major illness may feel unnatural (Miller, 1986). Formal role negotiation may be required so that family responsibilities become more equitable and decision-making becomes more collaborative. This process was described by one subject in the following interchange with the researcher:

SS: . . . And see, my family has always depended on me on both sides.
MH: . . . And how do we let our needs be known?
SS: I had to reverse.
MH: When you say "reverse," tell me more about that.
SS: Well, I sorta had to stop accepting so much responsibility and accepting more [from others], and not being . . . I was accused of being too independent. And I had to start taking a little more than trying to give it all.

Only one of the participants reported a major change in marital status after surgery; this participant divorced within a year of the surgery and believed her illness to have been a major factor in the deterioration of the relationship.

The experiences of other subjects illustrate the importance of intergenerational interdependence during illness and provide very positive examples of the potential help available to women who are alone. The help was generally received with gratitude; however, the gratitude was joined with a poignant sense of loss that accompanied the relinquishment of valued independence. Two subjects relocated to be nearer family who could provide such tangible supports as physical care and transportation, necessitating, however, the loss of irreplaceable emotional support from life-long friends.

This loss of emotional support suggests that extended families have difficulty with all five of the areas of work outlined by Corbin and Strauss (1988) for successful adjustment to chronic illness. In such families, patients' emotional needs appear to suffer most, not unlike the findings from studies of men as caregivers, in which men were reported to be better at providing tangible supports, such as medical regime or symptom management tasks, than in meeting emotional needs (Stollen 1990; Young & Kahana, 1989).

The women in this study also provide excellent examples of successful recovery aided by creativity and planning ahead whenever possible. One of the key aspects of success was having built in advance of the illness a network of dependable friends who were able and willing to help. Responsibilities were dispersed within the network, so that the burden was manageable for everyone involved. The subjects' stories indicated that these networks were reciprocal, ongoing arrangements, a way of living for women whose family members were few or chronically ill.

Theme #5

> Women and men associate different meanings and feelings with the surgical incision and scarring. Women may view the scar as a sign of mutilation and a threat to their identity, whereas men are more likely to view this bodily change as a badge of courage with the capacity for empowerment or enhancement of self-esteem.

Body image, or the somatic ego, is "the picture of our body that we form in our mind as the way that the body appears to ourselves" (Severyn, 1969, p. 234). Body image is thought to be a social construction "developed through the reflected perceptions about the surfaces of one's body and responses to sensations" (Norris, 1978, p. 5). This portion of the persona is an important component of one's self-concept, having significant impact upon one's self-esteem and sense of security (Roberts, 1986).

Changes in body image have been shown to constitute significant sources of emotional suffering and loss in surgical and trauma patients (Fitzgerald, 1989; Lee, 1970; Roberts, 1986). Wright (1987), in her study of 20 coronary artery surgery patients, found that most subjects expressed intense dissatisfaction with surgical incisions. Damage to body image is believed to be frightening and traumatic to most individuals as it threatens the sense of wholeness (Levine, 1960). Threats to wholeness are particularly significant in American society where physical beauty is valued almost to the point of obsession.

The meaning the individual assigns to assaults on the body, and the feelings of damage and loss that accompany this assault, are thought to be related to the individual's values and to personality traits such as self-esteem (Roberts, 1986). Also, since body image is a socially constructed phenomenon, perceived damage to one's body image is likely to be associated with gender-specific values assigned to physical appearance and the integrity of bodily functions. Fisher (1973) contends that men and women experience their bodies in radically different ways; women are more aware of what is occurring in their bodies, having had more contact with bodily phenomena with negative connotations such as menses and care of babies and young children, as well as more experiences with body change than men. Therefore, says Fisher, women are less anxious about their bodies being attacked. Data from this study, indicate that women are, to the contrary, very threatened by surgery and the potential for mutilation. Subjects' comments about their surgical incisions and scars revealed not only fear of mutilation, but also a great sense of having been damaged. One of the most poignant examples of this was a patient's dream that occurred either during the surgical procedure or during the postoperative period:

> . . . when they carried me to open heart surgery, it was like I had a nightmare . . . it was like I had a nightmare. I remember that. I remember that as good as anything . . . It's just like it was a field of people, people I knew . . . and they had houses built up on stilts, like target practice. And through the whole surgery . . . I was out there the whole time and people was out there shooting pellet guns and BB guns and they were all hitting me . . . and I was black and blue. I was feeling the pain and misery from all those shots.

The mutilation fears of female patients are not illogical: rather, they reflect an almost universal human response to threat of injury. In addition, however, living, in a society defined by male dominance, where sexual objectification is the primary process for the subjugation of women, such fears of mutilation are to a great extent justifiable (MacKinnon, 1982; Miller, 1986). Indeed, there is perhaps no better example of the mistreatment of women to be found than in the history of modern gynecological surgery in the United States. Sims, revered by many as the father of modern gynecological surgery, perfected the surgical correction of childbirth-related injuries (vaginal-vesicular fistulae) with repeated operations upon unanesthetized slave women (Scully, 1980). Abuse of patients in contemporary society is not as overt; there is, however, evidence of the persistence of abuse in less tangible forms:

> . . . as patients, women are considered primarily as physical bodies to be medicated by the physician who knows best what is good for them. Many of the medical procedures currently imposed on women are technologically complex, and highly profitable but of doubtful safety or even necessity. Since the 1960's for instance, the "pill" has become the most popular form of birth control; hysterectomy has become one of the most frequently performed surgeries and the numbers of births occurring through Caesarian-section has more than tripled since 1970 (Jagger, 1983, p. 188).

The findings of this study indicate that in addition to fears of mutilation, women have significant concerns about the cosmetic changes in their bodies and the way scarring may affect their sexual desirability and intimacy. Such patient concerns are consistent with the studies of burn patients, in which women have been found to be concerned about beauty and men about function (Fitzgerald, 1989). These findings are not surprising given the emphasis in our society upon beauty and designer bodies: physical attractiveness is considered a key indicator of one's value in society and one's ability to achieve love. Although both genders seem to suffer from this societal standard, women, as the targets of male dominance through sexual objectification, are more vulnerable to "not measuring up." One subject, a 62-year-old divorcee and grandmother, who continues to work full time in a textile mill, expressed her concerns in the following dialogue:

> SS: For the longest time, I was very much aware of it [the mediastinal incision]. It had a bad place right here that just stood up. A bad scar there, sort of a white looking scar . . . and, it finally went down. But still, I'm self conscious of that. I really am, very much so. I've always been a type of person that just . . . I guess appearance means a whole lot to me when I get out or something.

MH: I can understand why.
SS: Well, like I said, I'd go out and I'd go . . . and I used to love to dance. Oh God, I just loved to dance.
MH: Did you? Do you still dance?
SS: No, I haven't danced since my heart operation. I just don't have what I did have or something, I hadn't got that back.

Another subject felt that her surgical incision was a key factor in the dissolution of her marriage. This very attractive patient was quite concerned about the effect the incision might have upon a future sexual relationship:

SS: I have a hangup about this scar on my chest. I have a horrible scar . . . mine is gross. "Keloided" and it's gross. I've gone twice to the plastic surgeon and he says he can fix it . . . It's gross. You see?
MH: That's not gross.
SS: It is to me. And it was very noticeable to L. It was a bad turn-off for L. I noticed that right off. I tried to get him to discuss it but he wouldn't . . . I go to the beach and for the longest time I wore a T-shirt. Then this year I decided that I wasn't going to hide it. The first day on the beach, this guy goes, "gosh, what is that on your chest?" It is a hangup for me, I do hide it a lot.

These findings indicate that sex-role related values attached to the self concept influence patients' assignments of meaning to body image. These are likely to be important factors in the later stages of recovery. One subject from the author's previous study of men described the different gender responses to surgical incisions in the following dialogue:

MH: Do you think men worry about scars?
SS: Men, I don't think so. I can see it might become a macho thing [for men] and a problem for a female. It could be a real macho thing if it's not disfiguring . . . it could be a real ego booster. Yea, a little cut here, a scar there, something to show off, something to talk about, a conversation piece, you know "I was in the service, this that and another thing happened to me" (Hawthorne, 1990, p. 148).

Theme #6

> Women recovering from coronary bypass surgery report greater mediastinal incisional discomfort than men. Needed instructions and information were not given by nurses regarding wound care.

Most of the subjects in this study reported incisional discomfort associated with the need for breast support. Wound care as it related to this obvious problem for women was not discussed with any of the subjects by any of their caregivers. It seems obvious that a brassiere may in itself be very uncomfortable and wearing one may interfere with incisional healing; yet, the weight of breast tissue apparently is a source of great discomfort.

Women in this study also indicated that the location of the incision made it very difficult to perform self-care activities in the early postoperative phase. Chief among their complaints was inability to lift both arms at the same time, which is often necessary when a woman shampoos or combs her hair. Dressing was also a problem: again, fastening a brassiere was almost impossible if it fastened in the back, as was putting on panty hose. These activities may not present life threatening problems in the hospital setting, but may mushroom from the perspective of the unwell and vulnerable individual who lives alone. Lack of sensitivity to these problems by caregivers underscores the perception of cardiac disease as a problem of men, with care reflecting this perspective.

Theme #7

> Women attend to different signs and symptoms than men as cues to activity resumption during recovery and rehabilitation. Cues used reflect the "otherness" orientation of women's lives as well as a knowledge base consistent with women's alienation from the public sphere of science and men.

Subjects in this study used family and home responsibilities and level of fatigue to guide activity resumption and rehabilitation, rather than specific instructions from caregivers or physiologic parameters. In contrast, the men in the prior study followed specific discharge guidelines for activity resumption. This is consistent with Baker's (1989) findings that women recovering from gall bladder surgery resumed activities based upon family needs, which often superseded the physician's activity guidelines. Activities performed were limited primarily by the patient's level of fatigue and, hence, ability to perform perceived role responsibilities.

This method of gauging activity is consistent with the "otherness" orientation of women and the nature of woman's role in the family as the individual with major responsibility for caregiving. Their pragmatic approach to recovery may indicate that women are indeed more attuned to their bodies than men. From patient reports, using fatigue to monitor activity resumption during the early phases of recovery was effective, and may be better for older patients than relying upon externally set parameters for such activities as distance walking. The behavior of these women suggests that they are aware of two sets of guidelines for recovery: guidelines from caregivers (those from the public sphere), and guidelines that emerged from the woman's own judgment of her wellness (the private sphere).

In the early phases of recovery, women patients may feel very confident in this mode of activity progression and may be more relaxed about the recovery process than men. In later recovery and rehabilitation, however, two different sets of rehabilitation guidelines may remain unintegrated or even be in conflict. This is a problem, since in later phases of rehabilitation health outcomes may be dependent upon the patient's understanding of and attention to guidelines from medical science. For example, inclusion of aerobic exercise within a routine exercise program and monitoring of cardiovascular risk factors may significantly influence coronary disease progression. Most of these study subjects, however, had never participated in a formal cardiac rehabilitation program and indicated a lack of understanding of the importance of aerobic exercise to cardiovascular health. Their reports suggest that women may not view household and family activities as physical "work," and may underestimate the amount of cardiac energy required to accomplish such tasks. Women may also be unable to successfully integrate formal rehabilitation programs, which are constructed from an androcentric perspective, with the workload of managing the household. Indeed, this was one subject's specific complaint. More attention in both practice and research is needed to help women anticipate and remap activity expenditures so that cardiovascular health can be optimized while role responsibilities are met.

The women in this study did not discuss their health in terms of cardiac function or success in reducing risk factors, unlike the men in the author's previous study, who demonstrated an almost religious attention to physiologic parameters. This again reflects differences in orientation between genders to public and private spheres. Two of the women subjects, one a registered nurse, the other a teacher, said that they deferred to the physician for such activities as cholesterol level monitoring. As one said, "I let him watch things like that."

SUMMARY AND CONCLUSIONS

Examining the recovery of these women from coronary artery surgery, one is impressed with the power of this surgical procedure to positively affect health outcomes. Although the women in the study had been dangerously ill, their reports of recovery and wellness indicated that the surgical intervention was quite successful in attenuating symptoms; the patients were satisfied with the care they had received and the results of surgery.

The women also demonstrated amazing skill in orchestrating generally successful recovery within their home environments; this was in sharp contrast to their lack of success in obtaining timely recognition and treatment of life threatening cardiac disease. The data suggest that their difficulties reflect an apparent gender bias that cuts across all financial, educational, racial, and age lines.

Perhaps the most important lesson to be learned from these stories, however, is the importance of approaching patients from an interpretive framework that helps to determine their needs and to design appropriate care. This study clearly demonstrates that many women in this society exist in a subculture, and their needs differ from men in accordance with their societal roles and associated interactive skills. This has important implications for practice in light of the nurse's unique role in determining patient needs and particularly considering what is understood about the communication skills of the "expert" nurse (Paterson & Zderad, 1976; Shurpin, 1989). The nurse, already recognized as a skillful interpreter of the scientific world for the patient, with heightened awareness of how profoundly gender and role can impede communication between caregiver and patient, can anticipate such difficulties and use communication strategies that specifically counter patient passivity and reticence. Equally important, the nurse, who often functions as part of a multidisciplinary team, can assume an advocate role for those patients who may find more direct communication particularly difficult. In such circumstances, the nurse ensures that patient needs are clearly and expeditiously communicated and understood, and that patient needs for information from caregivers have been satisfied.

Gaining such appreciation for how a patient's perception of illness events and his/her ability to articulate needs may be significantly influenced by gender also underscores the importance of communication skills within nursing education. This is particularly poignant when one considers that gender is perhaps only one of multiple factors that could significantly affect the patient's interpretation of events. The themes from this study suggest that indeed factors other than gender are major influences upon patients' perceptions. Such findings attest to the importance of considering the synergy between illness trajectory and biography, as the meaning of illness is perceived to be profoundly different depending on lifespan stage and individual life experience. As these findings are carefully considered, it seems clear that the nurse needs to be equipped with both the understanding and the communication skills that enable her to consider each patient interaction as an interpretive event.

The results of this study also suggest that there are significant gaps in our knowledge as a result of the omission of women from major research investigations of coronary disease and treatment. Information is sorely needed about the presentation and symptom patterns of women with the disease. Research is also needed on the communication patterns and coping styles of women, for these are likely to have significant effects upon their interactions with physicians as they report illness.

The study has also generated many important research questions. For example, investigation is needed on the effects of postoperative family disruption and distress and the perceived need by women for greater social support upon recovery and achievement of long cardiovascular health. The results of this study also raise questions about women's apparent lack of concern for cardiac risk factor modification. Each question deserves careful and serious attention. The information gained will be critical as the nursing profession confronts and combats the gender bias that ultimately diminishes the quality of care provided to all patients.

REFERENCES

American Heart Association. (1989). *1990 heart facts.* Dallas, TX: Author.
Ayanian, J. Z., & Epstein, A. M. (1991). Differences in the use of procedures between women and men hospitalized for coronary heart disease. *New England Journal of Medicine, 325*(4), 221–225.
Baker, C. A. (1989). Recovery, A phenomenon extending beyond discharge. *Scholarly Inquiry for Nursing Practice, 3,* 181–194.
Becker, R. C., Corrao, J. M., & Alpert, J. S. (1988). The decision to perform coronary bypass surgery in women. What are the facts? *American Heart Journal, 116,* 891–893.
Bogdan, R. C., & Bilken, S. K. (1992). *Qualitative research for education: An introduction to theory and methods.* Boston: Allyn and Bacon, Inc.
Boogaard, M.A. K. (1984). Rehabilitation of the female patient after myocardial infarction. *Nursing Clinics of North America, 19,* 433–440.
Brown, P. (1975). Women and politeness: A new perspective on language and society. *Reviews in Anthropology, 3*(3), 240–249.
Carmen, E., Russo, N. F., & Miller, J. B. (1981). Inequality and women's mental health: An overview. *American Journal of Psychiatry, 138*(10), 1319–1330.
Cassell, E. J. (1986). The return to ideals. *Daedalus, 115,* 185–208.
Chodorow, N. (1978). *The reproduction of mothering.* Berkeley: The University of California Press.
Christakis, G. T., Ivanov, J., Weisel, R. D., Birnbaum, P., Tirone, E., Salerno, T. A. & the Cardiovascular Surgeons of the University of Toronto. (1989) . The changing pattern of coronary artery bypass surgery. *Circulation, 80*(supp I), I-151-I-161.
Corbin, M. & Strauss, A. (1988). *Unending work and care.* San Francisco: Jossey-Bass.
Davis, L. L. (1987). Convalescence and implications for nursing research. *Image: The Journal of Nursing Scholarship, 12,* 177–120.
Eaker, E. D., Packard, B., & Thom, E. J. (1989). Epidemiology and risk factors for coronary heart disease in women. *Cardiovascular Clinics, 19,* (3), 129–145.
Ehrenreich, B. & English, D. (1979). *For her own good: 150 years of the expert's advice to women.* London: Pluto Press.
Evart, C. K., Stewart, K. J., Gillian, R. E., Keleman, M. H., Valenti, S. A., Manley, J. D. & Keleman, M. D. (1986). Usefulness of self-efficacy in predicting over-exertion during programmed exercise in coronary artery disease. *American Journal of Cardiology, 57,* 557–561.
Fisher, S. (1973). *Body consciousness: You are what you feel.* Engelwood Cliffs: Prentice-Hall.
Fitzgerald, K. A. (1989). Burns. In B. Riegel & D. Ehrenreich (Eds.), *Psychological aspects of critical care nursing* (pp. 234–256). Rockville, MD: Aspen Publishers.
Gilligan, C. (1982). *In a different voice: Psychological theory and women's development.* Cambridge, MA: Harvard University Press.
Gilliss, C. L. (1984). Reducing family stress after coronary artery bypass surgery. *Nursing Clinics of North America, 19,* 103–112.
Glazer, M. D. & Hurst, J. W. (1987). Coronary ateriosclerotic disease: Some important

differences in men and women. *American Journal of Noninvasive Cardiology, 1,* 61–67.

Goody, E. N. (1978) . *Questions and politeness.* New York: Cambridge University Press.

Gove, W. R., & Tudor, J. F. (1973). Adult sex roles and mental illness. *American Journal of Sociology, 78*(4), 50–73.

Hawthorne, M. H. (1990). An interpretive study of the metaphors male coronary artery surgery patients use to describe the experience. (Doctoral Dissertation, Adelphi University, 1989). Ann Arbor, MI: *University Microfilms International.*

Hawthorne, M. H. (1991). Reconceptualizing cardiac illness: Using the trajectory framework. *Scholarly Inquiry for Nursing Practice, 5,* 185–195.

Hibbard, J. H., & Pope, C. R. (1983). Gender roles, illness orientation and use of medical services. *Social Science Medicine, 17,* 129–137.

Jagger, A. (1983). *Feminist politics and human nature.* Sussex: Rowman & Allanheld.

Khan, S. S., Nessin, S. Gray, Czer, L. S., Chaux, A., & Martloff, J. (1990). Increased mortality of women in coronary bypass surgery: Evidence for referral bias. *Annals of Internal Medicine, 712,* 561–567.

Lee, L. T. M. (1970). Emotional responses to trauma. *Nursing Clinics of North America, 4,* 579.

Levine, M. E. (1969). Pursuit of wholeness. *American Journal of Nursing, 69,* 98.

Lown, B. (1984). Cardiovascular collapse and sudden cardiac death. In B. Lown (Ed.), *A textbook of cardiovascular medicine* (pp. 778–808).

Kinney, M. R. & Craft, M. S. (1992). The person undergoing cardiac surgery. In C. E. Guzetta & B. M. Dossey (Eds.), *Cardiovascular nursing* (pp. 544–585). St. Louis: Mosby Year Book.

MacKinnon, C. A. (1982). Feminism, Marxism, method and the state: An agenda for theory. In N. O. Keohane, M. Z. Rosaldo & B. C. Gelpi (Eds.), *Feminist theory: A critique of ideology.* Chicago: University of Chicago Press.

Miller, J. B. (1986). *Towards a new psychology of women* (Second edition). Boston: Beacon Press.

Miller, J. F. (1983). *Coping with chronic illness.* Philadelphia: F. A. Davis.

Mishel, M. (1980). Perceived ambiguity of events associated with the experience of illness and hospitalization: Development and testing of a measurement tool. (Doctoral Dissertation, Claremont Graduate School, 1980). Ann Arbor, MI: *University Microfilms International.*

Murdaugh, C. (1986). Coronary heart disease in women. *Progress in Cardiovascular Nursing, 1,* 3–8.

Nathanson, C. A. (1975). Illness and the feminine role: A theoretical view. *Social Science & Medicine, 9,* 57–62.

Office on Women's Health, U. S. Public Health Service. (1991). *Action plan for Women's Health.* Washington, DC : Department of Health and Human Services.

Naunheim, K. S., Fiore, A. C., Wadley, J. J., McBride, L. R., Kanter, K. R., Pennington, D. G., Barner, H. B., Kaiser, G. C., & Willman, V. L. (1988) . The changing profile of the patient undergoing coronary artery bypass surgery. *Journal of the American College of Cardiology, 11,* 494–498.

Neugarten, B. L. (1979). Time, age and the life cycle. *American Journal of Psychiatry, 136,* 887–894.

Oakley, A. (1986). Feminism, motherhood and medicine. In J. Mitchell & A. Oakley, (Eds.), *What is feminism: A reexamination* (pp. 127–150). New York: Pantheon Books.

Parchert, M. A., & Creason, N. (1989). The role of nursing in the rehabilitation of women with cardiac disease. *Journal of Cardiovascular Nursing, 3*, 57–64.

Paterson, J,. & Zderad, L. (1976). *Humanistic nursing.* New York: John Wiley & Sons.

Peel, A., Semple, T., Wang, I., Lancaster, W. M., & Dall, J. L. G. (1962). A coronary prognostic index for grading the severity of infarction. *British Heart Journal, 24*, 745–760.

Penckofer, S. M., & Holm, K. (1990). Women undergoing coronary bypass surgery: Physiological and psychosocial perspectives. *Cardiovascular Nursing, 26*, 13–18.

Perlman, L. V., Ferguson, S., Bergeum, K., Isenberg, E. L., Hammerstein, J. F. (1971). Precipitation of congestive heart failure: Social and emotional factors. *Annals of Internal Medicine, 75*, 1–7.

Pollack, S. (1985). Refusing to take women seriously: The side effects, and politics of contraceptives. In R. Arditti, R. Klein, & S. Minden (Eds.), *Test tube women.* London: Pandora Press.

Rankin, S. H. (1990). Differences in recovery after heart surgery: A profile of male and female patients. *Heart & Lung, 19*, 481–485.

Rankin, S. H. (1989a). Women as patients and caregivers: Difficulties recovering from cardiac surgery. *Communicating Nursing Research, 22*, 9–15.

Rankin, S. H. (1989b). Women recovering from cardiac surgery. *Circulation, 80* (supp. II), II–391.

Richardson, J. V., & Cyrus, R. J. (1986). Reduced efficacy of coronary artery bypass grafting in women. *Annals of Thoracic Surgery, 42* (supp.), S16–S21.

Roberts, S. L. (1986). *Behavioral concepts and the critically ill patient* (Second Edition). Norwalk, CT: Appleton Century Crofts.

Rodin, J. (1980) Managing the stress of aging: The role of control and coping. In S. Levine & H. Ursin (Eds.), *Coping and Health* (pp. 172–202). New York: Plenum Press.

Russo, N. F. (1991). Reconstructing the psychology of women: An overview. In M. T. Notman & C. C. Nadelson (Eds.). *Women and men: New perspectives on gender differences* (pp. 43–61). Washington, DC: American Psychiatric Press.

Sandelowski, M., Davis, D. H., & Harris, B. G. (1989). Artful design: Writing the proposal for research in the naturalistic paradigm. *Research in Nursing and Health, 12*, 77–84.

Scully, D. (1980). *Men who control women's health.* Boston: Houghton Miflin Co.

Scully, D. & Bart, P. (1973). A funny thing happened on the way to the orifice. *American Journal of Sociology, 78*, 283–288.

Severyn, B. (1969). Nursing implications with a loss of body function, In *ANA clinical sessions* (p. 234). New York: Appleton Century Crofts.

Shurpin, K. M. (1989). An interpretive study of the nature and role of the talk of women in expert nurse practice. (Doctoral Dissertation, Adelphi University, 1989). Ann Arbor, MI: *University Microfilms International.*

Shutz, W. C. (1967). *Joy.* New York: Grove Press.

Spencer, F. C. (1989). A critique of emergency and urgent operations for complications of coronary heart disease. *Circulation, 79* (supp. I), I160.

Spradley, J. F. (1-979). *The ethnographic interview.* New York: Holt, Rinehart & Winston.
Stoller, E. P. (1990). Males as helpers: The role of sons, relatives and friends. *The Gerontologist, 30*(2), 228-234.
Thom, T. J. (1987). Cardiovascular disease mortality among United States women. In E. D. Eaker, B. Packard, N. K. Wenger, T. B. Clarkson, & H. A. Tyroler (Eds.), *Coronary heart disease in women* (pp. 33-41). New York: Haymarket Doyma.
Tobin, J. N., Wasserthiel-Sinoller, S., Wexler, J. P., Steingart, R. M., Budner, N., Lense, L., & Wachspress, J. (1987). Sex bias in considering coronary bypass surgery. *Annals of Internal Medicine, 107,* 19-25.
Young, R. F. & Kahana, E. (1989). Specifying caregiver outcomes: Gender and relationship aspects of caregiving strain. *The Gerontologist, 29*(5), 660-666.
Vavaro, F. F. (1991). Women with coronary heart disease. *Cardiovascular Nursing, 27*(6), 31-35.
Verbrugge, L. M. (1979). Female illness rates and illness behavior: Testing hypotheses about sex difference in health. *Women and Health, 4,* 61-79.
Wenger, N. K. (1990). Gender, coronary artery disease, and coronary bypass surgery. *Annals of Internal Medicine, 112,* 557-558.
Westbrook, M. T., & Viney, L. L. (1983). Age and sex differences in patient's reactions to illness. *Journal of Health and Social Behavior, 24 (December),* 313-324.
Wingate, S. (1991). Women and coronary heart disease: Implications for the critical care setting. *Focus on Critical Care, 18*(3), 212-218.
Wright, J. E. (1987). Self-perception alterations with coronary artery bypass surgery. *Heart & Lung, 16,* 483-490.

Acknowledgments. This study was supported by a grant from the American Nurses' Foundation. The author would also like to acknowledge Dr. Walter G. Wolfe, Professor of Surgery, Duke University Medical Center, for his support of this study.

Response
Sally H. Rankin

Hawthorne is to be commended for her extensive contribution to the burgeoning body of knowledge regarding gender differences and cardiac events in her study reporting the narratives of ten women who underwent coronary artery bypass surgery (CABS). This work has multiple implications for nursing practice during inpatient and outpatient recovery periods. By elaborating seven themes involved in recovery of women from CABS, Hawthorne juxtaposes her previous work with men recovering from CABS, as well as other published research, thus clarifying the unique counterpoint of women and cardiac surgery.

Hawthorne's use of an interpretive method to develop themes involved in CABS recovery is an appropriate approach to investigate the effects of major cardiac surgery on women's lives. She has chosen an intensive analysis of individual cases with a search for commonalities among them rather than establishing a priori a set of variables that might explain these effects. Mages and Mendelsohn (1979) refer to such analysis as a "personological" approach; in their study of the psychosocial effects of cancer they also noted certain themes, and, similar to Hawthorne's findings, many of them were mediated by age and gender. The following response discusses the seven themes, with comments on their utility for nursing practice and their relationship to other research regarding women and cardiac events.

Theme #1 notes that women understate the impact of cardiac surgery on their lives. This finding, supported by lifespan developmental theorists, may in part be explained by the older age at which women experience CABS, since the surgery is viewed as normative in terms of the aging process (Baltes, Reese, & Lipsett, 1980; Schaie, 1986). My own work indicated that not only did the oldest patients have the lowest levels of mood disturbance, but their caregiving husbands had even lower levels (Rankin, 1990; 1992) Although Hawthorne did not interview caregiving family members, it is possible that their low levels of distress mitigated the mood disturbances experienced by the women. The women who lived alone in Hawthorne's study lacked tangible assistance during their recovery, but they were not overwhelmed by the worry and anxiety characteristic of caregiving spouses (Biegel, Sales, & Schulz, 1991; Rankin, 1992).

Hawthorne's finding that more than half of her participants experienced angina a year after CABS suggests that the benefits of surgery do not persist as long for women as for men; this may be an additional reason that surgery does not have as great an impact on their lives. When female surgical participants in my study were questioned a year later about their willingness to repeat surgery, only 57% stated they would undergo a second surgery, whereas 88% of the men were willing to be revascularized (Rankin, 1991). This suggests that the benefits of surgery are calculated differently by women and men, and that the lack of positive dramatic changes influence women's evaluation of surgery.

Theme #2 is concerned with gender bias as an obstacle to surgery, not recognized as an impediment to the diagnosis of coronary heart disease (CHD) until 6 years ago. Tobin and associates (1987) were among the first to find that women were significantly less likely than men to be referred for further work-up following thallium scans. Apparently, cardiologists inferred a psychosomatic or other noncardiac related genesis to the presenting complaint. It is possible that ageism is also operative since, as noted earlier, women lag at least 10 years behind men in the development of CHD. Thus women are twice disadvantaged.

In addition to the above, women appear to present with different symptoms from men. For example, in our current study (Rankin, 1992–94), preliminary data analysis reveals that, of a group of women presenting with myocardial infarction, 46% had no chest pain at all and, of these, the primary presenting symptoms were shortness of breath (80%) or epigastric pain (20%). Of the 27% who had classic chest pain, epigastric, or abdominal pain was also found. Therefore, if women themselves are unaware of their vulnerability to CHD, and if their providers are unaware of the subtle differences in symptomatology, women may suffer unduly from CHD before diagnostic procedures are performed. In this scenario they are then older, sicker, and more likely to be suffering from comorbidities when CABS is finally performed. It is not surprising that their hospital stays are longer (Rankin, 1990), their mortality greater during the perioperative period (Becker, Corrao, & Alpert, 1988), and their participation in cardiac rehabilitation less frequent than that of men (Packard, 1992).

Studies are needed to ascertain cardiac profiles of women with CHD, and these should be based upon the women's own descriptions of clinical symptoms. Profiles derived solely through the language of physicians and nurses who have been exposed to a male model of heart disease will have questionable applicability to women.

Theme #3 deals with status differences noted between professional caregivers and women having CABS. Patterns of sex-role socialization and communication are cited by Hawthorne as being responsible for perceived inequity in patient/professional caregiver relationships. The implication is that such inequity results in less desirable treatment and care than that received by male CABS patients. This is an important topic and one that is infrequently discussed in clinical settings where medicocentrism prevails. Indeed, women patients are not alone in their risk for being poorly understood. Growing numbers of Hispanic, Asian, and other immigrant populations who approach professional health care providers with deference and passivity may also receive inadequate care during the perioperative period.

Women not qualifying for CABS because they are uninsured may be at even greater risk for status inequalities; their access to health care providers is so limited that they have not developed the necessary language to express their symptoms nor the skills to access the health care system in the first place. In my first study of recovery from cardiac surgery, minority group representation was poor, with no African-American women, two Hispanics, one Filipina, and one "none of the above; the remaining 19 women were Caucasian. Therefore, we might surmise that women who cannot gain access to CABS would represent greater status differentials than those participating in Hawthorne's study.

Theme #4 is concerned with women's remapping of relationships following cardiac surgery. This is not unique to CABS but is a feature of women's lives regardless of the type of illness, disability, or health transition. Kessler, McLeod, and Wethington's work (1985) suggests that because women "cast a wide net in their concern" they are more vulnerable to stresses experienced by their family members, friends, and even by others to whom they are less intimately related (p.498). The pivotal role played by women—whether in families with children, older families or as single women assisting other family members—continues whether they are ill or recovering from major surgery or childbirth.

Themes #5 and #6 are considered together as they relate to issues caused by the sternotomy incision, and are thus issues with which nursing can intervene. Hawthorne's recognition of differing meanings given to the scar by men and women is an important finding. Viewing the incision as mutilation (women) versus a badge of courage (men) suggests that women should be prepared differently for the surgery. Perhaps they would be better prepared if presented with photos so that they are informed regarding this surgical sequela. The parallel between women who undergo mastectomy and those who have CABS should not be overlooked in future research.

Theme #7 is related to the fourth, because the driving force during CABS recovery for women is comprised of relationships in which they are involved. Thus, instead of using guidelines for activity resumption given to them by their health care providers, women are more likely to use family environment cues. For example, women in my first study (1988) reported vacuuming or cooking large dinners for the family within 2 weeks of hospital discharge because "there was no one else to do it. My advice to women on hospital discharge is that they not remove their bathrobes or get dressed in street clothing until they know they are recovered—since wearing a bathrobe seems to authorize neglect of household responsibilities!

The fact that the scar is related to more mediastinal incisional discomfort in women than in men has implications for the ways in which nursing can intervene with anticipatory guidance—both before hospital discharge and at follow up during the first postoperative surgical visit. Since CABS patients are discharged from the hospital within a week following surgery, they should be prepared for the difficulties they may encounter at home. They should also be encouraged to have family members or friends available for assistance with activities of daily living.

Hawthorne has shared an "insider's view" of the experience of 10 women undergoing CABS. Her sensitive portrayal of the difficulties women encounter following surgery, as well as the contrasts with the experience of men, reinforces the importance of individualizing patient care and developing a more complete data base and "female model" of women and heart disease.

REFERENCES

Baltes, P. B., Reese, H. W., & Lipsitt, L. P. (1980). Life-span development psychology. *Annual Review of Psychology, 31,* 65–110.

Becker, R. C., Corrao, J. M., & Alpert, J. S. (1988). Coronary artery bypass surgery in women. *Clinical Cardiology, 11,* 443–448.

Biegel, D. E., Sales, E., & Schulz, R. (Eds.) (1991). Caregiving in heart disease. In *Family caregiving in chronic illness* (pp. 105–146). Newbury Park, CA: Sage.

Kessler, R. C., McLeod, J. D., & Wethington, E. (1985) The costs of caring: A perspective on the relationship between sex and psychological distress. In I. G. Sarason & B. R. Sarason (Eds.), *Social support: Theory, research and applications.*

Dordrecht, The Netherlands: Martinus Nijhoff.

Mages, N. L., & Mendelsohn, G. A. (1979). Effects of cancer on patients' lives: A personological approach. In G. C. Stone, F. Cohen, and N. E. Adler (Eds.), *Health psychology: A handbook* (pp. 255–284). San Francisco: Jossey-Bass.

Packard, B. (1992) Clinical aspects of coronary heart disease in women. In N. K. Wenger, & H. K. Hellerstein (Eds.), *Rehabilitation of the coronary patient* (pp. 217–230). New York: Churchill Livingstone.

Rankin, S. H. (1988) Gender, age, and caregiving as mediators of cardiovascular illness and recovery (Doctoral dissertation, University of California, San Francisco).

Rankin, S. H. (1991). Patient and caregiver trajectories one year after cardiac surgery. *Proceedings of the Western Institute of Nursing*. Albuquerque, NM: WSRN.

Rankin, S. H. (1992) Psychosocial adjustments of coronary artery disease patients and their spouses: Nursing implications. *Nursing Clinics of North America, 27,* 271–284.

Rankin, S. H. (1992–94). African- and Anglo-American women adapting to myocardial infarction. 1R55 NR 026170182.

Tobin, J. M., Wassertheil-Smoller, S., Wexler, J. P. et al. (1987). Sex bias in considering coronary bypass surgery. *Annals of Internal Medicine, 107,* 19–25.

Response
Jonathan N. Tobin

"Why Can't A Woman Be More Like A Man?"

It is remarkable that while the existence of gender differences or gender bias in diagnosis and treatment of coronary disease was seriously questioned by many until a few years ago, today its existence is generally accepted by most. How did we come to this point?

During the past few years a number of quantitative studies have examined gender differences in the prevalence, diagnosis, treatment, and outcome of coronary artery disease. These studies have been conducted in a variety of clinical settings and in different patient populations. It was previously observed that gender accounted for a significant proportion of variance in the decision to order cardiac catheterization and possible coronary bypass surgery among patients undergoing resting and exercise nuclear medicine studies (Wassertheil-Smoller, Steingart, Wexler, et al., 1987). Specifically for nuclear exercise study patients, a striking, tenfold gender difference was observed for patients with abnormal scans (Tobin et al., 1987). What are mechanisms that account for gender differences in treatment? Why were examining cardiac physicians of patients undergoing exercise nuclear medicine scans much more likely to attribute symptoms and complaints to non-cardiac and psychiatric causes in women than in men (Tobin et al., 1987)?

This observation suggests a higher threshold for convincing physicians that chest pain in women is cardiac in origin, and should be aggressively managed, even though equal proportions of patients had previous diagnoses of typical angina by their referring physicians, and equal rates were receiving anti-anginal drug therapy (Tobin et al., 1987). Until very recently, few studies reported about women cardiac patients, and many studies excluded women from study completely.

The early findings of gender bias have subsequently been validated and extended to patients in a number of different clinical settings along the continuum of diagnosis and treatment of heart disease. For example, a study of male and female patients undergoing coronary bypass surgery reported that higher operative mortality rates observed in women were due entirely to more advanced age and worse cardiac status and function (Khan et al., 1990). Among patients following myocardial infarction enrolled in the SAVE study, physicians were less aggressive in their prior management of coronary disease in women

(Steingart et al., 1991). After myocardial infarction, men and women are equally likely to undergo catheterization, when adjusted for age, but women are less likely to be referred for coronary bypass surgery (Krumholz et al., 1992). Gender differences have been observed in patients hospitalized for coronary disease (Ayanian & Epstein, 1991), along with both gender and ethnic differences for angiography patients undergoing bypass surgery (Ayanian et al., 1993) and patients admitted to hospitals for coronary disease (Wenneker & Epstein, 1989).

While severely symptomatic women are equally likely to be referred for coronary bypass surgery as men, minimally symptomatic or asymptomatic women are less likely to be referred for catheterization and surgery (Bickell et al., 1992). Similar differences have been observed for men and women referred for percutaneous transluminal coronary angioplasty (Hannan et al., 1992; Bell et al., 1993; Hillborne et al., 1993).

It has been reported previously that women present with worse functional status at surgery but have recovery patterns similar to men, with respect to sexuality, leisure activities, and occupational status (Rankin, 1990). The interesting study presented by Hawthorne extends the study of gender differences to a small group of female coronary bypass surgery patients after surgery. Hawthorne presents analyses of a series of focused interviews with female coronary artery bypass patients, and examines ways in which the experiences of women differs from those of men reported in a previous study (Hawthorne, 1991) following coronary artery bypass graft surgery.

Hawthorne identifies seven major themes which emerge and recur during her interviews with nine female bypass patients. These themes include: minimizing surgical experience, delay in diagnosis and treatment, gender role differences in interactions with caregivers, re-establishment of relations and family functions following surgery, meaning of incision and scarring, greater mediastinal and incisional discomfort for women, and patterns of self-care during recovery.

It is important to look for reasons for these post-surgical differences in recovery. A popular self-help book written by a surgeon who invented one of the precursors to bypass surgery stated

> ". . . the happiness and well-being of a person in the postcoronary period sometimes depends on his ability to handle his sexuality" (Vineberg, 1975:78) and that ". . . it's extremely important for the physician to include the wife in any counseling session with a heart patient. It is not sufficient just to tell the patient that he can have

sexual relations. It is important that the wife realizes that it is perfectly safe to do so." (Vineberg, 1975:85).

Even the way in which cardiac surgical facilities are structured reflect this male-centered perspective. One female bypass patient reported that

"[T]here were all men on my floor . . . When I realized their [postsurgical] exercises were geared to men, I asked for exercises for female Bypassers. They got very huffy. 'We're not prepared for female Bypassers. We don't have anything special for women. Most Bypassers are male' . . ." (Hoffman, 1985: 105).

Another female patient recounted

"[W]hen I'd complain about my chest, my doctor would say, 'You can't be having heart pain. At 48, still menstruating, a woman doesn't have heart disease'. My husband had Bypass, even my doctor had Bypass, but nobody figured I needed Bypass" (Hoffman, 1985: 315).

The hidden message contained in these studies and observations is the same: despite the epidemiologic evidence to the contrary, coronary disease is a man's disease and coronary bypass surgery is a man's operation. The issues raised in Hawthorne's article are significant for a number of reasons. If it is true that women tend to more often accept heart disease as an inevitable consequence of aging, then the message of risk factor reduction must be targeted especially to women through the mass media, and, in primary care settings, *before* they develop coronary disease. This is equally true in the setting where cardiac disease has already been diagnosed, since, according to Hawthorne, women report less concern than men with physiologic parameters, such as cholesterol and blood pressure in guiding their recovery following surgery. These two related facts suggest the critical role that the nursing profession, a profession historically dominated by women, can play in the prevention, diagnosis, and long-term management of coronary disease. These findings suggest the need for nurses to educate themselves, their physicians, and their patients concerning the prevalence and consequences of coronary disease in women.

Nurses are already a critical part of the health care teams caring for patients with suspected or proven heart disease at any point along their illness trajectory, ranging from primary care prevention, early intervention, and risk factor modification to diagnosis, management, and follow-up of patients after heart attacks and heart surgery. Hawthorne has identified a number of significant opportunities for nurses to contribute further to patient care.

Hopefully, changes such as the awareness of the underlying gender-based assumptions, recent popular books targeting women and heart disease (e.g., Diethrich & Cohan, 1993), revisions in health professional school curriculum, as well as activities such as the Women's Health Initiative (Healy, 1991) will have a positive impact on reducing gender bias in the diagnosis and treatment of all health problems, including coronary disease. Efforts must be made to reach all women from every ethnic and economic group to reduce risk factors and to prevent cardiac disease, where possible, and to diagnose and intervene with effective treatments early. In a situation where social artifact has masqueraded as scientific fact, nurses have a critical role to play, as educators and advocates for prevention and early intervention.

REFERENCES

Ayanian, J. Z., & Epstein, A. M. (1991). Differences in the use of procedures between women and men hospitalized for coronary heart disease. *New England Journal of Medicine, 325,* 221–225.

Ayanian, J. Z., Udvarhelyi, I. S., Gatsonis, C. A., Pashos, C. L., & Epstein, A. M. (1993). Racial differences in the use of revascularization procedures after coronary angiography. *Journal of the American Medical Association, 269,* 2642–2646.

Bell, M. R., Holmes, Jr., D. R., Berger, P. B., Garratt, K. N., Bailey, K. R., & Gersh, B. J. (1993). The changing in-hospital mortality of women undergoing percutaneous transluminal coronary angioplasty. *Journal of the American Medical Association, 269,* 2091–2095.

Bickell, N. A., Pieper, K. S., Lee, K. L., Mark, D. B., Glower, D. D., Pryor, D. B., & Califf, R. M. (1992). Referral patterns for coronary artery disease treatment: Gender bias or good clinical judgement? *Annals of Internal Medicine, 116,* 791–797.

Diethrich, E. B., & Cohan, C. (1992). What can you do to stop the number 1 killer of American women: Women and heart disease. New York: Random House, Inc.

Hannan, E. L., Arani, D. T., Johnson, L. W., Kemp, H. G., & Lukacik, G. (1992). Percutaneous Transluminal Coronary Angioplasty in New York State: Risk Factors and Outcomes. *Journal of the American Medical Association, 268,* 3092–3097.

Hawthorne, M. H. (1991) Reconceptualizing cardiac illness: Using the trajectory framework. *Scholarly Inquiry for Nursing Practice.*

Healy, B. (1991). The yentl syndrome. *New England Journal of Medicine, 325,* 274–276.
Hilborne, L. H., Leape, L. L., Bernstein, S. J., Park, R. E., Fiske, M. E., Kamberg, C. J., Roth, C. P., & Brook, R. H. (1993). The appropriateness of use of percutaneous transluminal coronary angioplasty in New York State. *Journal of the American Medical Association, 269,* 761–765.
Hoffman, N. Y. (1985). *Change of heart: The bypass experience.* Orlando, FL: Harcourt Brace Jovanovich Publishers.
Krumholz, H. M., Douglas, P. S., Lauer, M. S., & Pasternak, R. C. (1992). Selection of patients for coronary angiography and coronary revascularization early after myocardial infarction: Is there evidence for a gender bias? *Annals of Internal Medicine, 116,* 785–790.
Laskey, W. K. (1992). Gender differences in the management of coronary artery disease: Bias or good clinical judgement? *Annals of Internal Medicine, 116,* 869–871.
Rankin, S. H. (1990). Differences in recovery from cardiac surgery: A profile of male and female patients. *Heart & Lung, 19,* 481–485.
Steingart, R. M., Packer, M., Hamm, P., Coglianese, M. E., Gersh, B., Geltman, E. M., Lewis, S. J., Gottlieb, S. S., Bernstein, V., McEwan, P., Jacobson, K., Brown, E. J., Kukin, M. L., Kantrowitz, N. E., & Pfeffer, M. A. (1991). Sex differences in the management of coronary artery disease. *New England Journal of Medicine, 325,* 226–230.
Tobin, J. N., & Wassertheil-Smoller, S., Wexler, J. P., Steingart, R. M., Budner, N., Lense, L., Wachspress, J. (1987). Sex bias in considering coronary bypass surgery. *Annals of Internal Medicine, 107,* 19–25.
Vineberg, A. (1975). *How to live with your heart.* New York: Optimum Publishing Co., Lt.
Wassertheil-Smoller, S., Steingart, R. M., Wexler, J. P., et al. (1987). Nuclear scans: A clinical decision making tool that reduces the need for cardiac catheterization. *Journal of Chronic Disorders, 40,* 385–397.
Wenneker, M. B., & Epstein, A. M. (1989). Racial inequalities in the use of procedures for patients with ischemic heart disease in Massachusetts. *Journal of the American Medical Association, 261,* 253–257.

Chapter 4

Health-Promoting Behaviors and Quality of Life Among Individuals With Multiple Sclerosis

Alexa K. Stuifbergen

OVERVIEW

Chronic conditions have profound and pervasive effects on the quality of life of millions of Americans (USDHHS, 1991). The estimated one-quarter million Americans with MS face a unique set of stressors and challenges as they seek to adapt to a chronic illness with an unknown cause, few medical therapies, and an uncertain prognosis that almost always includes some degree of functional disability (Wasserman, 1988). The purpose of this study was to explore factors related to performance of health-promoting behaviors and to examine the relationship between the practice of health-promoting behaviors and perceived quality of life for individuals with MS. A general conceptual model was used as a framework for exploring the relationships among antecedent variables (demographic/disease factors, barriers, resources, perceptual factors), health-promoting behaviors, and perceived quality of life with a convenience sample of 61 individuals with MS. Analyses supported a hypothesized relationship between health-promoting behaviors and quality of life. Subsequent research with larger samples is needed to

Note: Originally published in *Scholarly Inquiry for Nursing Practice: An International Journal*, Vol. 9, No. 1, 1995. New York: Springer Publishing Company.

clearly address the relative strength and path of variables in the proposed model.

INTRODUCTION

The practice of health-promoting behaviors has been acknowledged as a valuable and important strategy to maintain the independence and quality of life of persons with chronic and/or disabling conditions (Parcel, Bartlett, & Bruhn, 1986; USDHHS, 1991). Despite recognition of health promotion activities as a form of symptom management for various chronic diseases, including multiple sclerosis (MS), persons with chronic and disabling conditions have been largely overlooked in investigations of health. Consequently, little is known about factors influencing their health-promoting behaviors and how participation in such behaviors may influence their quality of life.

Individuals diagnosed with a chronic disease must adapt to the experience of living with a long-term, incurable illness that imposes limitations on their functioning (Dimond & Jones, 1983; Woods, Yates, & Primomo, 1989). Current estimates indicate that approximately 250,000 to 350,000 persons in the United States have physician-diagnosed MS, a disease of the central nervous system in which the cells of the immune system destroy the myelin-insulating axons, thus interfering with the efficiency of electrical conduction within the central nervous system (Anderson et al., 1992). MS typically has its onset between the ages of 15 and 50, and is more common among women and descendents of northern Europeans. Primary symptoms of MS include weakness, numbness, gait disturbances, fatigue, visual disturbances, dizziness, ataxia, bladder and bowel problems, cognitive dysfunction, changes in sexual functioning, pain and muscle weakness, spasm, and spasticity (Schapiro, 1991). The onset and progression of symptoms is unpredictable and wide variations in the possible trajectory make it difficult if not impossible to predict disease course for a particular individual (Smeltzer, 1992). For some, the disease may be relatively benign, resulting in only mild neurological dysfunction. For others, the disease may progress or exacerbate, causing major neurological losses and disability. Although some will be severely disabled, two-thirds of those diagnosed with MS remain ambulatory after 20 years (Schapiro, 1991).

The uncertainty and unpredictability of MS, as well as the potentially progressive and disabling nature of the disease, make MS useful as a model for research designed to explore adjustment to chronic illness (Smeltzer, 1992). While extensive biomedical research efforts focus on finding a cause and a cure, individuals with this chronic condition continue their everyday struggle to manage their symptoms and maintain their quality of life. Optimal symptom management currently centers on client education, appropriate exercise, and the practice of positive health habits (Schapiro, 1991). Although previous studies have examined selected factors that may influence one or more components of quality of life for individuals with chronic illnesses, the relationship between health-promoting behaviors and quality of life has not been investigated.

Earlier studies have identified factors associated with health-promoting lifestyles among adults with disabilities (Becker, Stuifbergen, Ingalsbe, & Sands, 1989; Stuifbergen & Becker, 1994) and provided qualitative data about the use of health-promoting behaviors by individuals with MS as innovative coping strategies to manage the demands of illness (Stuifbergen, 1992). This exploratory study was designed to empirically examine the assumed relationship between health-promoting behaviors and quality of life and to serve as the first phase in refinement and testing of a conceptual model to predict quality of life among persons with MS. In this initial phase, zero-order and partial correlations between the components of the model were examined to determine if the relationships between variables observed in previous studies of other populations were similar to the correlations observed in a group of adults with MS. The specific purposes of this exploratory study were to: (1) identify the barriers; resources; perceptual; and demographic and disease factors that are related to performance of health-promoting behaviors among individuals with MS; (2) examine the relationship between the practice of health behaviors and quality of life for individuals with MS; and (3) refine a model of factors influencing quality of life in adults with MS.

CONCEPTUAL MODEL

The preliminary model (Figure 1) used to guide this study represents a synthesis of findings from the literature and the investigator's prior research. The model proposes four antecedent factors that influence the selection and use of health-promoting behaviors: Demographic/ Disease Factors, Resources, Barriers, and Perceptual Factors. Figure 4.1

includes the direction of the relationships reported in the literature between specific antecedent factors and health-promoting behaviors. Selection and use of health-promoting behaviors is posited to have a positive relationship with quality of life and to explain additional variance unaccounted for by the antecedent factors.

Demographic/Disease Factors

The associations between demographic factors (age, gender, education, employment) and disease-related variables (severity of illness/disability, length of illness) and the consequences of MS on individuals' lives have been explored in prior studies. In a longitudinal study designed to analyze the adjustment process of 103 individuals with MS, Brooks and Matson (1982) found being female, hours employed, living arrangement, and income to be significantly related to positive adjustment (improving self-concept). In a 5-year study of 211 subjects with MS, Gulick and Bugg (1992) reported higher levels of functioning in fine and gross motor activities and intimacy among the more recently diagnosed. Older age at diagnosis was related to decreased functioning in motor activities, socializing/recreation, and intimacy.

In a cross-sectional epidemiological survey of 256 individuals with MS, Harper, Harper, Chambers, Cino, and Singer (1986) found that the

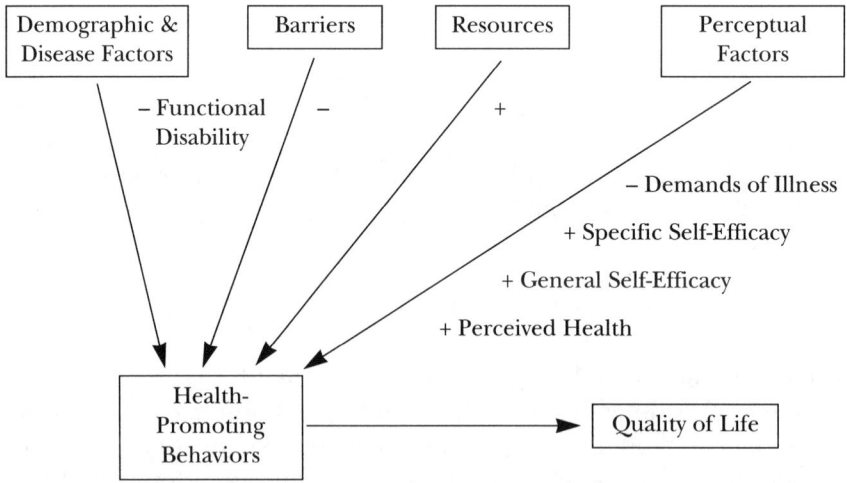

FIGURE 4.1 Preliminary Model and Predicted Relationships.

combination of disease and demographic variables accounted for 21% of the variance in Quality of Life scores. Greater severity of disease was related to decreased scores on measures of physical health, social health, and quality of life scores, but not emotional health. Age, employment status, and income were inversely related to physical health scores. Educational level was positively associated with social health, employment status, and mental health scores. Demographic/disease factors measured in this study included age, gender, severity of illness (functional disability), cognitive impairment, and length of time since diagnosis.

Resources

A variety of resources, including income and social support, is related to the selection and use of health-promoting behaviors and health outcomes. A substantial body of research suggests that social support as a resource may affect both physical and psychological health through its stress-mediating and/or stress-buffering role (Heitzmann & Kaplan, 1988). In particular, social support has been represented as a crucial factor in coping with the demands of physical illness and disability (Wallston, Alagna, DeVellis, & DeVellis, 1983). In a study of 149 families in which one spouse had MS, Weinert (1983) found social support had a consistent and positive impact on family functioning. Financial resources are also related to health behaviors and their outcomes. Low-income people, regardless of ethnicity, have a rate of disability, measured as activity limitation, twice that of whites and greater than all other ethnic groups (USDHHS, 1991). In studies of individuals with MS, higher family income has been related to positive adjustment (Brooks & Matson, 1982), and social status was significantly related to depression and functional disability (Wineman, 1990).

Barriers

Barriers are defined as perceptions regarding the unavailability, inconvenience, or difficulty of a particular health-promoting option (Pender, 1987). Barriers may arise from people's internal cognitions, from significant others, and from the environment. Existing literature documents barriers to health care services for both disabled and nondisabled persons; they include time, distance, cost, availability of services, and aspects of the provider-consumer relationship (Melnyk,

1988; Nosek, 1984). The concept of barriers, operationalized in different ways, has been related to participation in exercise programs (Dishman, Sallis, & Orenstein, 1985), the primary prevention behaviors of rest, nutrition, exercise (Duffy, 1986), and skin care (Dai & Catanzaro, 1987). Becker, Stuifbergen and Sands (1991) reported the development of a scale that measures barriers to health behaviors for disabled persons ($N = 135$). The participants rated lack of money, being too tired, the impairment, concern about crime, and lack of time as most frequently interfering with their ability to take care of their health. Scores on the barriers scale were negatively associated with general self-efficacy ($r = -.48$, $p < .01$), perceived health status ($r = -.29$, $p < .01$) and the likelihood of engaging in health-promoting behaviors ($r = -.29$, $p < .01$).

Perceptual Factors

A number of perceptual factors may influence health-promoting behaviors and the conceptualization of quality of life. Those considered here include perceived health, self-efficacy, and perceived demands of illness. The tendency for consumers to define health as a multidimensional concept, not limited to the absence of illness, is a common theme represented in previous findings (Stuifbergen, Becker, Ingalsbe, & Sands, 1990; Williams, 1983). Many individuals with chronic and disabling conditions perceive themselves as predominantly healthy; both Williams (1983) and Stuifbergen et al (1990) found that the majority of chronically ill or disabled participants rated their overall health as good or excellent ($N = 70$; $N = 135$, respectively).

The self-efficacy construct (Bandura, 1982) has emerged as an important predictor of behavioral actions. Bandura describes behavior as a joint function of outcome expectancies (beliefs about the consequences of that behavior) and personal efficacy expectancies (beliefs about one's ability to perform specific behaviors in specific situations). Self-efficacy varies according to the level of task difficulty, the generalizability of self-efficacy from other tasks, and the certainty of a person's perception of his or her ability to perform the task. Bandura also emphasized that judgments of self-efficacy can vary across activities and life circumstances. Although Bandura acknowledged the relatedness of general self-efficacy (a global disposition or characteristic) and specific self-efficacy, he argued that the most powerful measures focus on specific or particular self-efficacy and outcome expectations for particular behaviors. In a review of 21 studies aimed at enhancing good health practices, Strecher, DeVellis, Becker, and Rosenstock (1986) concluded that self-efficacy discriminated successful smoking quitters, effective weight losers, effective contraceptive users, and exercise persisters from those not successful in implementing these changes in their health behaviors.

An important predictor of response to chronic illness is the individual's perception of how that illness affects everyday life. The demands of illness are subjective judgments about the difficulties, problems or challenges inherent in day-to-day living with a chronic illness. These demands encompass the direct effects of a disease, personal disruption occurring as a consequence of illness, and environmental transactions necessitated by the illness (Woods, Haberman, & Packard, 1989). Demands of illness represent the product of individuals' appraisals and reappraisals of the impact of illness on their lives and will vary with the course of the illness (Woods, Yates, & Primomo, 1989). Descriptive studies of chronically ill individuals have related increasing severity of illness to decreased sexual activity (Sjorgren & Fugl-Meyer, 1982), severe restrictions in recreation and leisure activities (McSweeney, Grant, Heaton, Adams, & Timms, 1982), limitations in instrumental and nurturant roles for homemakers (Reisine, Goodenow, & Grady, 1987), and reduced labor-market activity and income (Paringer, 1983).

Health-Promoting Behaviors

Pender (1987) defines health-promoting behaviors as "activities directed toward increasing the level of well-being and actualizing the health potential of individuals, families, communities, and societies" (p.4). These ongoing behavioral activities include, but are not limited to, physical exercise, nutritional eating practices, social support, and stress-management techniques. Although health promotion activities have been investigated in a number of groups of "well" individuals, there has been little research on the health-related attitudes and behaviors of adults with long-term chronic illnesses and disabilities. Much of the work reported in the special education and rehabilitation literature has focused on the effects of training programs targeted at specific health behaviors, usually exercise. The results of these studies indicate that individuals with disabling conditions ranging from mild to severe can be taught to perform various exercises, and there is some indication that the effects of training generalize to other situations (Broadhead, 1981).

Selected studies document that chronically ill and disabled persons desire and choose health-promoting behaviors. Nosek (1984) found in persons with orthopedic impairments that level of independence was positively related to health status when defined as use of medical services and health-promoting practices. Warms (1987) found that individuals with a spinal cord injury desired health-promotion services more frequently than disability-related services, particularly access to services relating to exercise, nutrition, and stress management. In a study of the demands of illness experienced by individuals with MS, the most frequently reported activity for managing the physical demands of illness was exercise (Stuifbergen, 1992). Participants described a wide variety of fitness activities that had helped them cope with their symptoms—ranging from stretching exercises to swimming, jogging, and tennis. Gulick (1991) reported that persons with MS who performed self-assessments and monitoring of health behaviors and symptoms had fewer hospitalizations and office visits for health care than matched subjects who did not perform similar assessments.

Becker, Stuifbergen, Ingalsbe, and Sands (1989) reported that an adaptive definition of health, general self-efficacy, age, and barriers to health-promotion activities were statistically significant predictors of scores on a self-report measure of health-promoting behaviors for 135 disabled consumers of Independent Living Centers. In a correlational follow-up study with a second group of adults with disabilities ($N = 117$), Stuifbergen and Becker (1994) found that the likelihood of engaging in health-promoting behaviors was significantly ($p < .05$) related to decreased need for mechanical ($r = -.26$) and personal ($r = -.23$) assistance, fewer barriers ($r = -.25$), general self-efficacy ($r = .44$) and specific self-efficacy for health practices ($r = .62$). Multiple regression analyses revealed that adults with disabilities were more likely to engage in health-promoting behaviors if they had higher scores on the measures of general and specific self-efficacy, had a wellness-oriented definition of health, required less mechanical assistance with their daily activities, and were female.

Quality of Life

Quality of life has become a relevant measure of efficacy in clinical studies and a growing body of research literature suggests that people's health status is related to their perceptions of their quality of life (Burckhardt, Woods, Schultz, & Ziebarth, 1989; Dillard, Campbell, & Chisolm, 1984). Definitions and descriptions of quality of life have included both objective and subjective indicators of physical and psychological phenomena (Oleson, 1990). Purely objective indicators such as income, living situations, and physical functioning assume that a decrease in the indicator is analogous to a decrease in quality of life. These objective measures fail to consider that the importance ascribed to various domains of life, such as physical functioning, may vary among individuals and may be influenced by changes in life circumstances. Thus objective indicators of quality of life provide limited information about how individuals perceive their own lives.

In contrast, subjective evaluations of quality of life represent the individual's perception of important life domains and satisfaction with those domains (Oleson, 1990). Life domains include objective factors such as roles and activities believed to influence quality of life. It is the individual's satisfaction with these critical domains, rather than his/her particular level or status however, that is of central importance to subjective evaluations of quality of life. Measured subjectively, quality of life reflects an individual's sense of well-being and satisfaction with life.

Results of studies conducted with MS populations have suggested that contact with healthy people (Maybury & Brewin, 1984) and perceived support from family and friends (McIvor, Riklan, & Reznikoff, 1984) are related to better psychosocial adaptation. Wineman (1990) found that perceived supportiveness of interactions was directly related to purpose in life and that functional disability had a direct effect on the degree of psychosocial adaptation. Studies conducted with other chronically ill groups have identified linkages between quality of life and mastery, fatigue, dyspnea severity, self-help, self-esteem and perceived support (Braden, 1990; Burckhardt, 1985; Moody, McCormick, & Williams, 1991).

SUMMARY

Chronically ill individuals must manage a wide variety of disease-related, intrapersonal, and environmental demands to maintain their quality of life. Engaging in health-promoting behaviors is one strategy recommended to manage disease symptoms and enhance quality of life. Factors associated with the selection and use of health-promoting behaviors in other groups include demographic/disease factors, resources, barriers, and perceptual factors. Barriers and resources may be especially crucial for persons with chronic and disabling conditions whose life circumstances, even when they possess the necessary knowledge about good health practices, make it difficult for them to implement health-promoting behaviors. Few studies have explored health behaviors in individuals with MS and the presumed relationship between health-promoting behaviors and quality of life for persons with chronic and disabling conditions has not been empirically investigated. The specific research questions were:

1. What is the relationship between reported health-promoting behaviors and perceived quality of life among adults with MS?
2. What is the relationship of antecedents (demographic/disease factors, barriers, resources and perceptual factors) and health-promoting behaviors among adults with MS?
3. What combination of antecedents (demographic/disease factors, barriers, resources and perceptual factors) best predicts perceived quality of life among adults with MS?
4. Does frequency of reported health-promoting behaviors add significantly to the prediction of perceived quality of life among adults with MS after the effects of the antecedent factors have been accounted for?

METHOD

Sample

In this descriptive correlational study, subjects were recruited through a mailing to 200 individuals on the mailing list of the local chapter of the National Multiple Sclerosis Society. To protect the privacy of respondents, the mailing labels on the envelopes were affixed by staff at the MS office. Individuals who were interested in receiving more information about the study and possibly participating were asked to return a card providing name and phone number to the investigator. Seventy-five postcards were returned. A target sample size of 60 that would allow correlations greater than .25 to be detected as statistically significant at the .05 level was chosen for this study (Glass & Stanley, 1970).

Research staff contacted interested individuals by phone to explain study requirements and procedures. If the individual wished to participate, a data collection visit was scheduled at a mutually acceptable time at the investigator's research office. Calls continued until 61 subjects were recruited. Only two phone contacts declined to participate, one for transportation reasons; a second was too disabled to leave the home setting.

The mean age of participants was 42.5 years (range 20–76), and most were female (77%), Anglo (89%), married (67%), and college graduates (61%). Only two participants (3%) had not finished high school. Most participants (69%) had children; 43% had children under the age of 18. Almost half (46%) of the participants were unemployed and 21% worked 20 or fewer hours a week. When asked about job-related changes (multiple responses were possible), 26% indicated that they had retired for health reasons, 12% indicated they were fired for health reasons, and 16% had taken a less demanding job. A majority of the sample (54%) indicated that they had adequate financial resources to meet their needs, while 15% reported they had very few financial resources. Thirty-one percent of the participants were receiving some type of government assistance.

All subjects reported they had physician-diagnosed MS. When subjects were asked about their "type of MS," most (80%) were able to give a lengthy description of symptoms, but not state a particular type. The mean time since first experiencing symptoms (16.2 years) was almost double the mean length of time since diagnosis (8.5 years). Personal assistance with daily activities was needed some (57%), most (3%), or all (2%) of the time, and mechanical assistance (e.g., wheelchair, motorized cart) was required some (30%), most (13%) or all (11%) of the time.

Procedure

When participants arrived at the investigator's office, the study was explained and informed consent obtained. Self-report instruments were presented in a booklet format. Print size was enlarged and items were spaced to enhance readability and ease of completion. The questionnaire battery was self-administered in a quiet setting free of distractions. Incapacity Status scale ratings were obtained using a structured interview format. The Neuropsychological Screening Battery for MS (Rao, 1991) was administered to subjects by a certified rehabilitation nurse specifically trained to administer the battery by a consulting neuropsychologist. Data described here were collected at the first of three data collection contacts. Additional nutritional and fitness assessments and a mailed follow-up were later completed as part of the larger study to obtain data to support validity of instruments with a chronically ill population.

Instruments

Demographic/Disease Factors measured in this study included age, gender, length of illness, functional disability, and cognitive impairment. A background information sheet was used to collect demographic and disease-related information. The Neuropsychological Screening Battery for Multiple Sclerosis (NSBMS) (Rao, 1991) was used to identify cognitive dysfunction. The NSBMS provides measures of the cognitive functions most often affected by MS: sustained attention and concentration, verbal learning, visuospatial learning and semantic retrieval. Protocols for administration and scoring described by Rao (1991) were carefully followed. Rao (1991) includes four measures in the index for determining cognitive impairment: the score on Consistent Long-Term Retrieval of the Selective Reminding Test, the Total Recall (Trials 1–5) for the 7/24 Spatial Recall, the Total Correct from the hard form of the PASAT (PASAT2), and the number of total responses from the Word List Generation Test. Cognitive impairment is suspected if the individual fails (test performance falls below the 5th percentile of the normal control group) two or more tests.

The Incapacity Status Scale (ISS) (Kurtzke, 1981) provided an objective measure of functional disability—the physical limitation in ability to perform one's usual roles and activities. A trained rater used a structured interview to assess the degree of impairment in 16 aspects of personal functioning (e.g., ambulation, vision, bladder and bowel functioning) represented on this scale. Each of the 16 items is rated on a 5-point scale, with "0" indicating normal functioning and "4" indicating complete inability to perform the activity. The ISS was thoroughly evaluated by a panel of international MS experts for use as a minimal record for disability for MS. Evidence supporting the construct validity of the scale has been presented by Kurtzke (1981).

Barriers were measured by the Barriers to Health-Promoting Activities for Disabled Persons Scale (Becker et al., 1991) and responses to single items about the amount of personal and mechanical assistance required. The Barriers scale is an 18-item, 4-point scale that asks respondents to indicate how often the listed barriers (e.g., lack of time, being too tired) keep them from taking care of their health. Responses are scaled from 1 "Never" to 4 "Routinely." Higher scores on this summated rating scale indicate greater perceived barriers. Reported internal consistency reliability of the Barriers scale was .82 (Cronbach's alpha). Internal consistency in the present study was .81.

Resources such as perceived adequacy of financial resources and education were determined from the background information sheet. The Interpersonal Relationship Inventory (Tilden, Nelson, & May, 1990) was used to measure the multiple dimensions of interpersonal relationships within support networks. This instrument is unique in its extension of the usual measurement of social support to include less often measured aspects of reciprocity and conflict. This 39-item, 5-point scale yields three 13-item subscales:

1. social support: perceived availability or actual enactment of helping behaviors by members of the social network;
2. reciprocity: perceived availability or occurrence of an exchange of emotional or tangible resources or the returning of such goods or services;
3. conflict: perceived stress in relationships caused by behaviors of others.

Subscale scores range from 13 to 65, and scores are used separately and not combined. Internal consistency of subscales was reported to range from .78 to .89, and test-retest correlations ranged from .81 to .91. In the present study, internal consistency ranged from .74 for the Reciprocity subscale to .89 for the Conflict and Social Support scales.

Perceptual Factors assessed included perceived health status, specific self-efficacy for health practices, general self-efficacy, and perceived demands of illness. Perceived Health Status was measured by the 4-item Health Self-Rating scale, a subscale of the Multilevel Assessment Instrument (Lawton, Moss, Fulcomer, & Kleban, 1982). Subjects rate the overall quality of their health, with higher scores indicating better perceived health. Lawton et al. have reported a test/retest correlation of .92 over three weeks, internal consistency, measured by Cronbach's alpha, of .76, and correlations of .63 with clinicians' ratings of health status. The alpha reliability coefficient in the present study was .74.

Specific Self-Efficacy for Health-Promoting Behaviors was measured with the Self-Rated Abilities for Health Practices scale (SRAHP) (Becker, Stuifbergen, Oh, & Hall, 1993), which measures beliefs about one's abilities to perform health-promoting practices in the domains of nutrition, physical activity/exercise, psychological well-being, and responsible health practices. This 28-item scale asks respondents to rate how well they are able to perform each health practice on a 5-point scale from 0 "Not at All" to 4 "Completely." Ratings for the 28 items are summed to yield a total score on the SRAHP. Alpha internal consistency of the total scale is .92, and reliability of individual subscales ranges from .76 to .90. Two week test-retest reliability is .70. A principal components factor analysis with varimax rotation of responses from 188 subjects confirmed that the proposed four-factor solution accounted for 61% of the total variance (Becker et al., 1993). Internal consistency of the SRAHP in the present study was .94 for the total scale.

General self-efficacy was measured with the General Self-Efficacy subscale of the Self-Efficacy Scale (Sherer et al., 1982), a measure of beliefs about personal ability to affect outcomes in various situations. Scores on the 17-item, 5-point Likert scale range from 17 to 85, with higher scores indicating greater general self-efficacy. Sherer et al. reported a Cronbach alpha coefficient of .86 and construct validity is supported by the confirmation of expected relationships with other psychological constructs as well as success in vocational and educational settings. The alpha coefficient in the present study was .86.

A modified version of the Demands of Illness Inventory (Haberman, Woods, & Packard, 1989) was used to measure the events or experiences attributed to MS that tax personal and social resources, and thus well-being. This modified version consists of 61 statements that subjects score on a 5-point Likert scale measuring the extent to which each demand is attributed to the illness experience. Internal consistency of the total scale of this modified version was .95.

Health-Promoting Behavior was operationalized with the Health Promoting Lifestyle Profile (HPLP) (Walker, Sechrist, & Pender, 1987). This 48-item, 4-point scale assesses the frequency with which individuals report engaging in activities directed toward increasing their level of health and well-being. Responses are scaled from 1 "Never" to 4 "Routinely." This instrument is composed of six subscales identified through factor analysis:

1. self-actualization—having a sense of purpose, seeking personal development and satisfaction;
2. health responsibility—taking responsibility for one's own health practices and seeking professional assistance when needed;
3. exercise—engaging in regular physical exercise;
4. nutrition—establishing eating patterns and making healthy food choices;

5. interpersonal support—maintaining intimate and close relationships; and
6. stress management—recognizing and controlling stress to achieve relaxation.

Internal consistency alphas are reported to range from .70 to .90 for the subscales and .92 for the total scale. Internal consistency of the total scale was .92 in the present study. Data from nutrition and fitness assessments supported the validity of the HPLP in chronically ill populations.

The Quality of Life Index (QLI)—MS version (Ferrans & Powers, 1985) was originally developed to measure quality of life of "healthy persons" and specific versions have been developed for a number of patient groups, including hemodialysis patients, persons with MS, and persons with cancer. The QLI—MS version is a 72-item measure composed of two parts: Part 1 measures satisfaction with various domains of life (e.g., health, being able to get around, standard of living, achieving personal goals), and Part 2 measures the importance of the same domains. Subjects respond to each item on a 6-point scale, ranging from "very satisfied" to "very dissatisfied" for Part 1 and "very important" to "very unimportant" for Part 2. Total quality of life scores are calculated by weighting each satisfaction response with its paired importance response. Therefore, scores reflect individual values as well as satisfaction. The highest scores are produced by combinations of high satisfaction/high importance responses. Factor analysis revealed four dimensions underlying the QLI: health and functioning, socioeconomic, psychological/spiritual, and family. This four-factor solution explained 91% of the total variance (Ferrans & Powers, 1992). Internal consistency in use with individuals receiving dialysis was reported to be .90. Internal consistency of the QLI-MS version in this study was .87.

FINDINGS

Means, standard deviations, and the range of scores for each of the self-report variables measured in the study appear in Table 4.1. At a descriptive level, the majority of participants (56%) viewed their overall health as good or excellent. Fifty-one percent of the subjects passed all cognitive tests and 15% of the sample failed two or more tests; thus they were

TABLE 4.1 Scores of Adults with MS on Antecedent Variables and Health-Promoting Lifestyle Dimensions ($N = 61$)

Scale	M	SD	Possible Range of Scores	Actual Range of Scores
Incapacity Status Scale	12.38	7.14	0–48	0–34
Barriers	34.33	7.50	0–72	18–54
Interpersonal Relationships Inventory				
• Social support	51.95	8.33	13–65	30–64
• Reciprocity	50.02	5.60	13–65	36–61
• Conflict	37.22	9.61	13–65	14–61
Perceived health	7.16	2.11	4–13	4–13
Self-rated abilities	79.69	18.48	0–112	23–112
General self-efficacy	61.69	9.79	17–85	40–83
Demands of illness	111.38	40-19	0–244	8–192
Health Promoting Lifestyle Profile				
• Self-actualization	38.67	7.58	13–52	26–52
• Health responsibility	24.95	5.47	10–40	12–36
• Exercise	9.69	4.09	5–20	5–19
• Nutrition	17.34	3.91	6–24	7–23
• Stress management	19.39	4.46	7–28	10–28
• Interpersonal support	21.46	4.27	7–28	9–28
Total	**131.51**	**19.79**	**48–192**	**81–168**

designated as cognitively impaired. Responses for these subjects ($n = 9$) were examined separately. Subjects most frequently failed the PASAT1 and PASAT2, measures of sustained attention and information-processing speed. The scores of subjects with cognitive impairment on self-report scales were not significantly different from scores of the remaining subjects; therefore, responses from all 61 subjects were retained for the analyses.

This sample perceived being too tired, lack of convenient facilities, their impairment, lack of time, lack of money and interferences with other responsibilities as the most frequent problems (barriers) that interfered with their ability to take care of their health. Examination of item scores on the Self-Rated Abilities for Health Practices scale, a critical predictor of health-promoting behaviors in prior research with other groups with disabilities (Stuifbergen & Becker, 1994), revealed that five of the six items with the lowest mean ratings (indicating lower specific self-efficacy) are items from the exercise/physical activity subscale. An examination of the health-promoting lifestyle subscale patterns using average item subscale scores (mean subscale scores divided by the number of items) revealed that this sample of persons with MS scored highest on the subscales of interpersonal support and self-actualization and lowest on the exercise subscale.

Table 4.2 presents a matrix of the Pearson correlation measures of the antecedent factors and total scores on the HPLP and Quality of Life Index. As seen in Table 4.2, there was at least one measure in each antecedent factor that was significantly correlated ($p < .05$) with HPLP scores and Quality of Life Index scores. Higher scores on the HPLP (indicating greater frequency) were significantly ($p < .05$) associated with increasing age ($r = .28$), decreased barriers ($r = -.25$), higher social support ($r = .67$) and reciprocity ($r = .59$), lower conflict ($r = -.29$), and increased specific self-efficacy ($r = .67$) and general self-efficacy ($r = .37$). Higher quality of life index scores (indicating more positive perceptions) were associated with being female ($r = .37$), decreased functional disability ($r = .48$), decreased barriers ($r = -.60$), increased interpersonal support ($r = .52$) and reciprocity ($r = .50$), decreased conflict ($r = -.28$), better financial resources ($r = .45$), greater specific ($r = .62$) and general ($r = .41$) self-efficacy, fewer demands of illness ($r = -.48$), and positive perceptions of current health ($r = .57$). Reported frequency of engaging in health-promoting behaviors was significantly related to perceived quality of life ($r = .51$, $p < .01$).

After it was determined that the assumptions of linearity, normality and constant variance were met, stepwise multiple regression was performed to determine the best combination of variables for the prediction of scores on the Quality of Life Index. Due to the limited sample size, decision rules were used to reduce the large number of empirical referents. Strength of simple-order correlations of at least .30 was accepted as empirical evidence of the relationship of the particular variable with quality of life. To reflect the proposed conceptual model, at least one variable was selected from each antecedent factor. If more than two variables from an antecedent factor qualified for inclusion, evidence of multicollinearity and theoretical issues were used to select variables for inclusion as predictors. Using these rules,

TABLE 4.2 Correlations of Scores on Antecedent Variables with Health-Promoting Lifestyle Profile (HPLP) and Quality of Life Index (QLI) Scores ($N = 61$)

Antecedent Factors	HPLP	QLI
Demographic/Disease Factors		
Age	.28*	.11
Gender†	.18	.37**
Functional disability	.07	−.48**
Number cognitive tests failed	.18	.08
Length of illness	.14	.06
Barriers		
Barriers scale	−.25*	−.60**
Mechanical assist.††	−.10	.18
Personal assist.††	−.08	.31**
Resources		
Financial†††	.20	.45**
Education††††	−.02	.05
Social support	.67**	.52**
Reciprocity	.59**	.50**
Conflict	−.29*	−.28*
Perceptual Factors		
Perceived health	.08	.57**
Self-rated abilities	.67**	.62**
General self-efficacy	.37**	.41**
Demands of illness	.01	−.48**
Health-Promoting Lifestyle Profile—Total		.51**

*$p < .05$ **$p < .01$
†(1 = Female, 0 = Male)
††(0 = Needed all of the time; 3 = Does not need any assistance)
†††(3 = Adequate; 0 = Very Few)
††††(1 = Grade school or less, 6 = Post graduate degree)

TABLE 4.3 Multiple Regression to Predict Total Score on Quality of Life Index ($N = 61$)

Explanatory Variables	R^2	R^2 Change	Beta	F Change	Significance of Change
Antecedent Factors					
Self-rated abilities	.38	.38	.62	36.72	<.001
Perceived health	.57	.19	.45	25.46	<.001
Financial resources	.62	.05	.24	7.41	<.009
Reciprocity	.68	.06	.28	11.27	<.001
Health-Promoting Lifestyle Profile	.69*	.01	.15	1.63	.207

*Adjusted R^2 = .67 $F = 24.89$ ($df = 5/55$) $p < .001$

the antecedents of gender, severity of illness, barriers, financial resources, reciprocity, specific self-efficacy, perceived demands of illness and perceived health were entered into a first block using stepwise selection. The combination of the self-rated abilities, perceived health, financial resources and reciprocity accounted for 66% of the variance in Quality of Life Index scores. HPLP scores were entered in a second block, but did not add significantly to the explained variance in Quality of Life Index scores.

DISCUSSION

Although no causal relationships can be established with this correlational design, this study has identified factors associated with health-promoting behaviors and quality of life in this group. Reports of engaging in health-promoting behaviors were significantly related ($r = .51$, $p < .01$) to the measure of quality of life and these two measures shared significant correlates among the measures of barriers, resources, and perceptual factors. There were no common significant correlates among the demographic/disease factors for HPLP and QLI scores. The combination of specific self-efficacy (a consistent predictor of health behaviors), perceived health, financial resources, and reciprocity explained 68% of the variance in Quality of Life scores. Although scores on the HPLP were moderately related to scores on the Quality of Life Index, this variable did not significantly add to the variance accounted for in QLI scores after the other antecedent factors had been entered.

Findings from this study were consistent with the limited research regarding health behaviors of adults with chronic and disabling conditions. As in other groups (Stuifbergen et al., 1990; Stuifbergen & Becker, 1994; Williams, 1983), participants reported generally positive perceptions of their current health, despite living with a chronic, potentially disabling condition. The barriers of impairment, lack of money and being too tired were among the four highest ranking barriers for this sample and earlier samples of adults with disabilities (Becker et al., 1991). The correlations between health-promoting behaviors and demographic factors, barriers, financial resources, and perceptual factors of general and specific self-efficacy observed in this sample of persons with MS were similar to correlations observed in earlier studies of adults with a wide range of disabilities (Stuifbergen & Becker, 1994).

In an earlier study (Stuifbergen, 1992), individuals with MS described health-promoting behaviors, particularly exercise, as the most frequent strategy used for "coping with" the physical demands of illness. Therefore, the finding in this study that participants felt they were least able to complete related to physical activity and exercise is of particular concern. Low efficacy expectations for physical activity/exercise in this sample may be related to the increased difficulty of motor behaviors for these individuals. Since perceptions of ability were strongly related to reports of engaging in health-promoting behaviors ($r = .67$, $p < .01$), health-care professionals should consider the serious implications of this finding for this population. In "healthy" populations a large percentage of the physical deterioration that occurs with aging is related to inactivity. The impact of inactivity on physical changes of aging may be even more significant for a group of individuals already experiencing some physical limitation.

Pearson correlations among major study variables provided general support for the model proposed in Figure 4.1. It should be noted that objective measures of functional disability (Incapacity Status Scale) and subjective measures of illness severity (Demands of Illness) were not related to health-promoting behaviors, but were significantly associated with perceived quality of life. Perhaps moderate increases in illness severity may motivate individuals to engage in health-promoting behaviors, while individuals at the extremes may be uninterested or unable to participate in health-promoting behaviors. A revision of the model that considers demographic and disease characteristics as contextual variables with direct and indirect influences on quality of life may be appropriate.

Several limitations must be acknowledged and carefully considered when drawing conclusions from this study. The convenience sample was obtained by using a mailing list of one office of the National Multiple Sclerosis Society. Recruitment of participants who belong to groups such as the MS Society introduces its own selection bias into results. Individuals not affiliated with any group for persons with MS may perceive themselves, their health and their quality of life quite differently. The practice of health behaviors reported in this study may also be influenced by the geographic location of the study sample. The hot humid summers and mild winters may have introduced environmental factors not found in other settings. Although virtually all individuals contacted by the investigator agreed to participate, one must suspect that those most interested in health issues responded to the original mailout from the MS Society. In addition, the small sample size limited the multivariate analysis of the data. Specifically, the power of multivariate analyses would be seriously reduced with such a small sample. Therefore, use of path analytic techniques to specify direct and indirect influences of variables on quality of life was not possible in this study. Consequently, findings from this study must be viewed as exploratory, interpreted with caution, and replicated in larger samples and in other settings.

Certainly this study suggests as many questions as it answers. An empirical relationship between reports of health-promoting behaviors and subjective quality of life was demonstrated for this group of chronically ill adults. Important predictors and their paths of influence, however, remain unclear. Qualitative methods are currently being used in a follow-up study to extend understanding of the key model concepts, search for possible additional concepts, and ensure that the measurement instruments for use in subsequent studies are valid representations of the concepts as viewed from the frame of reference of the person with MS. This type of qualitative study is essential to ensure that relevant and important concepts are not omitted from the refined and fully specified model that will subsequently be tested in a much larger sample using quantitative methods (e.g., LISREL). A fully specified model, if statistically confirmed, may then be used to guide future studies of specific interventions designed to enhance quality of life for individuals with MS.

REFERENCES

Anderson, D. W., Ellenberg, J. H., Leventhal, C. M., Reingold, S. C., Rodriquez, M., & Silberberg, D. H. (1992). Revised estimate of the prevalence of multiple sclerosis in the United States. *Annals of Neurology, 31,* 333–336.

Bandura, A. (1982). Self-efficacy mechanism in human agency. *American Psychologist, 37,* 122–147.

Becker, H. A., Stuifbergen, A. K., Ingalsbe, K., & Sands, D. (1989). Health promoting attitudes and behaviors among persons with disabilities. *International Journal of Rehabilitation Research, 12,* 235–250.

Becker, H. A., Stuifbergen, A. K., Oh, H., & Hall, S. (1993). The self-rated abilities for health practices scale: A health self-efficacy measure. *Health Values, 17,* 42–50.

Becker, H. A., Stuifbergen, A., & Sands, D. (1991). Development of a scale to measure barriers to health promotion activities among persons with disabilities. *American Journal of Health Promotion, 5,* 449–454.

Braden, C. J. (1990). A test of the self-help model: Learned response to chronic illness experience. *Nursing Research, 39,* 42–47.

Broadhead, G. D., (1981). Physical education for previously unserved severely handicapped children. *Rehabilitation Literature, 42,* 86–89.

Brooks, N. A., & Matson, R. R. (1982). Social-psychological adjustment to multiple sclerosis: A longitudinal study. *Social Science & Medicine, 16,* 2129–2135.

Burckhardt, C. (1985). The impact of arthritis on quality of life. *Nursing Research, 34,* 11–16.

Burckhardt, C., Woods, S., Schultz, A., & Ziebarth, D. (1989). Quality of life of adults with chronic illness: A psychometric study. *Research in Nursing & Health, 12,* 347–354.

Dai, Y. T., & Catanzaro, M. (1987). Health beliefs and compliance with a skin care regimen. *Rehabilitation Nursing, 12,* 13–16.

Dillard, J. M., Campbell, N. J., & Chisolm, G. B. (1984). Correlates of life satisfaction of aged persons. *Psychological Reports, 54,* 977–978.

Dimond, M., & Jones, S. (1983). *Chronic illness across the life span.* Norwalk, CT: Appleton-Century-Crofts.

Dishman, R., Sallis, J., & Orenstein, D. (1985). The determinants of physical activity and exercise. *Public Health Reports, 100,* 158–171.

Duffy, M. E. (1986). Primary prevention behaviors: The female-headed, one parent family. *Research in Nursing and Health, 9,* 115–122.

Ferrans, C., & Powers, M. (1985). Quality of life index: Development and psychometric properties. *Advances in Nursing Science, 8,* 15–24.

Ferrans, C., & Powers. (1992). Psychometric assessment of the quality of life index. *Research in Nursing & Health, 15,* 29–38.

Glass, G., & Stanley, J. (1970). *Statistical methods in education and psychology.* Englewood Cliffs, NJ: Prentice Hall.

Gulick, E. E., (1991). Self-assessed health and use of health services. *Western Journal of Nursing Research, 13,* 195–219.

Gulick, E. E., & Bugg, A. (1992). Holistic health patterning in multiple sclerosis. *Research in Nursing & Health, 15,* 175–185.

Haberman, M. R., Woods, N. F., & Packard, N. J. (1989). *Demands of illness inventory: Reliability and construct validity assessment.* Unpublished manuscript.

Harper, A. C., Harper, D. A., Chambers, L. W., Cino, P. M., & Singer, J. (1986). An epidemiological description of physical, social and psychological problems in multiple sclerosis. *Journal of Chronic Disease, 39*, 305–310.

Heitzmann, C. A., & Kaplan, R. M. (1988). Assessment of methods for measuring social support. *Health Psychology, 7*, 75–109.

Kurtzke, J. F. (1981). A proposal for a uniform minimal record of disability in multiple sclerosis. *Acta Neurologica Scandinavica, 64* (Suppl. 87), 110–129.

Lawton, M. P., Moss, M., Fucomer, M., & Kleban, M. H. (1982). A research and service oriented multilevel assessment instrument. *Journal of Gerontology, 37*, 91–99.

Maybury, C. P., & Brewin, C. R. (1984). Social relationships, knowledge, and adjustment to multiple sclerosis. *Journal of Neurology, Neurosurgery, and Psychiatry, 47*, 372–376.

McIvor, G. P., Riklan, M., & Reznikoff, M. (1984). Depression in multiple sclerosis as a function of length and severity of illness, age, remissions, and perceived social support. *Journal of Clinical Psychology, 40*, 1028–1033.

McSweeney, J., Grant, I., Heaton, R., Adams, K., & Timms, R. (1982). Life quality of patients with chronic obstructive pulmonary disease. *Archives of Internal Medicine, 142*, 473–478.

Melnyk, A. (1988). Barriers: A critical review of recent literature. *Nursing Research, 37*, 196–201.

Moody, L., McCormick, K., & Williams, A. R. (1991). Psychophysiologic correlates of quality of life in chronic bronchitis and emphysema. *Western Journal of Nursing Research, 13*, 336–352.

Nosek, M. (1984). *Relationships among measures of social independence, psychological independence, and functional abilities in adults with severe orthopedic impairments.* Unpublished doctoral dissertation, The University of Texas at Austin.

Oleson, M. (1990). Subjectively perceived quality of life. *Image, 22*, 187–190.

Parcel, G. S., Bartlett, E. E., & Bruhn, J. G. (1986). The role of health education in self-management. In K. A. Holroyd & T. L. Creer (Eds.), *Self-management of chronic disease* (pp. 3–27). Orlando FL: Academic Press.

Paringer, L. (1983). Women and absenteeism: Health or economics. *American Economic Review, 73*, 123–127.

Pender, N. J. (1987). *Health promotion in nursing practice.* Norwalk, CT: Appleton and Lange.

Rao, S. M. (1991). *Neuropsychological Screening Battery for Multiple Sclerosis.* Unpublished Manuscript.

Reisine, S. T., Goodenow, C., & Grady, K. E. (1987). The impact of rheumatoid arthritis on the homemaker. *Social Science and Medicine, 25*, 89–95.

Schapiro, R. (1991) *Multiple sclerosis: A rehabilitation approach to management.* New York: Demos Publications.

Sherer, M., Maddux, J. E., Mercandante, B., Prentice-Dunn, S. Jacobs, B., & Rogers, R. W. (1982). The self-efficacy scale: Construction and validation. *Psychological Reports, 51*, 663–671.

Sjorgren, K., & Fugl-Meyer, A. R. (1982). Adjustment to life after stroke with special reference to sexual intercourse and leisure. *Journal of Psychosomatic Research, 26,* 409–417.

Smeltzer, S. (1992). Use of the trajectory model of nursing in multiple sclerosis. In P. Woog (Ed.). *The chronic illness trajectory framework: The Corbin and Strauss nursing model* (pp. 73–88). New York: Springer Publishing Co.

Strecher, V. J., DeVellis, B. M., Becker, M. H., & Rosenstock, I. M. (1986). *Health Education Quarterly, 13,* 73–91.

Stuifbergen, A., Becker, H., Ingalsbe, K., & Sands, D. (1990). Perceptions of health among adults with disabilities. *Health Values, 14*(2), 18–26.

Stuifbergen, A. (1992). Meeting the demands of illness: Types and sources of support for individuals with MS and their partners. *Rehabilitation Nursing Research., 1,* 14–23.

Stuifbergen, A., & Becker, H. A. (1994). Predictors of health-promoting lifestyles in persons with disabilities. *Research in Nursing & Health, 17,* 3–13.

Tilden, V., Nelson, C., & May, B. (1990). The IPR Inventory: Development and psychometric characteristics. *Nursing Research, 39,* 337–343.

U.S. Department of Health Human Services Public Health Services. (1991). *Healthy people 2000.* (DHHS Publication No. PHS 91–50212). Washington, DC: U.S. Government Printing Office.

Walker, S. N., Sechrist, K. R., & Pender, N. J. (1987). The health-promoting lifestyle profile: Development and psychometric characteristics. *Nursing Research, 36*(2), 76–81.

Walker, S. N., Volkan, K., Sechrist, K., & Pender, N. (1988). Health-promoting life styles of older adults: Comparisons with young and middle-aged adults, correlates and patterns. *Advances in Nursing Science, 11,* 76–90.

Wallston, B. S., Alagna, S. W., DeVellis, B. M., & DeVellis, R. F. (1983). Social support and physical health. *Health Psychology, 2,* 367–391.

Warms, C. A. (1987). Health promotion services in post-rehabilitation spinal cord injury health care. *Rehabilitation Nursing, 12,* 304–308.

Weinert, C. (1983). The physiological and psychosocial stress of long-term illness and the effects of social support on the "healthy" functioning of families. *Western Journal of Nursing Research, 5*(3), 34.

Williams, R. (1983). Concepts of health: An analysis of lay logic. *Sociology, 17,* 185–205.

Wineman, N. M. (1990). Adaptation to multiple sclerosis: The role of social support, functional disability, and perceived uncertainty. *Nursing Research, 39,* 294–299.

Woods, N. F., Haberman, M. R., & Packard, N. J. (1989). *Demands of illness: Relationships to individual, dyadic, and family adaptation.* Unpublished manuscript.

Woods, N. F., Yates, B. C., & Primomo, J. (1989). Supporting families during chronic illness. *Image, 21,* 46–50.

Acknowledgments. The project was supported by a grant from the National Multiple Sclerosis Society. The investigator gratefully acknowledges the contributions and assistance of the following persons and organizations: Sheri Allen Wright, R.N., C.R.R.N., Valerie Jacobson, R.N., B.S.N., Research Assistant, and Vicki Larue, Executive Director, Southeast Texas Chapter, The National Multiple Sclerosis Society, The Center for Health Care Research and Evaluation, The University of Texas at Austin School of Nursing.

Response

N. Margaret Wineman
Kathleen M. Schwetz

Care for individuals with chronic disabling conditions must emphasize keeping them at the highest level of functioning possible, with the goals of minimizing the development of secondary functional limitations and increasing the number of years without disability (Pope & Tarlov, 1991). These goals are particularly important for individuals with multiple sclerosis (MS) because treatments for MS are limited; the life span is not usually prematurely shortened, and the illness trajectory is unpredictable. Stuifbergen's research examines key variables that may affect health-promoting behaviors and quality of life in this population. Our response to Stuifbergen's research focuses on its clinical implications for nurses practicing in the advanced role. Specifically, we will discuss how this research may be used by nurses to directly affect client outcomes and indirectly affect clients by advocating for social policy and health care reform.

A healthy degree of skepticism on the part of the researcher about changing clinical practice based on one study is appropriate and in keeping with the basic tenets and mores of science. Stuifbergen rightfully cautions us that findings from her study need to be viewed within the limitations of the research. Individuals with chronic progressive illnesses, and specifically MS, however, must live and cope today with the limitations imposed by the illness. These individuals and their families must learn how to incorporate the disability into life patterns, roles, and relationships, often with little, if any, help from health care professionals. Although, as Stuifbergen indicates, a fully specified and tested model is desirable for guiding nursing interventions in this area, researchers need to interpret and apply research findings for use by clinicians now, with full awareness that we will continue to develop, test, and refine models for guiding future clinical practice.

Many nursing research studies with individuals who have a chronic illness have focused on quality of life, health, and well-being. Stuifbergen's research makes a significant contribution to this expanding scientific body of knowledge upon which nursing practice may be based. Her work includes less frequently examined health-promotion activities aimed at improving well-being, such as seeking personal development, pursuing professional assistance, engaging in regular exercise, making healthy nutritional decisions, and managing stress responses. The antecedent and intervening variables studied by other nurse researchers have included, for example, social support (Gulick, 1994; Stuifbergen, 1992; Wineman, 1990), coping and illness uncertainty (Wineman, Durand, & Steiner, 1994; Wineman, Schwetz, Goodkin, & Rudick, 1994), and hope (Foote, Piazza, Holcombe, Paul, & Daffin, 1990). The factors investigated by Stuifbergen and other researchers depict nurses' holistic/wellness orientation and their awareness of the importance of primary and preventive care for individuals with chronic unpredictable, disabling conditions.

Based on this research, we now know that functional disability, although making a significant impact on client outcomes, is only one of several variables that influences the individual's quality of life, health, and well-being. Stuifbergen found, for example, that fatigue, time and financial constraints, competing responsibilities, diminished physical abilities, and decreased access to facilities were the most frequent barriers to the ability to care for oneself. Functional disability was not even related to subjects' health-promoting lifestyle profile ($r = .07$), and it was only one of many variables that was significantly correlated with quality of life. In fact, when compared to functional ability, barriers ($r = -.60$), reciprocity ($r = .50$), perceived health ($r = .57$), self-rated abilities ($r = .62$), general self-efficacy ($r = .41$), and the demands of illness ($r = -.48$) were all about as strongly or more strongly associated with quality of life. These findings are important for nurses practicing in the advanced role because they provide further evidence regarding the client's need for primary and preventive care and the need for a multidisciplinary health care team that is fully equipped to provide this care.

The advanced practice nurse's role as part of the multidisciplinary team is to identify the needs and problems that develop as a result of the illness, directly intervene where appropriate, and refer to other providers when necessary. For example, nurses may intervene directly to help individuals minimize barriers to care by developing new strategies to combat fatigue, restructuring daily activities to conserve energy, and enlisting the aid of family members to better manage time. Nurses may indirectly intervene to remove barriers to health-promoting behaviors by making referrals to home-care agencies when the client needs additional assistance in meeting personal care requirements. Stuifbergen's research suggests that if nurses intervene to bring about positive change by minimizing these barriers, subjective quality of life will be enhanced.

Stuifbergen also indicates that the unpredictability of MS makes it "a model for research designed to explore adjustment to chronic illness" (p. 2). The fact that MS does have an unpredictable illness course may make it an uncommonly stressful chronic illness. Convincing evidence in the literature indicates that high levels of perceived illness uncertainty result in greater disturbances in emotional well-being (e.g., Mishel, Padilla, Grant, & Sorenson, 1991; Wineman, 1990; Wineman et al., 1994). This empirical relationship may be used as a basis for intervention. For example, the nurse is in a pivotal position to minimize illness uncertainty by providing ongoing health education regarding diagnosis, prognosis, and the rationale for symptom and illness management. These educational interventions have the potential to reduce some, but not all, illness uncertainty. The remaining uncertainty that is inherent in the illness trajectory may be effectively managed through the trusting relationship between nurse and client. The nurse may be, and is often, the one consistent element in a frequently changing illness environment. Understanding how this perceptual factor, perceived illness uncertainty, relates to health-promoting behaviors and quality of life is important for the identification and refinement of a fully specified model to guide nursing practice.

To meet the highly specialized, complex, and changing needs of clients with MS, an interdisciplinary approach founded on rehabilitative principles forms the basis of a comprehensive model of health care delivery. This approach is designed to provide clients with access to the services needed to maintain an active role in maximizing autonomy and quality of life (Ahearn & Schwetz, 1985). The interdisciplinary team, usually comprised of neurologists, advanced practice nurses, physical and occupational therapists, social workers, recreational therapists, vocational counselors, and psychologists, is best prepared to provide comprehensive care. For example, according to Stuifbergen's research, study participants "were least able to complete behaviors related to physical activity and exercise" (p.18). This finding may be due to motor limitations. Alternatively, Stuifbergen's findings may be the result of poor community access to an exercise program designed with the person's functional limitations in mind. In situations where an individualized exercise protocol is desirable, the advanced practice nurse might intervene by referring the client to a physical therapist within a specific health network to design an individualized exercise program. The nurse may also help the physical therapist identify realistic goals and outcomes to maximize the client's compliance. In this way, different team members complement each other to meet the specialized needs of the client with MS.

Stuifbergen's findings also have implications for social policy and health care reform. The present care for individuals with a chronic disability is fragmented; there is limited accessibility because of financial and geographic barriers; and our health care and insurance systems are disease-focused, rather than wellness-focused. Stuifbergen found that for individuals with MS, fatigue, poor accessibility to facilities, their impairment, lack of time, and interference with other responsibilities were barriers to taking care of their own health. Nursing's aim is to help individuals deal with these barriers to maintain health and the highest level of functioning possible. Our present health care system, however, is not designed to facilitate health promotion and preventive nursing interventions. Many legislators and clients are not aware of the roles and responsibilities of nurses in primary and preventive health care systems (New York State Nurses Association, 1994). Insurance coverage for rehabilitative services is usually limited to the acute care setting and only continues as long as functional improvements are observable (Pope & Tarlov, 1991). These restrictions are antithetical to the health promotion and preventive goals of nursing care in long-term-care situations. They ignore both the goal of maintaining well-being for people with MS and the fact that functional improvement may not be observable for a long time. For the person with MS, the result may be the development of secondary functional limitations that lead to further costly disability.

Nurses need to actively work to remove barriers to health-promoting behaviors by ensuring that health insurance is accessible and affordable. According to the Committee on a National Agenda for the Prevention of Disabilities (Pope & Tarlov, 1991), the primary source of health care coverage in the United States is employer-provided insurance. Since many people with a disability are unemployed, it is common that they have difficulty obtaining adequate coverage. In addition, insurance companies often deny coverage to individuals with a chronic illness or provide coverage with an exclusion clause for preexisting conditions. Even when coverage is available, it is mainly limited to acute illness situations, excluding essential secondary and tertiary services. It is also worth noting ". . . that a multitude of restrictive reimbursement schemes either refuse to pay (advanced nurses) for their services or funnel their payment through physicians or hospitals or other institutions" (*"Advance Practice Nursing,"* 1992, p. 75). The potential outcome of poor access to primary and preventive nursing care and other services for people with MS is the development of equally disabling complications. Stuifbergen's research suggests that nurses need to be available and accessible to clients in the community so that they can work directly with clients to augment abilities, minimize disabilities, and preserve roles and relationships.

It is to nursing's credit and our clients' benefit that our scientific knowledge base has quickly developed, even though we have not yet fully specified, tested, and refined our clinical models. Clients have a right to the best of nursing research, and we must actively examine the implications of that research for practice so nurses can utilize it as a basis for intervention and as a foundation for social policy and health care reform. Stuifbergen's work makes an important contribution to this knowledge, emphasizing, as it does, the factors affecting health-promoting behaviors as important strategies for maintaining autonomy and promoting the quality of life of individuals with chronic disabling conditions.

REFERENCES

Advanced practice nursing article provides compelling reasons for legislative reform. (1992, October). *Nurse Practitioner, 17*(10), 71, 75–78.

Ahearn, J. P., & Schwetz, K. M. (1985). Comprehensive supportive therapy in multiple sclerosis. *Seminar in Neurology, 5,* 146–154.

Foote, A. W., Piazza, D., Holcombe, J., Paul, P., & Daffin, P. (1990). Hope, self-esteem and social support in persons with multiple sclerosis. *The Journal of Neuroscience Nursing, 22,* 155–159.

Gulick, E. E. (1994). Social support among persons with multiple sclerosis. *Research in Nursing & Health, 17,* 195–206.

Mishel, M. H., Padilla, G., Grant, M., & Sorenson, D. S. (1991). Uncertainty in illness theory: A replication of the mediating effects of mastery and coping. *Nursing Research, 40,* 236–240.

New York State Nurses Association. (1994). *Expanding the nation's understanding of primary and preventive care services within a reformed health care system.* (American Nurses Association House of Delegates Report). (Available from the New York State Nurses Association, 2113 Western Avenue, Guilderland, New York 12084-9501).

Pope, A. M., & Tarlov, A. R. (Eds.) (1991). *Disability in America: Toward a national agenda for prevention.* Washington, DC: National Academy Press.

Stuifbergen, A. (in press). Health promoting behaviors and quality of life among individuals with multiple sclerosis. *Scholarly Inquiry for Nursing Practice.*

Stuifbergen, A. (1992). Meeting the demands of illness: Types of support for individuals with MS and their partners. *Rehabilitation Nursing Research, 1,* 14–23.

Wineman, N. M. (1990). Adaptation to multiple sclerosis: The role of social support, functional disability, and perceived uncertainty. *Nursing Research, 39,* 294–299.

Wineman, N. M., Durand, E. J., & Steiner, R. P. (1994). A comparative analysis of coping behaviors in persons with multiple sclerosis or a spinal cord injury. *Research in Nursing & Health, 17,* 185–194.

Wineman, N. M., Schwetz, K. M., Goodkin, D. E., & Rudick, R. A. (1994). *Effects of illness uncertainty, stress, and coping on emotional well-being upon entry into a clinical drug trial.* Manuscript submitted for publication.

Chapter 5

Families and Children's Chronic Conditions: Knowledge Development and Methodological Considerations

Virginia E. Hayes

OVERVIEW

The complexity of studying families has been a deterrent in the development of knowledge about families as the unit of care. When chronicity in childhood is combined with family study, research and theory development is particularly challenging. Although publication in the field of chronic illness in childhood has been quite prolific, there are few comprehensive, recognizably organized ways to think about providing care for the family as a whole. This is profoundly important as increasing responsibility of day-to-day care for children with long-term health conditions shifts to the family and to community-based care. This chapter presents a synthesis of what is known about families in health care when one member is a child with a long-term health concern, identifies gaps in knowledge that potentially compromise optimal health care delivery, and suggests methods for expanding and deepening our understanding so that we might improve the quality of our efforts to assist families that live with a child with a chronic condition.

Note: Originally published in *Scholarly Inquiry for Nursing Practice: An International Journal*, Vol. 11, No. 4, 1997. New York: Springer Publishing Company.

INTRODUCTION

That families are complex to understand and study is undebatable (Ganong, 1995; Gilgun, 1992; Hayes, 1993). It follows that families and chronic health conditions together are complex and challenging to understand and to study (Eiser, 1993; Kazak, 1989; Newby, 1996; Patterson, 1988; Patterson & Garwick, 1994; Rolland, 1987; Stuifbergen, 1987). How frequently do nurses working with families with chronically ill youngsters hear the statement—accusatory or resigned—that others simply cannot understand these families' experiences unless they are in similar situations? Family life is *so* complex and so varied, how *could* its interplay with childhood chronicity possibly be apprehended well enough by others to apply sensitive, comprehensive health care?

Knowledge development in the area of children, families, and chronicity has been at once prolific and dissipated, with the result that although we know quite a lot about how families respond and manage a child's chronic illness, there are few comprehensive, recognizably organized ways to think about providing care for the family as a whole. This is profoundly important as increasing responsibility of day-to-day care for children with long-term health conditions shifts to the family and to community-based care. Within the caregiving family, the health condition and its management has implications for each individual member as well as the family as a whole, that is, as an aggregate (Doherty & Campbell, 1988; Eiser, 1993; Jessop & Stein, 1989; Perrin, Shayne, & Bloom, 1993).

The purpose of this chapter is to present a synthesis of what is known about families in health care when one member is a child with a long-term health concern, to identify gaps in knowledge that potentially compromise optimal health care delivery (particularly nursing interventions), and to suggest methods for expanding and deepening our understanding so that we might improve the quality of our efforts to assist families with the everyday challenges of living with a child with a chronic condition. What is actually known about what it's like to live every day when one of the family is a child with a chronic health problem? What responses assist families to deal with the extra demands of a long-term condition or disability? What have family researchers discovered about health promotion, health maintenance, and health improvement practices that are (or could be) part of daily life when a child has a chronic condition? I believe that better understanding of what it is like to be a family with such a youngster could help us aim, plan, and carry out better care for this group of families, from specific interventions in hospital or community to policy formulation and program planning. The chapter starts with a brief introduction to the significance of pediatric chronicity and some related terminology; critically reviews selected, important research literature in two sections, as well as the impact on individuals and on families; and ends with a few thoughts on methods for future family study.

SIGNIFICANCE OF PEDIATRIC CHRONICITY

Defining the Problem

A generally held definition of a pediatric chronic health condition is one that interferes with a child's daily functioning for more than 3 months a year, causes hospitalization for more than 1 month a year, or is likely to do either of these (Gale, 1989). Definitional problems, however, have compromised the epidemiological picture of the issues, research, policies, and programs for children and their families (Perrin et al., 1993). Perrin and her colleagues recommend two levels of definition: duration and the impact of the condition on the child. (The review that follows encompasses both of these, adding the impact on the family as well as the child.) A confounding factor concerning terminology in pediatric chronicity, in both the literature and in practice, is debate and sensitivity around the terms chronic illness, developmental delay, disability, long-term health condition, special needs, and so forth. In this chapter, I use the term 'children with chronic conditions' as a consistent all-inclusive term. (In practice, I have always found it best to wait until family members themselves voice a term, and use theirs.) This term encompasses children with chronic illnesses, disabilities, and long-term health conditions that include physical conditions, developmental delay, psychosocial problems, and the complex combinations of these that often require technological interventions. A chronic condition is one that is not only long term, but is either not curable or has residual features that result in limitation(s) requiring special assistance or adaptation in function (Eiser, 1993; Jackson, 1992; Jessop & Stein, 1988). Such conditions include, for example, speech, hearing and visual disabilities; arthritis; autism; cancer; diabetes; cerebral palsy; a wide range of congenital conditions such as spina bifida, heart, lung, liver, kidney disease, and cystic fibrosis; and a variety of acquired conditions such as brain injury, neurological diseases, and so on. Thus, the term covers a broad range: some conditions do not render the child "ill" at all, while others impose a severe handicap or are associated with significant health and developmental outcomes. Frequently, serious chronic conditions occur in multiples and require complex or technically demanding care and hence, respite care if these children are cared for at home.

In this review, I have taken a noncategorical approach to the children's conditions (Stein, Bauman, Westbrook, Coupey, & Ireys, 1993), acknowledging that families' responses to them have elements in common as well as aspects that are unique. The present review is limited to childhood conditions and/or behavior(s) that are persistent and severe enough to result in unusual demands on parents and other caregivers when providing appropriate care. These conditions or behaviors require that the parents and/or caregivers receive extra support in supervising, assisting, or facilitating the child's development.

Scope of Chronicity in Childhood

Total numbers of children with chronic conditions are imprecise. Statistical information is not kept in ways that make estimates accurate or accessible. In addition to the problems related to definition, there are issues related to reporting and methodology. The result is figures for pediatric chronicity that range from 5%–30% (Newacheck & Taylor, 1992). Using the American National Health Interview Survey on Child Health, however, Newacheck and Taylor estimate that 31% of children are affected by one or more chronic conditions, and that 21% of these have two, and 9%, three or more. According to these authors, 22% of these conditions bother the children often or all the time, and 25% of parents report that the conditions cause a great deal of bother.

Newacheck and Taylor also estimate that 5% of American children with a chronic condition are severely affected, or about 2% of all children. In the U.S. this small number of children (up to the age of 19 years) accounts for 24% of all school absences, 19% of all physician contacts, and 33% of all hospital days related to chronic conditions. Despite progressive improvement in children's health in this century and recent technological advancements in health care, the number of children and adolescents with chronic conditions continues to rise (Thompson & Gustafson, 1996). "Dramatic medical advances in the past few decades have resulted in many chronically ill children, who previously would have died much earlier from their illnesses, now surviving into adulthood"

(Newachek & Taylor, 1992, p. 364). And what do we know of the impact on them, their siblings, parents, families, and communities?

"STATE OF THE SCIENCE": RESEARCH ABOUT CHILDREN, CHRONICITY, AND FAMILIES

Health professionals and families have focused more on chronicity in childhood since pediatric infections and many acute health problems have become more easily managed. Responding to trends in survival, treatment, and care, theoretical and research work has proliferated. In the past three decades, we have learned much about the conditions and their management, and about the effects on parents, the affected children, and to some extent, the well siblings. Social science knowledge development has primarily documented the stressful effects for the children and family members (Jessop & Stein, 1989; Kazak, 1987; McCubbin, 1988; Midence, 1994; Sharkey, 1995), with less attention being paid to the many families that cope effectively and creatively, thriving despite the extra tasks and adaptations (Abbott & Meredith, 1986; Clawson, 1996; Eiser, 1990; McCubbin, 1989; Patterson, 1988). In fact, except for anecdotal accounts, little is known about *family* responses and adaptation to chronic illnesses in general (Gilliss, 1989; Hayes, 1993; O'Neill & Sorensen, 1991; Rolland, 1988; Whall & Loveland-Cherry, 1993). Primarily, the research and theory published to date is family *related* and focuses on selected specific aspects of family life, such as parental attributes, attitudes, stress, coping behaviors, management style, or resources, or children's developmental, educational, or psychosocial responses. Usually, even when the family is the stated focus of study, *individual* informants are used to try to understand *family* responses (Ganong, 1995; Gilliss, 1991; Hayes, 1993; Moriarty, 1990; Sidani & Jones, 1995). Systematic evaluation of the day-to-day effects of living with a chronically ill child on the whole family—that is, research with the family as the unit of analysis remains extremely rare, this at a time when there is movement toward considering the family as the unit of care across health disciplines and greater acknowledgment that the family affects and is affected by the child's illness (Doherty & Campbell, 1988; Eiser, 1993; Jessop & Stein, 1989; Perrin et al., 1993; Wallace, Biehl, MacQueen, & Blackman, 1997).

Individual Effects of Pediatric Chronicity

There is substantial literature concerning the impact of chronicity on peoples' lives, but it principally describes effects with the family as context for the individual, for example, in the case of studies of young families, using parents (usually mothers) as informants or observations from researcher/health care professionals. I have found it useful to categorize the rather fragmented literature in the area of pediatric chronicity into two broad groups: (1) theory and research that informs us about individuals' responses to the conditions, and (2) work that informs us about families as units.

Children with Chronic Conditions

Clinical observations and analyses dominate the literature about children's responses to their chronic conditions. It is widely held, for example, that having a chronic condition touches the affected child and siblings developmentally, socially, cognitively, and emotionally, and that outcomes depend on a wide variety of factors such as the nature and severity of the condition, socioeconomic factors, vulnerability, and temperament (Eiser, 1993; Jessop & Stein, 1988; Midence, 1994; Rose, 1987; Schraeder, 1995; Thompson, Curtner, & O'Rear, 1994; Yoos, 1987). Support for understanding specific effects on children, however, comes from small studies of particular diagnostic groups of children that primarily use parents as informants rather than the children themselves. Generally speaking, consequences for the affected child are thought to be related to separation from home and family; facing frustration, fear, and boredom; and the obstacles to making and keeping friends. Anxiety and guilt dominate the theoretical accounts of child consequences, although the existing research-based evidence is sometimes conflicting. In fact, little direct empirical support can be found for *either* the effects of the chronic condition on the ill child or the child's view of the effect of the condition on her or his family (Eiser, 1993; Hobbs, Perrin, & Ireys, 1985; Rose, 1987).

Psychosocial or mental health effects of children's chronic conditions are frequently studied (see reviews by Eiser, 1993; Midence, 1994; Steinhauer, Mushin, & Rae-Grant, 1974; Thompson & Gustafson, 1996). In general, these studies show affected children at risk for behavioral and emotional difficulties. "Specifically, on the basis of structured diagnostic interviews, it appears that anxiety-based disorders are the most frequent, although milder forms of externalizing problems . . . are evident in some illnesses and age groups" (Thompson & Gustafson, 1996, p. 86). Although there are few longitudinal studies that demonstrate the stability of such findings over time, Thompson and Gustafson conclude that there is no direct relationship between chronicity and psychosocial adjustment, but rather a wide range of psychological and behavioral responses.

Two important longitudinal studies *are* reported by Stein and Jessop (1991) and Pless and Wadsworth (1989). Stein and Jessop, in evaluating a pediatric ambulatory care treatment/support project and refining a data collection instrument called the Personal Adjustment and Role Skills Scale (PARS II), followed families for about 5 years in an experimental design. Mothers supplied the data about their children of more than 5 years of age. Children in the intervention group were rated as significantly less withdrawn, anxious, depressed, and hostile and as more productive. There were no differences in peer relationships or dependency. Pless and Wadsworth conducted a cohort study of 500 children born in 1946 in the United Kingdom with chronic physical disorders, comparing them with 3,500 well people in the same cohort when they were then 40 years old. Among other findings, the level of risk for psychosocial problems in the disabled group was estimated to be 30%–50% compared with an estimate of 6% for the general population, a figure that has not, to my knowledge, been examined in modern cohorts. Without recent comparisons, such work continues to foster the negative attitudes associated with pediatric chronicity, and without strong challenges to the contrary, the negative-effects model continues to dominate both clinical management and research approaches to children's chronicity (Steinhausen, 1994).

Examples of the "deficit model" are prevalent: Wallander, Varni, Babani, Banis, and Wilcox (1988) demonstrated that mothers reported their children to have more behavioral and social competence problems than the norms for the instrument used in the research, when clinically their children were not exhibiting problems. Breitmayer, Gallo, Knafl, and Zoeller (1992) agree. Using a sample of children ($N = 67$) and parents as informants, they found that both mothers and fathers indicated a significantly greater (though modest) incidence of social competence difficulties among their children with chronic conditions, with the largest deficit being in social relationships. In contrast, and using children, parents, and teachers as informants, Nassau and Drotar (1995), in a study of 25 children with insulin-dependent diabetes, 19 children with asthma, and 24 healthy children, describe those with chronic illnesses as resilient in their social competence when compared to healthy peers, since they showed no statistically significant differences in social adjustment, social performance, and social skills from any of the groups of informants. Similarly, Sterling and Friedman (1996) report 54 children with diabetes to be more empathic than their 54 healthy peers. In response to filmed vignettes, the chronically ill group "provided qualitatively different and more sophisticated empathic responses than healthy peers" (p. 53). A final example comes from a cross-sectional study by Wolman, Resnick, Harris, and Blum (1994), who compared 1,683 chronically ill adolescents' Adolescent Health Surveys with those of 1,650 healthy adolescents, finding emotional well-being to be more a function of family connectedness than of having a chronic condition, though the latter is associated with lower well-being scores.

Feeman and Hagen (1990), using mothers' assessments, examined the intellectual ability, academic performance, behavior, and social perceptions of 48 children, comparing those with seizure disorders to an equal number who were "healthy." The data suggested that both the ill children and their siblings were at risk for developmental lags and related problems. Among the very few published studies that have used data from the children themselves, Ritchie, Caty, and Ellerton (1984) analyzed narrative recordings of play interviews with 42 chronically ill and 40 acutely ill and well 2- to 5-year-old children. Investigating their hospital-related concerns, these researchers found that being ill provides fewer opportunities for play with peers and adults. Strength and agility, which are linked with competence and self confidence, may be affected by prolonged periods of inactivity. Kazak and Clark (1986) report that children with myelomeningocele have a significantly lower Piers-Harris self-concept than a group of healthy peers, and Walsh and Ryan-Wenger (1992) report that children with asthma experience stressors related to self-concept as well as school, family, and peer relationships, the children explaining that they feel left out of the group and inferior in sports.

In a complex study using child, parent, and teacher subjects to glean an understanding of the correlates of pediatric illness, Perrin, Ayoub, and Willett (1993) found children's adjustment to depend on health status, verbal intelligence, gender, family environment, and mother's locus of control. Specifically, the 187 healthy and chronically ill children attributed their adjustment mostly to family environment, their own health status, and verbal intelligence. Parents rated their children quite similarly, with maternal locus of control entering the explanatory "parent model." In the "teacher model" tested in this study, teachers also associated children's adjustment with family environment, but gender and verbal intelligence contributed more strongly. These authors conclude that most children with the chronic conditions studied (cerebral palsy, seizures, and orthopedic problems) function quite well, but in the eyes of all three sets of observers, perhaps not quite as well as healthy children.

In a recent review of risk and resilience in children with disabilities, Patterson and Blum (1996) conclude that conditions that are invisible, have remitting-relenting courses, and have an uncertain prognosis are associated with the greatest emotional problems. Males exceed females in terms of emotional sequelae. Sociability, flexibility, and physical characteristics of attractiveness are protective. It seems then, that there is evidence of both risk and resilience among children with chronic conditions and that a wide range of factors can influence outcomes. In some ways our presuppositions and current theoretical notions of negativity are upheld, and in some ways they are challenged. There is much yet to understand about children's own responses to chronicity and disability.

Siblings

Negative-impact assumptions are more tempered in investigations of well siblings' responses to living with a sister or brother with a chronic condition, and there is a small but growing literature in this area (for an excellent chronological review that covers sibling relationship over the lifespan, see Faux, 1993). The children themselves are informants in proportionately more of these studies, frequently in combination with their parents. Whereas some researchers report findings associated with the "downside" (Lobato, Faust, & Spirito, 1988; Reynolds, Garralda, Jameson, & Postlethwaite, 1988), other results have been more positive (Clements, Copeland, & Loftus, 1990), and some simply neutral. For example, Williaams, Lorenzo, and Borja (1993) found that 100 siblings' housekeeping and caretaking activities were significantly increased in the presence of pediatric chronicity (see also Gallo, Breitmayer, Knafl, & Zoeller, 1991). This study also demonstrated that siblings' social and school activities decreased and that they received less caregiving from their mothers, findings supported by Davies (1993) in a descriptive study of 19 mothers. Using parents' data, Lavigne and Ryan (1979) and Tritt and Esses (1988) report siblings of chronically ill children to be irritable and socially withdrawn, and to have significantly more behavior problems than a "healthy" sample, whereas other work (Dyson, 1989; Gallo, Breitmeyer, Knafl, & Zoeller, 1992; Thompson et al., 1994) demonstrates that psychosocial adjustment and self-concept may be similar to that of normative samples according to parent report. Conclusions drawn by researchers from siblings' own responses are much the same: mixed. Faux (1993), Gallo and her colleagues (1991), Kazak and Clark (1986), and Pinyerd (1983) found that siblings did not express overwhelming needs or concerns themselves; worried about their brothers or sisters; thought their play and school activities were not affected; played with, protected, and helped out with their affected sibling; and had good friends. Though they noted differences in household chores, siblings did not attribute these to favoritism (parent data and observations of the children's behavior were sometimes inconsistent with these findings, however). Sometimes, siblings want more information about the health condition but may not ask (Canam, 1986; Eiser, 1993; Kruger, Shawver, & Jones, 1980). Adverse outcomes documented are: increased aggression, poor peer relations, anxiety, somatization, decline in school performance, and depression (Dyson, 1989; Simeonsson & McHale, 1981).

Perhaps due to changing societal beliefs and mores, older, pessimistic outlooks about well siblings' responses to pediatric chronicity such as anger, jealousy, fear, maladjustment, emotional and behavioral difficulties are moderating (Perrin, 1993; Pless, 1972; Poznanski, 1969). These *are* concerns, of course, but siblings are also reported to benefit emotionally and psychologically from their experiences with their brother's or sister's chronic condition and its management: they are reported to have a greater understanding of people and a more positive outlook, and to be well adjusted, more compassionate, more sensitive, more appreciative of their own health, more socially competent. As Drotar and Crawford (1985) and Gallo et al. (1992) discern, there is no one-to-one link between the presence of the chronic condition and siblings' responses; age, gender, type and controllability of the illness, and other family members' responses to it and its management are contributing factors. Although much sibling research has been conducted recently (especially in the 1980s), threads and trends are not really discernible, and there continue to be inconsistencies. Lobato, Faust and Spirito (1988) note that further research is needed, "but an understanding of these interactions will occur only if their family context is fully appreciated both conceptually and methodologically" (p. 404). Hence, qualitative methods offer excellent means to understand more about both ill children's and siblings' responses to chronicity.

Research With Children

In summary, what little information is available about children with chronic conditions and their siblings is derived from clinical reports and case studies, small samples, and personal accounts published in the general press. Frequently, these are small, uncontrolled, cross-sectional studies with methodological problems that make generalizations difficult (Brett, 1988; Lobato et al., 1988). Partly, this is due to the small numbers of children in diagnostic groups, which strengthens the case for considering noncategorical approaches in order to pool results, make samples larger, and have more confidence in the findings. Research about children frequently depends on parents as informants, although this is changing somewhat in sibling studies. When children are informants, there is selection preference for older children and those whose parents choose to give permission on their behalf. While it can be argued that these are practical necessities, the result is underdeveloped understanding about the responses of *young* children and those whose parents protect them from participation in research. There is acute need for the development of methodological approaches suitable to study children, particularly suitable data gathering techniques. Since practicing nurses are skilled in establishing good rapport with children of all ages, their skills could be applied to research efforts. We need to increase our knowledge about the effective coping strategies employed by some children and families (Eiser, 1990; Gallo et al., 1992), and apply it in fostering and strengthening coping. Children *are* at risk; knowing more about those risks from their own perspective would guide families, communities, and health professionals to better prevent or ameliorate them.

Parents

Reports of parents' responses to chronicity are now prolific in the child health care literature. Like many assumptions about their children, the "received view" about parental outcomes is rather negative; it has been held that they are stressed and burdened, in direct relation to the severity of the child's condition, the demands of management, and the amount of support available (Hobbs et al., 1985; Holroyd & Guthrie, 1986; Kazak & Marvin, 1984; Whyte, 1992; Wilton & Renaut, 1986). Mothers are thought to be more distressed and vulnerable than fathers, sometimes to the level of being at-risk for psychopathology (Eiser, 1993; Kazak, 1987; Mardiros, 1982; Tavormina, Boll, Dunn, Luscomb, & Taylor, 1981). Divorce is *thought* to be higher among marriages with a child's chronic illness present, but recent reviews have demonstrated how equivocal this is; many marriage relationships are strengthened (for an excellent review and critique of the divorce literature in the area and the research methods used, see Eiser, 1993, pp. 134–138).

To illustrate the variation and breadth in the published research concerning parental impact, I have sampled the following studies simply as examples. The picture of impact is often framed as parental 'perceptions' or 'experiences,' and often these are interpretive studies of parents of children with specific or mixed (noncategorical) diagnoses. Simon and Smith (1992) describe 11 parents' accounts of living with children with liver disease as six processual themes: beginning (discovery of the diagnosis), guilt and parenting inadequacy, pain and stress, uncertainty and fear of the future, lack of control and taking control, and developing a personal philosophy and family adaptation. These themes are similar to those described by Messias, Gilliss, Sparacino, Tong, and Foote (1995), of parents' recall 13 to 25 years after the birth of a baby with a congenital heart defect. The diagnostic process is described as: something is wrong, illusive normality, rude awakening, managing uncertainty, making new meaning, and taking stock. Similar as well is Howard's (1992) naturalistic inquiry/grounded theory of mothers dealing with life-long schizophrenia: perceiving the problem, searching for solutions, enduring the situation, surviving the experience. Scharer and Dixon (1989) used a more structured approach to interviewing 10 "families" with ventilator-dependent children, actually 5 sets of parents during their child's hospitalization, and 5 at home. An initial set of 18 categories was combined into three main themes concerning the management of their lives in the presence of their children's conditions and care: barriers (e.g., dealing with the health care system, finances), resources (e.g., significant others, health care personnel, services), and parenting (e.g., normalization, active or passive strategies). Qualitative accounts such as these tell stories that tend to "ring true" in clinical practice with parents, and do assist in understanding the context-bound experiences of parents' everyday lives and the "constant-ness" of living with a child's chronic condition. Stories always seem to start with the diagnostic or entrance process, and continue with ongoing adaptations as parents change over time.

McKeever, Angus, and Thaha (1994) depict more depth and complexity in their critical social theory approach to 33 mothers' and 29 foster mothers' characteristics, activities, and circumstances as they care for children with disabilities. Interviews; personal, privately recorded accounts; and a structured questionnaire describe the many additional-to-regular-parenting activities these mothers carry out; the almost constant vigilance the (noncategorical) children require; their compromised leisure, sleep, and rest; some gratifications, unpleasantness, and distress; and the physical arduousness of caregiving and its impact on their health. These authors conclude that caregiving, even in the Canadian Medicare system, has significant negative financial consequences, since unpaid mothers work as an alternative to paid health services and have inadequate community and governmental support.

Another way researchers access the impact of parenting chronically ill children is by assaying parents' needs. Parents are described as needing: (1) more information, given in a more timely, respectful manner, and devoid of health care jargon; (2) more instrumental, emotional, and financial support; (3) more leisure and sleep; (4) more time for partners, other children, and friends; (5) more understanding of family, friends and the general public; (6) more energy; greater sense of control; and sometimes, (7) more skills (Bailey, Blasco, & Simeonsson, 1992; Canam, 1993; Cosper & Erickson, 1985; Diehl, Moffitt, & Wade, 1991; Graves & Hayes, 1996; Knox & Hayes, 1983; McAnear, 1990; Perrin et al., 1993; Robinson, 1985; Young, Creighton, & Sauve, 1988). Parents have also been polled about their service delivery needs, which are often expressed as being different from those provided by health care professionals: less fragmentation, better collaboration, more integrated management of their child's care, more available counseling and support services, better equipment, better trained health care personnel, better and more available respite and child care; better educational services, better assessment and referral mechanisms, better medication and pain management, and better relationships with health professionals (Diehl et al., 1991; Horner, Rawlins, & Giles, 1987; Thorne & Robinson, 1988; Walker, Epstein, Taylor, Crocker, & Tuttle, 1989). One report highlights mothers' perceptions of the environments (communities) in which they lived (Turner-Henson, 1993), finding that their perceptions of the neighborhood as resourceful, safe, and accessible interacted statistically with environmental variables such as median family income, degree of poverty, number of women workers (outside the home), educational level of women in the community, population density. These needs-based investigations are of particular interest to nurse investigators as they assist to frame interventions and direct policy influence.

The nature of parenting-with-caregiving is another thrust of health-related research with young families. Methods are both quantitative and qualitative. For example, Seideman and Kleine's (1995) grounded theory captures parents' entrance and subsequent, ongoing performance process in "transforming" parenting when a child is developmentally delayed or mentally retarded. Like Messias and her colleagues (1995), Seideman and Kleine tap into participants' long-term perspectives, interviewing 42 parents whose children were 10 months to 69 years. Parents describe moving from their initial reactions and responses to transforming their notions of parenting and the activities that they expected to be part of it, gradually construing reality differently. Christian's (1993) findings agree; she calls this "shifting gears." Miles, who has a large program of research focused on mothers of life-threatened infants and children, investigated mothers' role changes (Miles, D'Auria, Hart, Sedlack, & Watral, 1993). These researchers used quantitative and qualitative approaches to uncover 31 mothers' role changes as they responded to their children's condition, each a special response related to a common element of a "normal" parent role: advocating, caregiving, protecting, nurturing, and stress. The concepts mapped in both these interpretations have a confirming ring for those of us who work with families with children with special needs and must be appealing to parents as well.

A large ($N = 367$), theory-driven investigation of school-aged children's families has been conducted by Holaday and Turner-Henson (Holaday, Turner-Henson, Harkins, & Swan, 1993; Turner-Hensen, Holaday, & Swan, 1992). Caregiving responsibilities were examined for several factors: medical treatment time use, children's domestic chores, and family dinner patterns. Three quarters of the children, who were all well enough to attend school, received some form of medical treatment at home, usually the responsibility of the mother as an add-on to her time. As some children are unable to accomplish the chores commonly done by healthy children, parents may shoulder this work as well. Parenting the chronically ill child *is* different; additional work, demands, or burden, are the terms commonly found in this literature.

Application of Knafl, Gallo, Breitmayer, Zoeller, and Ayres' (1993) findings, however, warn us to be cautious in overgeneralizing or oversimplifying. In what may look like similar situations to an outsider's eye, parents (sometimes even within the same family) vary in their responses to the chronic illness, its management, care, and interpretations of its effect on the family and their parenting philosophies.

Parents' stress and coping comprises a large body of literature. Indications of stress may be measured or obtained by interview. One of the difficulties here is being sure parents and researcher have the same or similar notions of what is meant by stress. Frequently its meaning is taken for granted, and researchers focus beyond, on factors that contribute to or ameliorate stress. For example, maternal adjustment to children's chronic conditions is said to vary with appraised daily stress, palliative coping, level of family support, illness severity, child psychological development, and family conflict (Thompson, et al., 1994), and with uncertainty, loneliness, socioeconomic status, religious affiliation, chronic illness in a family member other than the affected child, and other concurrent stressors (Van Dongen-Melman et al., 1995). Cohen (1995) has found parental uncertainty, itself associated with heightened distress, to be associated with seven commonly occurring triggers such as routine medical appointments, being exposed to negative outcomes in children with the same or similar condition, or changes in the treatment regimen. In the published research concerning parental stress and coping, particularly in the subsection of studies examining the effects of home care of the medically fragile or technology-dependent child, the deficit model of distress predominates. Home care is associated with high distress (Hazlett, 1989; Joyce, Singer, & Isralowitz, 1983; Leonard, Brust, & Nelson, 1993; Montgomery, Gonyea, & Hooyman, 1985; Snowdon, Cameron, & Dunham, 1994; Teague et al., 1993).

Sometimes to researchers' surprise, findings about the quantity and quality of parental stress have been inconclusive or contradictory, and current research activity has shifted from documenting deficits to focusing on how stressors are handled. Thus, the marital discord, anxiety, depression, feelings of entrapment, fatigue, chronic grief, fear, financial pressures, and isolation (Gallagher, Beckman, & Cross, 1983; Kazak & Marvin, 1984; McCubbin, 1988; Worthington, 1989) are considered much less definitive than was once believed and are coming to be seen as being mediated by complex responses and situations within families, and therefore as highly varied among parents. Characteristics of the care situation, parent, and family resources clearly mediate parental stress and burden (Fagan & Schor, 1993; Gallagher et al., 1983; Gibson, 1995; McCubbin, 1988, 1989; Ray & Ritchie, 1993; Wegener & Aday, 1989). Barriers to effective coping include obstacles associated with the health care system, including relationships with professionals (Robinson, 1987; Scharer & Dixon, 1989; Stewart, Ritchie, McGrath, Thompson, & Bruce, 1994; Wuest & Stern, 1990), finances (Scharer & Dixon, 1989), and severity and course of the child's illness (Goldberg & Simmons, 1988). Effective management of the situation and parental coping have been shown to be associated with: (1) maintaining a positive outlook (Austin & McDermott, 1988; Barbarin & Chesler, 1984; Gibson, 1988, 1995; McCubbin, 1989; Ray & Ritchie, 1993), (2) parents' attitudes toward their affected children and their conditions (Austin & McDermott, 1988), (3) information seeking and problem solving (Barbarin & Chesler, 1984; Deatrick, Knafl, & Walsh, 1988; Hayes & Knox, 1984), (4) parental confidence or self-efficacy in ability to competently care for the child (Deatrick et al., 1988; Gibson, 1988, 1995; Goldberg & Simmons, 1988; Ray & Ritchie, 1993), (5) support from the health team (Gibson, 1988; Scharer & Dixon, 1989; Wuest & Stern, 1990), (6) family stability or strengths (Gallagher et al., 1983; Gibson, 1988; McCubbin, 1989; Ray & Ritchie, 1993), and especially, (7) maintaining self esteem and social support, including contacts with parents dealing with similar situations (Austin & McDermott, 1988; Gibson, 1988, 1995; McCubbin, 1989; Scharer & Dixon, 1989). Slowly, caring for a child with a long-term health problem, in the literature at least, is shaking off the stigma of being associated with family "dysfunction" that has characterized previous approaches, and has been associated with negative outcomes for children and families (Eiser, 1993; McCubbin, 1989).

Research With Parents

A caution about the parents-and-pediatric-chronicity literature: Either stated or not, much of the research is actually about *mothers*, sometimes this is evident in titles and abstracts and sometimes it is not. The small number of studies about differences between mothers and fathers alert us to be careful about carrying assumptions from one gender and role to the other. Parents seem to respond both the same and differently (Copeland & Clements, 1993; Eiser & Havermans, 1992; Eiser, Havermans, Kirby, Eiser, & Pancer, 1993; Krauss, 1993). Eiser (1993) notes that partly this is due to: mothers shouldering more care, being the parent who takes the child to places where research is conducted (such as health centers and clinics), possibly being more interested in cooperating with research, or simply being more available. Some researchers, however, have a particular interest in mothering, and focus their studies on female parents for particular reasons (e.g., Fagan & Schor, 1993; McKeever et al., 1994). There has been little interest in studying fathering per se; more research in *both* mothering and fathering is needed.

This parent-related body of literature, though substantial in size, is still limited in terms of the development of cohesive theory to understand parent responses to chronicity. It is plagued by small samples, diagnostic specificity, few comparison studies or replications, and methodological flaws, even though it is clinically grounded for the most part. Though intuitively appealing qualitative studies are becoming prevalent, they lack "generalizability" in the positivist sense, and therefore require replications, comparisons, or published accounts of others' uses of the developed theory in order to demonstrate practical applicability in the care of children and families. Most important, in many parent-related studies, there is frequent conceptual "hazing" between parental and family responses; that is, parents are assumed to be the best/only informants for *family-level* responses to chronicity in childhood. Hence I have come to separate out studies that unequivocally investigate *family* concepts, though they are few in number. Mainly, these also use individual informants to tell about families.

Family Effects of Pediatric Chronicity

Clinically focused and theoretical publications address families as units rather better than research reports. Families are complex and difficult to study whole (Adams, 1988; Nye, 1988), and little research is undertaken with the family as the unit of analysis. But researchers have been fascinated by families since the turn of the century and have devised many empirical indicators to access family life. Several of these are seen in the health care literature, though proportionately few appear in the substantive field of pediatric chronicity, where children, sibling, and parent data *represent* family.

Children

With children (including well siblings), interviews (Kruger et al., 1980), observation (Murphy, 1992), and projective techniques such as drawings (Bossert & Martinson, 1990) and story-telling (Faulkner, 1996) have revealed children's awareness of the effects of health problems and their management on themselves and other family members, their perceptions of their families as "different," and their expressions of some anxiety and concern about their families. This work is rudimentary; *much* more needs to be learned about children from their own points of view.

Parents

As noted earlier, there is considerably more access to the understanding of families through parent report. To a large degree, such studies are quantitative. Some support the idea that children's chronic conditions do have an impact on the family and attempt to quantify it. For example, Schlomann (1988) found associations between children's developmental delays and family functioning; cognitive-psychosocial delays were associated with negative, while motor delays were associated with positive, family effects; and Cowen and colleagues (1986) found "well-functioning" interaction in families living with cystic fibrosis, even though there were individual disturbances related to the condition. Generally, the impact on family life is said to increase with increasing severity of the child's condition (McCubbin, 1988; Reynolds et al., 1988; Teague et al., 1993).

Family functioning, particularly in terms of cohesion and adaptability, is a frequent area of investigation through parental report. In comparing a group of families with children with chronic conditions with a "healthy children" group or standardization group, many researchers document no significant differences (e.g., Dyson, 1993; Kazak, Reber, & Snitzer, 1988; McCubbin, 1988). For example, McCubbin (1989) found no differences between single- and two-parent families dealing with a child with cerebral palsy, and Kazak (1987) found three groups of families dealing with various long-term children's conditions not to be isolated and to be similar to matched families with a healthy child in terms of personal stress, marital satisfaction, and social network size and density. An epidemiological study using a randomly selected sample of 3,294 Ontario families (Cadman, Rosenbaum, Boyle, & Offord, 1991) found increased rates of parental treatment for "nerves" and increased maternal negative affect scores but no difference in family "dysfunction" when comparing families with children with long-term conditions and those with healthy children, nor any difference in alcohol use.

Overall, family functioning has been found to have little to do with specific characteristics of the affected child (Trute, 1990). An important and consistent finding is that though individually there may be problems in marriages where there is a child with special needs, generally marital satisfaction and breakdown appear to be no different than in the general population (Barbarin & Chesler, 1984; Cadman et al., 1991; Kazak, 1987; Kazak & Clark, 1986; Patterson, 1985; Sabbeth & Leventhall, 1984; Walker, Van Slyke, & Newbrough, 1992).

Factors that ameliorate stressful conditions are called coping, and various elements of family coping, such as resources and social support are the subject of many studies. Finances, a sense of mastery over life events, mutuality, and members' overall physical and mental health have been shown to be positively associated with families' coping with pediatric chronicity (McCubbin, 1988; Snowdon et al., 1994). The financial aspects are more than the family-borne costs of health care; they are the outcomes of children's care frequently requiring a parent to give up part- or full-time paid employment. Social support is clearly a strong mediator in living with a pediatric chronic illness. For example, Kazak and Marvin (1984), McCubbin (1988), Reynolds (1988), and Snowden et al. (1994) have demonstrated that support networks were more dense and family dominated in more severe and long-term conditions, so that social support may not be as effective or easy to access in the presence of more demands. Kazak (1987) found mothers' and fathers' social networks to be significantly different in size and density. Walker and colleagues (1992), using the Questionnaire of Resources and Stress, found that some stress is associated with specific aspects of a child's disability, but not with increasing age of the child. Indeed, age of the child with the condition often affects parental stress in the *other* direction: as children with asthma get older, the family stress associated with their condition decreases as they become better able to report and manage symptoms themselves (Meyerhoff, Hayes, & Canam, 1997).

What quantitative studies of family responses to childhood chronicity do not do well yet is get at family interaction (Shonkoff & Hauser-Cram, 1987), and qualitative approaches that use only parents as informants, though they tap these elements better, naturally get parent-only perspectives. Canam (1987), for example, using content analysis, explored the ways parents view communication within families where a child has cystic fibrosis or epilepsy, identifying negative emotions that operated in parental decisions about talking about the condition, either to help themselves or others. Intra-familial communication, along with alterations in routine, problem solving, information seeking, and future planning are some of the ways chronic uncertainty infiltrates many aspects of family functioning, operating continuously, it would seem (Cohen, 1989, 1993; Sharkey, 1995). Dominant communication patterns may shift during critical periods of living with a pediatric chronic condition; Clements et al. (1990) explore these stressors and responses as parents articulate them.

Taking a broader view of the interaction between families and chronicity, Hamlett, Pellegrini, and Katz (1992) demonstrated quantitatively that family functioning, maternal social support, and children's chronic illnesses were significantly related to psychological adjustment of children with asthma and diabetes, both conditions associated with periodic stressful life events. In the same diagnostic groups and adding sibling assessment to their analyses, Hilliard, Fritz, and Lewiston (1985) found an association between parental aspirations or goals for their chronically ill child and the children's goals for themselves. This study found that parents were generally less controlling of their children with asthma or diabetes than with siblings, not more so, as is sometimes believed.

Management of the child's chronic condition within the family context is an area of particular interest among nurse researchers at present. Although family is often the focus in these studies, parents are frequently the primary informants for the family as a whole. For example, Cohen (1993) articulates the multidimensional yet universal aspects of managing uncertainty when living with a child's life-threatening condition. Concepts arising from interpretive studies like Cohen's, such as managing time, social interaction, information, awareness, the environment, and the outcomes of the illness within the family, are intuitively appealing and are easily applicable to practice. Christian's (1993) study adds ways of managing diabetes, asthma, and spina bifida within the family to our understanding of family "management" (minimizing, normalizing, and advocating). Edwards-Beckett and Cedargren (1995) describe parents' notions of how sharing information, interpersonal interactions, and supports and hindrances operate within their families; and Clements et al. (1990) outline elements of families' critical times when members' needs are increased: at diagnosis, when symptoms increase, when the child must be relocated, when parents must be absent, and when there are developmental changes.

The assessments of family outcomes (such as family functioning, stress, and so on) that were built into currently published quantitative studies were oriented by explicit or implicit researcher perspectives, rather than by those of family members themselves. That is, much research is theory driven rather than theory generating, and in efforts to control variables, rarely attempts to study whole-family dynamics. Qualitative studies seem to hold the best promise for helping us understand families as units, but only when the whole family becomes the unit of analysis. Although many of the researchers in the forgoing part of this review are making a genuine attempt to capture a *family* picture, the following summarizes the published studies I have been able to locate that analyze data that are, from my perspective, at the conceptual level of families and pediatric chronicity.

Family-as-Unit of Analysis Studies

Incredible strides have been made recently in trying to capture *family* in research. I think it is significant that most of these studies have used qualitative methods. Informants were primarily parents, but in each of these, data were also obtained directly from or by observation of all family members and integrated in analysis to address family-level understandings.

Snowden and her colleagues (1994) combined quantitative measures for family resources, functioning, and hardiness, and individual social support, in assessing family responses to having respite care. Both statistical and content analyses were used to obtain a combined family picture. These authors conclude that internal and external coping resources are important for families that have children with developmental disabilities. They report an association between sources of support and family hardiness. Descriptive correlation was similarly used by Cornman (1993) to capture the effects of childhood cancer on 20 families. Using individual, dyadic, and family techniques, she found that there were varied responses across instruments (life stress, self-esteem, marital satisfaction, and perception of family environment) and family members (mother, father, patient, sibling). Although the conclusions of this study—the importance of the family as social environment for the child, its key role in the child's response to therapy, and the reciprocal nature of the relationship between family members—are drawn at the family level, it is imperative to keep in mind that all data used individual informants.

Family interaction, functioning, and adjustment were examined longitudinally following the diagnosis of diabetes in an adolescent by

Hauser et al. (1986, 1988) using direct observations and multivariable analyses. The emphasis on observation of interactions between members and the conceptual definitions of interaction behaviors and styles are strengths of this work; parents and their diabetic children expressed significantly more enabling (focusing, problem solving, active understanding) behaviors than a comparison group of families whose children experienced a serious acute illness. Case studies are described by Desmond (1980) and Pollner and McDonald-Wikler (1985). Desmond visited two families of children with cancer longitudinally and used multiple ethnographic methods. She describes the troubled lives of these families, enriched by liberal reporting of narrative data. Pollner and McDonald-Wikler report a multiple-observations case study of an unusual family whose youngest child is persistently seen by her family as being competent, although she is severely mentally retarded. These authors document the family's "reality work" as their processes operate to process the "torrent of ostensibly discrediting and disconfirming information" about their daughter/sister.

In a now classic work, Davis (1963) also used longitudinal, ethnographic methods to portray 14 families' coping with the diagnosis, treatment and management of a child's poliomyelitis. He mapped interactional strategies he called passing (attempting to eradicate or disguise the visible signs of handicap in order to "pass" as normal), normalization, and disassociation, a response set where families avoided or insulated themselves from events that might make them acknowledge their differentness. Likewise, Ablon (1988) used multiple anthropological methods in her study of dwarf children, their families, and networks, tracing the means, methods, and courage of children and families in learning to live with a highly visible physical difference. This work eloquently illustrates the reciprocity of the impact of the condition and the family on each other. Another rich account of family life is presented by Burton (1975), who studied parents, children with cystic fibrosis, and their siblings in Northern Ireland. She traces the now familiar processes of obtaining a diagnosis, learning about the disease, coping, emotions, and advocacy. In a more recent and much larger work, Knoll (1992), using both qualitative and quantitative analyses, studied families' responses to a variety of developmental disabilities and chronic health conditions. He describes daily routines; caregiving; relationships with family, friends, and neighbors; financial implications; securing services; and family support, among other things, taking care to explain findings at the family level conceptually. On a much narrower scale, but with similar findings, Hurtig (1994) describes relations in families of children and adolescents with sickle cell disease.

Knafl and Deatrick and their colleagues have a well-established program of research around families' management of their child's chronic condition, wherein families are sometimes the unit of analysis (Deatrick & Knafl, 1990; Gallo, 1990; Knafl, Breitmayer, Gallo, & Zoeller, 1996; Knafl et al., 1993; Knafl, Gallo, Zoeller, Breitmayer, & Ayers, 1993; Kodadek & Haylor, 1990; Murphy, 1990). Derived from grounded theory with parents, siblings, and the child with the long-term condition, they focus on management behaviors directed toward the "special" child, the family system, and the social system, and direct us to think about family processes and interactions concerning a family's management of an ill child as a taken-for-granted part of everyday existence. These authors' methods and findings provide exciting direction for future studies: multimethod (triangulated), multimember, multidiagnostic group, cross-sectional and longitudinal approaches, carefully developed in a *program* of research are composed into constructions of family-level responses to children's chronic illnesses. Their current publications describe five family management styles (thriving, accommodating, enduring, struggling, floundering), each including a definition of the illness experience, management goals and approaches, and illness consequences. Hayes (1992) describes managing the child's condition as only one of five concepts descriptive of families "working things out" around pediatric chronicity at home; the others are: balancing, adapting, tolerating, and maintaining the family image.

Much earlier, and also using grounded theory, Benoliel (1970, 1975) used triangulation of methods in studying families of adolescents and adults with diabetes. Her work is important in the field for, among other things, its use of conjoint family interviews and data collected from people in a wide variety of roles both inside and outside the family. She described two essential tasks of families in her study of adolescents with diabetes: management of time and control of food become central in the lives of all family members. Tiller, Ekert, and Rickards (1977) describe another study in which whole family interviews were conducted. These authors conceptualized the responses of various members to acute lymphoblastic leukemia over time, then tied these to family functioning and relationships, noting greater stability in families where there were close relationships, the presence of teenagers, and stable external factors such as professional support. Family functioning and cancer are issues explored by Barbarin (1986) as well, though the family as unit selected for this review addresses the concept of stigma rather than of family per se. He describes, using data gleaned from several studies in his own and others' research and clinical experiences, how stigma operates to touch the family, its subsystems, individual members, and their interactions in social encounters and the community at large, how ambivalence and ambiguity confound family life and the dynamic aspects of stigma as a shared experience, ironically an outcome of the family's attempt to cope with the illness and its uncertainties.

Anderson and her colleagues (Anderson, 1981, 1990; Anderson & Chung, 1982; Anderson & Elfert, 1989) took a phenomenological approach to research with Chinese, Indo-Canadian, and Caucasian families with chronically ill children. Extensive observation and interviewing of families at home contribute to a family picture of "normalization," which varies in interpretation and operation among these cultural groups of parents. These authors also explore the implications of their findings for women as caretakers and for related health care and social policy.

Families and Pediatric Chronicity

Together, these studies contribute significantly to our understanding of family life with a chronically ill child, but the pieces do not comprise a complete enough knowledge base for comprehensive health care intervention and policy planning. Knowledge in no single conceptual area even scratches the surface of what health care professionals and families themselves need to know to design effective, sensitive care. Researchers and clinicians are working in relative isolation from one another, so we run the risk of encountering similar issues and repeating the same mistakes in research design and theory construction (Campbell, 1986; Ganong, 1995). At the family level, supposedly pivotal in the planning and delivery of reformed health care, we know very little about how families function in the presence of pediatric chronicity—how they react, adapt, become, and remain healthy families. In our clinical practice as well as our research, families themselves challenge us to intensify our attempts to understand their situations better and therefore plan, deliver, and educate about better family care (Hayes, 1992). Only then will cost-effective family interventions, programs, and policies become better suited to families' perceived needs, particularly in home care. What can be done to strengthen family study as it relates to health care for children and their families?

MOVING ON AND STRETCHING OUT

This paper critically reviews the "state of the science" in the interface between family (as a concept, as a functioning unit of society, and a focus of health interventions) and childhood chronicity. Published work tends to reflect health professionals' perspectives rather than those of families themselves and has been based on anecdotal accounts or small samples without replication. Frequently, there is cross-level inference from individual members' data to family-level conceptual conclusions (Feetham, 1984; Gilliss, 1991; Moriarty, 1990). Deficit models or negative responses to children's chronicity dominate, extending received views and restricting more open questions that might lead to broader views of chronicity and family impact. Although publication in the field is substantial (especially where parents have served as informants about the impact of children's chronic conditions on families), there has to date been little cohesive theory development. There is much need for research in the field of family nursing that specifically targets the family level of response and intervention. In short, we know very little about the interrelationships between families and chronic illness, particularly when the ill member is a child (Campbell, 1986). Were research, theory building, and knowledge development about families as units to be more comprehensive, practicing nurses would have better direction for family-level interventions, including policy development and cost-effective, high-quality community-based care. Nursing practice cannot be optimal without articulated, "tested" research and theory on which to base it, albeit in many domains: objective, subjective, practical, and speculative (Johnson & Ratner, 1997). What do we need to add to family nursing knowledge and how will we continue to generate that knowledge?

Much of the research reported here has resulted in information "snippets" highly relevant for families and their care. Replication studies and studies that build on previous findings are absolutely essential. Within established programs of research and in teams that are working on the development of specific phenomena, master's, predoctoral, doctoral, and post doctoral work can be organized to systematically build conceptual understanding of childhood chronicity and its impact within families and communities. Both cross-sectional and longitudinal designs, and qualitative, quantitative, and triangulated methods are critical to tapping into families' experiences with children's chronic conditions, and the resultant needs for preventive, health-promoting, and therapeutic interventions. Funding for longitudinal work remains relatively rare. Since adaptation to chronic illness occurs over time, affected by growth, development, and change in children, families, *and* health conditions, there is a need for sustained lobbying and fund-raising efforts aimed at increasing funders' understanding of, and support for, data collection over time. To capture the complexity of family life *and* maximize the often small samples possible from pediatric chronic illness populations, projects that overlap one another, or use continuous or the same participants and/or multiple sites could contribute to clinically and statistically significant findings over time. Sometimes it is justified, for efficiency and cost effectiveness, to design studies to simultaneously achieve multiple purposes using multiple methods.

This raises the topic of respondent burden, a very real consideration with busy, sometimes overbusy, families with a chronically ill child. At times, researchers assume too much responsibility for deciding what constitutes an unacceptable "burden" for potential research informants, without consulting *them*. It has been my experience that parents and older children in particular are very pleased to know they are contributing to the development of knowledge that will help others like themselves. In addition, creativity in the design and implementation of data collection strategies could minimize participant burden. For example, more use could be made of observational techniques, which are ideal for analyzing family interaction. Participant observation is particularly effective, since the individual collecting data can simultaneously help with caregiving in a home or an agency setting, using audio- or videotaping, and/or making notes later. Other examples are: having family members provide research "data" while they are engaged in another, concurrent activity; using monetary or other tangible remuneration; and viewing some aspects of data collection as at least partially therapeutic and something that families *gain* in doing, such as conversational interviews (Hutchinson & Wilson, 1994).

As intuition and practical wisdom already direct much family nursing care (Hayes, 1997), more well-designed intervention studies are needed to document the relative success of practices and policies. Specifically targeted policy background research is not commonly undertaken by nurse researchers, nor is the documentation of the outcomes of policy change. In this, nurses, with their first-hand, most-exposure-to-the-client knowledge of children and families, can work as important contributors to interdisciplinary research teams.

Research about the concept of family requires abstract thinking and an ability to embrace complexity. Data collection will require new instruments or interpretive approaches that address "family" rather than elements of family life that are family *related*. Since individuals are our informants about family, we need analytic techniques (quantitative and qualitative) that produce conceptual understanding about families as units. Family-level research requires both sophistication *and* gumption. Proportionately more researchers will require postdoctoral training to enable them to gain the skills necessary to design and analyze family data. At the same time, creative, "right-brain" thinking is increasingly needed to conceptualize and solve research problems that tap into *family* responses to chronic conditions. Add doses of confidence, risk-taking, "moxey," and tenacity, and the ideal family researcher emerges! This researcher will use case studies, projective techniques, and secondary analyses more often, design ingenious new ways to make the most of small samples, think of fun and ethically sound ways of involving children in research, design instruments and methods that enable whole families to provide data for family concepts, and advance statistical designs in ways that compose family concepts from combinations of individual and family measures. Rather than designing new ones, existing measures could be used in new ways (Birenbaum, 1995). We need research in all paradigms: postpositivist, interpretive, and critical. Thus, the "new age" family researcher will be able to use currently tried, and as yet untried, measurement, interpretive, and participatory approaches to elicit knowledge about families that may be unlike what we now know, yet very much from families' standpoints. To adequately explain these to others in writing, journals and electronic media will need to shift requirements to accommodate the longer articles that such reports require. More publication in lay language for lay readers is essential to families' gaining from, and utilizing research pertinent to their responses to chronicity and its management.

To date, much of the research and tentative theory building concerning families and pediatric chronicity has concentrated substantively on received notions and popular topics: stress, burden, coping, adaptation, impact on family functioning, and "clinical" families. For example, interactions and communication—between family members in the presence of chronicity, and between chronicity and families—require further investigation and theory development (Faux, 1993). Family members' shared experiences of children's chronicity (what they are and how they develop) are essentially uninvestigated. As noted earlier, the positive effects of living with pediatric chronicity are underresearched as well (Eiser, 1993). Ganong (1995) challenges us to broaden out, to think and design research laterally, considering both our epistemic and nonepistemic values, and considering families in all their diversity, contextualization, and *health*. His and others' challenges force family nursing researchers to grapple with family complexity, and to tackle gender, cultural, and paradigmatic issues such as postmodern and poststructural approaches. I think we need to continue investigation of individual responses to chronicity with the family as context or background, but as well to consider the family as foreground with individuals as background (Robinson, 1995). We need to address primary and secondary prevention as well as tertiary, and to investigate risk factors (Agee, Boyce, & Innocenti, 1995) and family health promotion (Maxwell, 1997).

It remains for health researchers to face the challenges of family-as-unit research, band with strong collaborators and take on the complexities and rewards of family-level research. The results can only be more, better-articulated knowledge, that is more easily applicable to practice and that is relevant to the care of families who live every day with children's chronic conditions and disabilities.

REFERENCES

Abbott, D., & Meredith, W. (1986). Strengths of parents with retarded children. *Family Relations, 35,* 371–375.

Ablon, J. (1988). *Living with difference: Families with dwarf children.* New York: Praeger.

Adams, B. N. (1988). Fifty years of family research: What does it mean? *Journal of Marriage and the Family, 59,* 5–17.

Agee, L. C., Boyce, G. C., & Innocenti, M. S. (1995, November 18). *Children at risk: The effects of multiple risk factors on children with disabilities.* Paper presented at the National Council for Family Relations, Portland, OR.

Anderson, J. M. (1981). The social construction of illness experience: Families with a chronically-ill child. *Journal of Advanced Nursing, 6,* 427–234.

Anderson, J. M. (1990). Home care management in chronic illness and the self-care movement: An analysis of ideologies and economic processes influencing policy decisions. *Advances in Nursing Science, 12*(2), 71–83.

Anderson, J. M., & Chung, J. (1982). Culture and illness: Parent's perception of their child's long term illness. *Nursing Papers, 14*(4), 40–52.

Anderson, J. M., & Elfert, H. (1989). Managing chronic illness in the family: Women as caretakers. *Journal of Advanced Nursing, 14,* 735–743.

Austin, J. K., & McDermott, N. (1988). Parental attitude and coping behaviors in families of children with epilepsy. *Journal of Neuroscience Nursing, 20,* 174–179.

Bailey, D. B., Blasco, P. M., & Simeonsson, R. J. (1992). Needs expressed by mothers and fathers of young children with disabilities. *American Journal on Mental Retardation, 97*(1), 1–10.

Barbarin, O. A. (1986). Family experience of stigma in childhood cancer. In S. C. Ainlay, G. Becker, & L. M. Coleman (Eds.), *The dilemma of difference*. New York: Plenum.

Barbarin, O. A., & Chesler, M. A. (1984). Coping as interpersonal strategy: Families with childhood cancer. *Family Systems Medicine, 2*, 279–289.

Benoliel, J. Q. (1970). The developing diabetic identity: A study of family influence, *Communicating nursing research. Vol. 3: Methodological issues in research*. Boulder, CO: Western Interstate Commission for Higher Education.

Benoliel, J. Q. (1975). Childhood diabetes: The commonplace in living becomes uncommon. In B. G. Glaser & A. L. Strauss (Eds.), *Chronic illness and the quality of life*. St. Louis: Mosby.

Birenbaum, L. K. (1995). Family research in pediatric oncology nursing. *Journal of Pediatric Oncology Nursing, 12*(1), 25–38.

Bossert, E., & Martinson, I. M. (1990). Kinetic Family Drawings-Revised: A method of determining the impact of cancer on the family as perceived by the child with cancer. *Journal of Pediatric Nursing, 5*, 204–213.

Breitmayer, B. J., Gallo, A. M., Knafl, K. A., & Zoeller, L. H. (1992). Social competence of school-aged children with chronic illnesses. *Journal of Pediatric Nursing, 7*, 181–188.

Brett, K. M. (1988). Sibling response to chronic childhood disorders: Research perspectives and practice implications. *Issues in Comprehensive Pediatric Nursing, 11*, 43–57.

Burton, L. (1975). *The family life of sick children*. London: Routledge & Kegan Paul.

Cadman, D., Rosenbaum, P., Boyle, M., & Offord, D. R. (1991). Children with chronic illness: Family and parent demographic characteristics and psychosocial adjustment. *Pediatrics, 87*, 884–889.

Campbell, T. L. (1986). Family's impact on health: A critical review. *Family Systems Medicine, 4*, 135–200.

Canam, C. (1986). Talking about cystic fibrosis within the family—What parents need to know. *Issues in Comprehensive Pediatric Nursing, 9*, 167–178.

Canam, C. (1987). Coping with feelings: Chronically ill children and their families. *Nursing Papers, 19*(3), 9–21.

Canam, C. (1993). Common adaptive tasks facing parents of children with chronic conditions. *Journal of Advanced Nursing, 18*, 46–53.

Christian, B. J. (1993). Quality of life and family relationships in families coping with their child's chronic illness. In S. G. Funk, E. M. Tornquist, M. T. Champagne, & R. A. Wiese (Eds.), *Key aspects of caring for the chronically ill: Hospital and home* (pp. 304–313). New York: Springer.

Clawson, J. A. (1996). A child with a chronic illness and the process of family adaptation. *Journal of Pediatric Nursing, 11*, 52–61.

Clements, D. B., Copeland, L. G., & Loftus, M. (1990). Critical times for families with a chronically ill child. *Pediatric Nursing, 16*, 157–224.

Cohen, M. H. (1989). The sources of management of uncertainty in life-threatening, chronic illness. *Communicating nursing research: Choices within challenges* (Vol. 22, pp. 155). Boulder, Colorado: Western Institute of Nursing.

Cohen, M. H. (1993). The unknown and the unknowable-Managing sustained uncertainty. *Western Journal of Nursing Research, 15,* 77–96.

Cohen, M. H. (1995). The triggers of heightened parental uncertainty in chronic, life-threatening childhood illness. *Qualitative Health Research, 5,* 63–77.

Copeland, L. G., & Clements, D. B. (1993). Parental perceptions and support strategies in caring for a child with a chronic condition. *Issues in Comprehensive Pediatric Nursing, 16,* 109–121.

Cornman, B. J. (1993). Childhood cancer: Differential effects on the family members. *Oncology Nursing Forum, 20,* 1559–1566.

Cosper, M. R., & Erickson, M. T. (1985). The psychological, social, and medical needs of lower socioeconomic status mothers of asthmatic children. *Journal of Asthma, 22,* 145–158.

Cowen, L., Mok, J., Corey, M., MacMillan, H., Simmons, R., & Levison, H. (1986). Psychologic adjustment of the family with a member who has cystic fibrosis. *Pediatrics, 77,* 745–753.

Davies, L. K. (1993). Comparison of dependent-care activities for well siblings of children with cystic fibrosis and well siblings in families without children with chronic illness. *Issues in Comprehensive Pediatric Nursing, 16,* 91–98.

Davis, F. (1963). *Passage through crisis.* Indianapolis: Bobbs-Merrill.

Deatrick, J. A., & Knafl, K. A. (1990). Management behaviors: Day-to-day adjustments to childhood chronic illness. *Journal of Pediatric Nursing, 5,* 15–22.

Deatrick, J. A., Knafl, K. A., & Walsh, M. (1988). The process of parenting a child with a disability: Normalization through accommodation. *Journal of Advanced Nursing, 13,* 15–21.

Desmond, H. (1980). Two families: An intensive observational study. In J. Kellerman (Ed.), *Psychological aspects of childhood cancer* (pp. 100–127). Springfield, IL: Charles C. Thomas.

Diehl, S. F., Moffitt, K. A., & Wade, S. M. (1991). Focus group interview with parents of children with medically complex needs: An intimate look at their perceptions and feelings. *Children's Health Care, 20,* 170–178.

Doherty, W. J., & Campbell, T. L. (1988). *Families and health.* Newbury Park, CA: Sage.

Drotar, D., & Crawford, P. (1985). Psychological adaptation of siblings of chronically ill children: Research and practice implications. *Journal of Developmental & Behavioral Pediatrics, 6,* 355–362.

Dyson, L. L. (1989). Adjustment of siblings of handicapped children: A comparison. *Journal of Pediatric Psychology, 14,* 215–229.

Dyson, L. L. (1993). Response to the presence of a child with disabilities: Parental stress and family functioning over time. *American Journal on Mental Retardation, 98,* 207–218.

Edwards-Beckett, J., & Cedargren, D. (1995). The sociocultural context of families with a child with myelomeningocele. *Issues in Comprehensive Pediatric Nursing, 18,* 27–42.

Eiser, C. (1990). Psychological effects of chronic illness. *Journal of Child Psychology and Psychiatry, 31,* 85–98.

Eiser, C. (1993). *Growing up with a chronic disease: The impact on children and their families.* London: Jessica Kingsley.

Eiser, C., & Havermans, T. (1992). Mothers' and fathers' coping with chronic childhood disease. *Psychology and Health, 7,* 249–257.

Eiser, C., Havermans, T., Kirby, R., Eiser, J. R., & Pancer, M. (1993). Coping and confidence among parents of children with diabetes. *Disability and Rehabilitation, 15,* 10–18.

Fagan, J., & Schor, D. (1993). Mothers of children with spina bifida: Factors related to maternal psychosocial functioning. *American Journal of Orthopsychiatry, 63,* 146–152.

Faulkner, M. S. (1996). Family responses to children with diabetes and their influence on self-care. *Journal of Pediatric Nursing, 11,* 82–93.

Faux, S. A. (1993). Siblings of children with chronic physical and cognitive disabilities. *Journal of Pediatric Nursing, 8,* 305–317.

Feeman, D. J., & Hagen, J. W. (1990). Effects of childhood chronic illness on families. *Social Work in Health Care, 14*(3), 37–53.

Feetham, S. L. (1984). Family research: Issues and directions for nursing. In H. H. Werley & J. J. Fitzpatrick (Eds.), *Annual Review of Nursing Research,* Vol. 2 (pp. 3–25). New York: Springer Publishing Company.

Gale, C. A. (1989). Inadequacy of health care for the nation's chronically ill children. *Journal of Pediatric Health Care, 3,* 20–27.

Gallagher, J. J., Beckman, P., & Cross, A. H. (1983). Families of handicapped children: Sources of stress and its amelioration. *Exceptional Children, 50,* 10–19.

Gallo, A. M. (1990). Family management style in juvenile diabetes: A case illustration. *Journal of Pediatric Nursing, 5,* 23–32.

Gallo, A. M., Breitmayer, B. J., Knafl, K. A., & Zoeller, L. H. (1991). Stigma in childhood chronic illness: A well sibling perspective. *Pediatric Nursing, 17,* 21–25.

Gallo, A. M., Breitmayer, B. J., Knafl, K. A., & Zoeller, L. H. (1992). Well siblings of children with chronic illness: Parents' reports of their psychologic adjustment. *Pediatric Nursing, 18,* 23–27.

Ganong, L. H. (1995). Current trends and issues in family nursing research. *Journal of Family Nursing, 1,* 171–206.

Gibson, C. (1988). Perspective in parental coping with a chronically ill child: The case of cystic fibrosis. *Issues in Comprehensive Pediatric Nursing, 11,* 33–41.

Gibson, C. H. (1995). The process of empowerment in mothers of chronically ill children. *Journal of Advanced Nursing, 21,* 1201–1210.

Gilgun, J. F. (1992). Definitions, methodologies, and methods in qualitative family research. In J. F. Gilgun, K. Daly, & G. Handel (Eds.), *Qualitative methods in family research* (pp. 22–39). Newbury Park, CA: Sage.

Gilliss, C. L. (1989). Family research in nursing. In C. L. Gilliss, B. L. Highley, B. M. Roberts, & I. M. Martinson (Eds.), *Toward a science of family nursing* (pp. 37–63). Menlo Park, California: Addison-Wesley.

Gilliss, C. L. (1991). Family nursing research, theory and practice. *Image, 23*(1), 19–22.

Goldberg, S., & Simmons, R. J. (1988). Chronic illness and early development. *Pediatrician, 15,* 13–20.

Graves, C. M., & Hayes, V. E. (1996). Do nurses and parents of children with chronic conditions agree on parental needs? *Journal of Pediatric Nursing, 11,* 288–299.

Hamlett, K. W., Pellegrini, D. S., & Katz, K. S. (1992). Childhood chronic illness as a family stressor. *Journal of Pediatric Psychology, 17*, 33–47.
Hauser, S. T., Jacobson, A. A., Wertlieb, D., Weiss-Perry, B., Follansbee, D., Wolsdorf, J. I., Herskowitz, R. D., Houlihan, J., & Rajapark, D. C. (1986). Children with recently diagnosed diabetes: Interactions within their families. *Health Psychology, 5*, 273–296.
Hauser, S. T., Paul, E. L., Jacobson, A. A., Weiss-Perry, B., Vieyra, M. A., Rufo, P., Spetter, L. D., DiPlacido, J., Wertlieb, D., & Wolfsdorf, J. (1988). How families cope with diabetes in adolescence. *Pediatrician, 15*, 80–94.
Hayes, V. E. (1992). *The impact of a child's chronic illness on the family system.* Unpublished doctoral dissertation, University of California, San Francisco.
Hayes, V. E. (1993). Nursing science in family care, 1984–1990. In S. L. Feetham, S. B. Meister, J. M. Bell, & C. L. Gilliss (Eds.), *Advances in the nursing of families* (pp. 18–29). Newbury Park, CA: Sage.
Hayes, V. E. (1997). Searching for family nursing practice knowledge. In S. E. Thorne & V. E. Hayes (Eds.), *Nursing praxis: Knowledge and action* (pp. 54–68). Thousand Oaks, CA: Sage.
Hayes, V. E., & Knox, J. E. (1984). The experience of stress in parents of children with long-term disability. *Journal of Advanced Nursing, 9*, 333–341.
Hazlett, D. E. (1989). A study of pediatric home ventilator management: Medical, psychosocial and financial aspects. *Journal of Pediatric Nursing, 4*, 284–293.
Hilliard, J. P., Fritz, G. K., & Lewiston, N. J. (1985). Levels of aspiration of parents for their asthmatic, diabetic, and healthy children. *Journal of Clinical Psychology, 41*, 587–597.
Hobbs, N., Perrin, J. M., & Ireys, H. T. (1985). Effects of chronic illness on children, families, and communities, *Chronically ill children and their families* (pp. 62–101). San Francisco: Jossey-Bass.
Holaday, B., Turner-Henson, A., Harkins, A., & Swan, J. (1993). Chronically ill children in self-care: Issues for pediatric nurses. *Journal of Pediatric Health Care, 7*(6), 256–263.
Holroyd, J., & Guthrie, D. (1986). Family stress with chronic childhood illness: Cystic Fibrosis, neuromuscular disease, and renal disease. *Journal of Clinical Psychology, 42*, 552–561.
Horner, M. M., Rawlins, P., & Giles, K. (1987). How parents of children with chronic conditions perceive their own needs. *MCN, 12*, 40–43.
Howard, P. B. (1992). *Lifelong maternal caregiving: learning to live with a child who has schizophrenia.* Unpublished PhD, University of Kentucky.
Hurtig, A. L. (1994). Relationships in families of children and adolescents with sickle cell disease. *Journal of Health and Social Policy, 5*, 161–183.
Hutchinson, S., & Wilson, H. (1994). Research and therapeutic interviews: A post structuralist perspective. In J. M. Morse (Ed.), *Critical issues in qualitative research methods* (pp. 300–315). Thousand Oaks, CA: Sage.
Jackson, P. L. (1992). The primary care provider and children with chronic conditions. In P. L. Jackson & J. A. Vessey (Eds.), *Primary care of the child with a chronic condition* (pp. 3–11). St. Louis: Mosby.
Jessop, D. J., & Stein, R. E. K. (1988). Essential concepts in the care of children with chronic illness. *Pediatrician, 15*, 5–12.

Jessop, D. J., & Stein, R. E. K. (1989). Meeting the needs of individuals and families. In R. E. K. Stein (Ed.), *Caring for children with chronic illness: Issues and strategies* (pp. 63–74). New York: Springer Publishing Co.

Johnson, J. L., & Ratner, P. A. (1997). The nature of the knowledge used in nursing practice. In S. E. Thorne & V. E. Hayes (Eds.), *Nursing praxis: Knowledge and action* (pp. 3–22). Thousand Oaks, CA: Sage.

Joyce, K., Singer, M., & Isralowitz, R. (1983). Impact of respite care on patients' perceptions of quality of life. *Mental Retardation, 21*, 153–156.

Kazak, A. E. (1987). Families with disabled children: Stress and social networks in three samples. *Journal of Abnormal Child Psychology, 15*, 137–146.

Kazak, A. E. (1989). Families of chronically ill children: A systems and social-ecological model of adaptation and challenge. *Journal of Consulting and Clinical Psychology, 57*, 25–30.

Kazak, A. E., & Clark, M. W. (1986). Stress in families of children with myelomeningocele. *Developmental Medicine and Child Neurology, 28*, 220–228.

Kazak, A. E., & Marvin, R. S. (1984). Differences, difficulties, and adaptation: Stress and social networks in families with a handicapped child. *Family Relations, 33*, 67–77.

Kazak, A. E., Reber, M., & Snitzer, L. (1988). Childhood chronic disease and family functioning: A study of Phenylketonuria. *Pediatrics, 81*, 224–230.

Knafl, K., Breitmayer, B., Gallo, A., & Zoeller, L. (1996). Family response to childhood chronic illness: Description of management styles. *Journal of Pediatric Nursing, 11*, 315–326.

Knafl, K. A., Gallo, A. M., Breitmayer, B. J., Zoeller, L. H., & Ayres, L. (1993). Family response to a child's chronic illness: A description of major defining themes. In S. G. Funk, E. M. Tornquist, M. T. Champagne, & R. A. Wiese (Eds.), *Key aspects of caring for the chronically ill: Hospital and home.* (pp. 290–303). New York: Springer.

Knafl, K. A., Gallo, A. M., Zoeller, L. H., Breitmayer, B. J., & Ayers, L. (1993). One approach to conceptualizing family response to illness. In S. L. Feetham, S. B. Meister, J. M. Bell, & C. L. Gilliss (Eds.), *The nursing of families: Theory/research/education/practice* (pp. 70–78). Newbury Park, CA: Sage.

Knoll, J. (1992). Being a family: The experience of raising a child with a disability or chronic illness. *Monographs of the American Association on Mental Retardation, 18*, 9–56.

Knox, J. E., & Hayes, V. E. (1983). Hospitalization of a chronically ill child: A stressful time for parents. *Issues in Comprehensive Pediatric Nursing, 6*, 217–226.

Kodadek, S. M., & Haylor, M. J. (1990). Using interpretive methods to understand family caregiving when a child is blind. *Journal of Pediatric Nursing, 5*, 42–49.

Krauss, M. W. (1993). Child-related and parenting stress: Similarities and differences between mothers and fathers of children with disabilities. *American Journal on Mental Retardation, 97*, 393–404.

Kruger, S., Shawver, M., & Jones, L. (1980). Reactions of families to the child with cystic fibrosis. *Image, 12*, 67–72.

Lavigne, J. V., & Ryan, M. (1979). Psychologic adjustment of siblings of children with chronic illness. *Pediatrics, 63*, 616–627.

Leonard, B. J., Brust, J. D., & Nelson, R. P. (1993). Parental distress: Caring for medically fragile children at home. *Journal of Pediatric Nursing, 8*, 22–30.

Lobato, D., Faust, D., & Spirito, A. (1988). Examining the effects of chronic disease and disability on children's sibling relationships. *Journal of Pediatric Psychology, 13*, 389–407.

Mardiros, M. (1982). Mothers of disabled children: A study of parental stress. *Nursing Papers (now Canadian Journal of Nursing Research), 14*(2), 47–56.

Maxwell, L. E. (1997). *Family processes and individual health-related decisions in response to heart-health initiatives.* Unpublished doctoral dissertation, University of British Columbia, Vancouver, BC.

McAnear, S. (1990). Parental reaction to a chronically ill child. *Home Healthcare Nurse, 8*, 35–40.

McCubbin, M. A. (1988). Family stress, resources, and family types: Chronic illness in children. *Family Relations, 37*, 203–210.

McCubbin, M. A. (1989). Family stress and family strengths: A comparison of single- and two-parent families with handicapped children. *Research in Nursing and Health, 12*, 101–110.

McKeever, P., Angus, J., & Thaha, S. (1994). *Raising disabled children in Canada: The characteristics, activities, and circumstances of biological and foster mothers.* Unpublished final report, University of Toronto.

Messias, D. K. H., Gilliss, C. L., Sparacino, P. S. A., Tong, E. M., & Foote, D. (1995). Stories of transition: Parents recall the diagnosis of congenital heart defect. *Family Systems Medicine, 13*, 367–377.

Meyerhoff, H., Hayes, V. E., & Canam, C. (1997). *Parenting the pre-school aged child with asthma: A secondary analysis using the Canam Adaptive Task Framework.* Unpublished manuscript, Vancouver, BC.

Midence, K. (1994). The effects of chronic illness on children and their families: An overview. *Genetic, Social and General Psychology Monographs, 120*, 311–326.

Miles, M. S., D'Auria, J. P., Hart, E. M., Sedlack, D. A., & Watral, M. A. (1993). Parental role alterations experienced by mothers of children with a life-threatening chronic illness. In S. G. Funk, E. M. Tornquist, M. T. Champagne, & R. A. Wiese (Eds.), *Key aspects of caring for the chronically ill: Hospital and home* (pp. 281–289). New York: Springer.

Montgomery, R. J., Gonyea, J. G., & Hooyman, N. R. (1985). Caregiving and the experience of subjective and objective burden. *Family Relations, 34*, 19–26.

Moriarty, H. J. (1990). Key issues in the family research process: Strategies for nurse researchers. *Advances in Nursing Science, 12*(3), 1–14.

Murphy, K. M. (1990). Interactional styles of parents following the birth of a high-risk infant. *Journal of Pediatric Nursing, 5*, 33–41.

Murphy, S. O. (1992). Using multiple forms of family data: Identifying pattern and meaning in sibling-infant relationships. In J. F. Gilgun, K. Daly, & G. Handel (Eds.), *Qualitative methods in family research* (pp. 146–171). Newbury Park: Sage.

Nassau, J. H., & Drotar, D. (1995). Social competence in children with IDDM and asthma: Child, teacher, and parent reports of children's social adjustment, social performance, and social skills. *Journal of Pediatric Psychology, 20*, 187–204.

Newacheck, P. W., & Taylor, W. R. (1992). Childhood chronic illness: Prevalence, severity, and impact. *American Journal of Public Health, 82*, 364–371.

Newby, N. M. (1996). Chronic illness and the family life-cycle. *Journal of Advanced Nursing, 23*, 786–791.

Nye, F. I. (1988). Fifty years of family research, 1937–1987. *Journal of Marriage and the Family, 50,* 305–316.

O'Neill, C., & Sorensen, E. S. (1991). Home care of the elderly: A family perspective. *Advances in Nursing Science, 13*(4), 28–37.

Patterson, J., & Blum, R. W. (1996). Risk and resilience among children and youth with disabilities. *Archives of Pediatrics & Adolescent Medicine, 150,* 692–698.

Patterson, J. M. (1985). Critical factors affecting family compliance with home treatment for children with cystic fibrosis. *Family Relations, 34,* 79–89.

Patterson, J. M. (1988). Chronic illness in children and the impact on families. In C. S. Chilman, E. W. Nunnally, & F. M. Cox (Eds.), *Chronic illness and disability* (pp. 69–107). Newbury Park: Sage.

Patterson, J. M., & Garwick, A. W. (1994). The impact of chronic illness on families: A family systems perspective. *Annals of Behavioral Medicine, 16*(2), 131–142.

Perrin, E. C., Ayoub, C. C., & Willett, J. B. (1993). In the eyes of the beholder: Family and maternal influences on perceptions of adjustment of children with a chronic illness. *Developmental and Behavioral Pediatrics, 14,* 94–105.

Perrin, E. C., Newacheck, P., Pless, I. B., Drotar, D., Gortmaker, S. L., Leventhal, J., Perrin, J. M., Stein, R. E. K., Walker, D. K., & Weitzman, M. (1993). Issues involved in the definition and classification of chronic health conditions. *Pediatrics, 91,* 787–793.

Perrin, J. M., Shayne, M. W., & Bloom, S. R. (1993). *Home and community care for chronically ill children.* New York: Oxford University Press.

Pinyerd, B. J. (1983). Siblings of children with myelomeningocele: Examining their perceptions. *Maternal-Child Nursing Journal, 12,* 61–70.

Pless, I., Roughmann, K., & Haggerty, R. (1972). Chronic illness, family functioning, and psychological adjustment: A model for the allocation of prevention mental health services. *International Journal of Epidemiology, 1,* 217–134.

Pless, I. B., & Wadsworth, M. E. J. (1989). Long-term effects of chronic illness on young adults. In R. E. K. Stein (Ed.), *Caring for children with chronic illness: Issues and strategies* (pp. 147–158). New York: Springer Publishing Co.

Pollner, M., & McDonald-Wikler, L. (1985). The social construction of unreality: A case study of a family's attribution of competence to a severely retarded child. *Family Process, 24,* 241–257.

Poznanski, E. (1969). Psychiatric difficulties in siblings of handicapped children. *Clinical Pediatrics, 8,* 232–234.

Ray, L. D., & Ritchie, J. A. (1993). Caring for chronically ill children at home: Factors that influence parents' coping. *Journal of Pediatric Nursing, 8,* 217–225.

Reynolds, J. M., Garralda, M. E., Jameson, R. A., & Postlethwaite, R. J. (1988). How parents and families cope with chronic renal failure. *Archives of Diseases in Childhood, 63,* 821–826.

Ritchie, J. A., Caty, S., & Ellerton, M. L. (1984). Concerns of acutely ill, chronically ill, and healthy preschool children. *Research in Nursing and Health, 7,* 265–274.

Robinson, C. A. (1985). The wrong kind of information. *The Canadian Nurse, 81,* 23–24.

Robinson, C. A. (1987). Roadblocks to family centered care when a chronically ill child is hospitalized. *Maternal-Child Nursing Journal, 16,* 181–193.

Robinson, C. A. (1995). Beyond dichotomies in the nursing of persons and families. *Image: Journal of Nursing Scholarship, 27,* 116–120.

Rolland, J. S. (1987). Chronic illness and the life cycle: A conceptual framework. *Family Process, 26*, 203–221.
Rolland, J. S. (1988). Family systems and chronic illness: A typological model. In F. Walsh & C. Anderson (Eds.), *Chronic disorders and the family* (pp. 143–169). New York: Haworth.
Rose, M. H. (1987). Individual adaptations of children with chronic conditions. In M. H. Rose & R. B. Thomas (Eds.), *Children with chronic conditions: Nursing in a family and community context* (pp. 13–28). Orlando: Grune and Stratton.
Sabbeth, B. F., & Leventhall, J. M. (1984). Marital adjustment to chronic childhood illness: A critique of the literature. *Pediatrics, 73*, 762–768.
Scharer, K., & Dixon, D. M. (1989). Managing chronic illness: Parents with a ventilator-dependent child. *Journal of Pediatric Nursing, 4*, 236–247.
Schlomann, P. (1988). Developmental gaps of children with a chronic condition and their impact on the family. *Journal of Pediatric Nursing, 3*, 190–187.
Schraeder, B. D. (1995). Children with disabilities. *Journal of Pediatric Nursing, 10*, 166–172.
Seideman, R. Y., & Kleine, P. F. (1995). A theory of transformed parenting: Parenting a child with developmental delay/mental retardation. *Nursing Research, 44*, 38–44.
Sharkey, T. (1995). The effects of uncertainty in families with children who are chronically ill. *Home Healthcare Nursing, 13*(4), 37–42.
Shonkoff, J. P., & Hauser-Cram, P. (1987). Early intervention for disabled infants and their families: A quantitative analysis. *Pediatrics, 80*, 650–658.
Sidani, S., & Jones, E. (1995). Use of the multitrait multimethod (MTMM) to analyze family relational data. *Western Journal of Nursing Research, 17*, 556–570.
Simeonsson, R. J., & McHale, S. M. (1981). Review: Research on handicapped children: Sibling relationships. *Child: Care, Health, and Development, 7*, 153–171.
Simon, N. B., & Smith, D. (1992). Living with chronic pediatric liver disease: The parents' experience. *Pediatric Nursing, 18*, 453–458.
Snowdon, A. W., Cameron, S., & Dunham, K. (1994). Relationships between stress, coping, resources, and satisfaction with family functioning in families of children with disabilities. *Canadian Journal of Nursing Research, 26*(3), 63–76.
Stein, R. E. K., Bauman, L. J., Westbrook, L. E., Coupey, S. M., & Ireys, H. T. (1993). Framework for identifying children who have chronic conditions: The case for a new definition. *Journal of Pediatrics, 122*, 342–347.
Stein, R. E. K., & Jessop, D. J. (1991). Long-term mental health effects of a pediatric chronic home care program. *Pediatrics, 88*, 490–496.
Steinhauer, P. D., Mushin, D. N., Rae-Grant, Q. (1974). Psychological aspects of chronic illness. *Pediatric Clinics of North America, 21*(4), 825–840
Steinhausen, H.-C. (1994). Psychological aspects of chronic disease in children and adolescents. *Hormone Research, 41 (Suppl. 2)*, 36–41.
Sterling, C. M., & Friedman, A. G. (1996). Empathic responding in children with a chronic illness. *Children's Health Care, 25*, 53–69.
Stewart, M. J., Ritchie, J. A., McGrath, P., Thompson, D., & Bruce, B. (1994). Mothers of children with chronic conditions: Supportive and stressful interactions with partners and professionals regarding caregiving burdens. *Canadian Journal of Nursing Research, 26*(4), 61–82.

Stuifbergen, A. K. (1987). The impact of chronic illness on families. *Family and Community Health, 9*(4), 43–51.

Tavormina, J. B., Boll, T. J., Dunn, N. J., Luscomb, R. L., & Taylor, J. R. (1981). Psychosocial effects on parents of raising a physically handicapped child. *Journal of Abnormal Child Psychology, 9,* 121–131.

Teague, B. R., Fleming, J. W., Castle, A., Kiernan, B. S., Lobo, M. L., Riggs, S., & Wolfe, J. G. (1993). "High-tech" home care for children with chronic health conditions: A pilot study. *Journal of Pediatric Nursing, 8,* 226–232.

Thompson, A. B., Curtner, M. E., & O'Rear, M. R. (1994). The psychosocial adjustment of well siblings of chronically ill children. *Children's Health Care, 23,* 211–226.

Thompson, R. J., Gil, K. M., Gustafson, K. E., George, L. K., Keith, B. R., Spock, A., & Kinney, T. R. (1994). Stability and change in the psychological adjustment of mothers of children and adolescents with cystic fibrosis and sickle cell disease. *Journal of Pediatric Psychology, 19,* 171–188.

Thompson, R. J., & Gustafson, K. E. (1996). *Adaptation to chronic childhood illness.* Washington, DC: American Psychological Association.

Thorne, S. E., & Robinson, C. A. (1988). Health care relationships: The chronic illness perspective. *Research in Nursing & Health, 11,* 293–300.

Tiller, J. W. G., Ekert, H., & Rickards, W. S. (1977). Family reactions in childhood acute lymphoblastic leukemia in remission. *Australian Paediatrics Journal, 13,* 176–181.

Tritt, S. G., & Esses, L. M. (1988). Psychosocial adaptation of siblings of children with chronic medical illnesses. *American Journal of Orthopsychiatry, 58,* 211–220.

Trute, B. (1990). Child and parent predictors of family adjustment in households containing young developmentally disabled children. *Family Relations, 39,* 292–297.

Turner-Hensen, A., Holaday, B., & Swan, J. H. (1992). When parenting becomes caregiving: Caring for the chronically ill child. *Family and Community Health, 15*(2), 19–30.

Turner-Henson, A. (1993). Mothers of chronically ill children and perceptions of environmental variables. *Issues in Comprehensive Pediatric Nursing, 16,* 63–76.

Van Dongen-Melman, J. E. W. M., Pruyn, J. F. A., De Groot, A., Koot, H. M., Hahlen, K., & Verhulst, F. C. (1995). Late psychosocial consequences for parents of children who survived cancer. *Journal of Pediatric Psychology, 20,* 567–586.

Walker, D. K., Epstein, S. G., Taylor, A. B., Crocker, A. C., & Tuttle, G. A. (1989). Perceived needs of families with children who have chronic health conditions. *Children's Health Care, 18,* 196–201.

Walker, L. S., Van Slyke, D. A., & Newbrough, J. R. (1992). Family resources and stress: A comparison of families of children with cystic fibrosis, diabetes, and mental retardation. *Journal of Pediatric Psychology, 17,* 327–343.

Wallace, H. M., Biehl, R. F., MacQueen, J. C., & Blackman, J. A. (Eds.). (1997). *Home care for children with technologic needs.* St. Louis: Mosby.

Wallander, J. L., Varni, J. W., Babani, L., Banis, H. T., & Wilcox, K. T. (1988). Children with chronic physical disorders: Maternal reports of their psychological adjustment. *Journal of Pediatric Psychology, 13*(197–212).

Walsh, M., & Ryan-Wenger, N. M. (1992). Sources of stress in children with asthma. *Journal of School Health, 62,* 459–463.

Wegener, D. H., & Aday, L. A. (1989). Home care for ventilator-assisted children: Predicting family stress. *Pediatric Nursing, 15,* 371–376.

Whall, A. L., & Loveland-Cherry, C. J. (1993). Family unit-focused research: 1984–1991. In J. J. Fitzpatrick, R. L. Taunton, & A. S. Jacox (Eds.), *Annual Review of Nursing Research* (pp. 227–247). New York: Springer.

Whyte, D. A. (1992). A family nursing approach to the care of a child with a chronic illness. *Journal of Advanced Nursing, 17,* 317–327.

Williaams, P. D., Lorenzo, F. D., & Borja, M. (1993). Pediatric chronic illness: Effects on siblings and mothers. *Maternal-Child Nursing Journal, 21,* 111–121.

Wilton, K., & Renaut, J. (1986). Stress levels in families with intellectually handicapped preschool children and families with nonhandicapped preschool children. *Journal of Mental Deficiency Research, 30,* 163–169.

Wolman, C., Resnick, M. D., Harris, L. J., & Blum, R. W. (1994). Emotional well-being among adolescents with and without chronic conditions. *Journal of Adolescent Health, 15,* 199–204.

Worthington, R. C. (1989). The chronically ill child and recurring family grief. *Journal of Family Practice, 29,* 397–400.

Wuest, J., & Stern, P. N. (1990). The impact of fluctuating relationships with the Canadian health care system on family management of otitis media with effusion. *Journal of Advanced Nursing, 15,* 556–563.

Yoos, L. (1987). Chronic childhood illnesses: Developmental issues. *Pediatric Nursing, 13,* 25–28.

Young, L. Y., Creighton, D. E., & Sauve, R. S. (1988). The needs of families of infants discharged home with continuous oxygen therapy. *JOGNN, 17,* 187–193.

Acknowledgment. This research was partially supported by an operating grant from the British Columbia Medical Services Foundation and to the researcher by a pre-doctoral fellowship from the National Health Research Development Program.

Response
Bonnie Holaday

ECOLOGICAL PERSPECTIVES ON KNOWLEDGE DEVELOPMENT AND FAMILIES AND CHILDREN WITH CHRONIC CONDITIONS

This response comments on the theoretically divergent and widely dispersed body of research on families with children with chronic conditions that Hayes has so ably summarized. This commentary uses Bronfenbrenner's (1979, 1989) ecological perspective to focus attention on what Hayes has identified as known about external environments and the functioning of families with children with chronic conditions and aspects of the internal environment that play a role in both the family's and the child's development.

Perhaps the most salient feature of the Bronfenbrenner model lies in its assumption that ecological variables affecting both the family and the child operate at multiple levels. A range of ecological variables is identified, from those directly affecting the family in daily interactions to those that operate more indirectly through the functions of social institutions and through cultural values and beliefs. Bronfenbrenner proposes four specific levels of ecological analysis: the microsystem, mesosystem, ecosystem, and macrosystem. These are conceptualized as being nested within each other like Russian dolls, and influences across levels are assumed to operate transactionally (Bronfenbrenner, 1989).

Macrosystem Influences

Bronfenbrenner (1979) defines the macrosystem as "consistencies in the form and content of lower-order systems (micro-, meso-, exo-) that exist, or could exist, at the level of the subculture or the culture as a whole, along with any belief systems or ideology underlying such consistencies" (p. 26). The macrosystem perspective suggests that cultural values and ideology shape human relationships at every level such as exchanges taking place between families and hospitals or schools to social exchanges between parents and health care providers. With respect to family issues, this level of analysis is useful in identifying some of the cultural beliefs and values that underlie organizational structures in health care systems, professional practices, and daily interactions that affect the lives of families of children with chronic conditions. Hayes cites several studies that demonstrate how stigma operates to impact families and children in terms of fundamental beliefs, assumptions, and values. Together, these comprise an ideology in which families and/or the ill child are viewed in negative ways or as experiencing problems or deficits. Hayes' review of the literature indicates that very few studies have examined transactions between the families and their environments or examined properties of environments as they are perceived by the family and how this affects the development of the family as a unit. Nursing research that will assist us in understanding these issues may be one of the most powerful avenues for moving forward with the development of more integrated interventions for these families.

Exosystem Influences

An exosystem is defined as "one or more settings that do not involve the developing person (or family) as an active participant, but one in which events occur that affect, or are affected by, what happens in the setting containing the developing person (or family)" (Bronfenbrenner, 1979, p. 25). Examples include legislative settings, school boards, or boards of directors for managed care organizations. Events occurring in these settings are strongly influenced by macrosystem variables and directly affect events taking place in the family's daily life. For example, a managed care organization can enhance or diminish a family's access to needed services depending on its organization and incentives. Networks of managed care providers can provide more coordinated care or they can sharply reduce a family's access to needed specialists. Another example of an exosystem variable relevant to family life is the organization of the school. Traditional beliefs concerning differences among children are reflected in the creation of separate structures, programs, or activities for serving children with and without disabilities. These structures and programs dramatically affect the nature and extent of interaction between children with disabilities and their nondisabled peers. As Hayes notes in her review, more research needs to focus on the family as a unit and on contextual issues. The lack of research is disturbing, given the fundamental importance of decisions made in these organizational contexts.

Mesosystem Influences

A mesosystem consists of "the interrelations of two or more settings in which the developing person (family) actively participates" (such as relations with neighbors, school teachers, health care settings, extended family members, and work) (Bronfenbrenner, 1979, p. 25). Influences at this level that are particularly relevant include the nature and extent of relationships among parents and extended family members, relationships among parents and teachers, and among parents and health care providers. Each of these constitute supportive links across settings for the family and the developing child.

Bronfenbrenner's focus on importance of social relationships across settings raises important questions about the extent to which the family's (or parents') participation in neighborhood programs as opposed to "special" programs at the hospital or at the school, may contribute to the family's lack of success in dealing with the community. Other important research, as cited by Hayes, is the testing of interventions that mediate the experiences of families and the children in a fashion that creates supportive links between settings and therefore contributes to positive outcomes.

Nursing research on mesosystem variables has been more extensive than work at either the exo- or macrosystem levels. Although it is clear that relationships among families and professionals are important, however, it is much less clear how they can be changed. More intervention-oriented research that yields effective strategies for improving relationships among people in the many settings in which the family participates is needed.

Microsystem Influences

Bronfenbrenner defines a microsystem as "a pattern of activities, roles, and interpersonal relations, experienced by the developing person (family) in a given setting with particular physical and material characteristics" (1979, p. 22). The majority of nursing research reviewed by Hayes focused on this level. In particular, there is a wealth of research describing interactions between the ill child and family members.

As summarized by Hayes, nursing research, at this level has yielded valuable information about parenting/caregiving challenges, normalization strategies, identification of effective intra-familial communication patterns, and family-level responses to stress. This body of research has made valuable contributions to the development of nursing interventions.

What is needed is more research that focuses on potentially important interactions among microsystem variables and ecological variables operating within higher order systems (e.g., exo- and macrosystem factors). Ecological contexts can vary for families and these can influence the outcomes of interventions focused on aspects of the microsystem. The ecological perspectives discussed in this commentary and in Dr. Hayes' review could add to the progress nursing has already made in addressing the challenges faced by families with children with chronic illnesses.

REFERENCES

Bronfenbrenner, U. (1979). *The ecology of human development.* Cambridge, MA: Harvard University Press.

Bronfenbrenner, U. (1989). The ecology of the family as a context for human development: Research perspectives. *Developmental Psychology*, pp. 22, 723–742.

Response
Janet A. Deatrick

The privilege of studying families and their children who have chronic conditions creates a moral imperative for us as researchers to perfect our science so that families and children benefit from our understandings. While those benefits may be far removed from the families and children being studied, we can at least indirectly repay our debt; by doing the best possible research, we respect our social contract with them.

Tanner, Benner, Chesla, and Gordon (1996, p. 217–218), however, remind us of the difficulties in translating research into clinical practice. In their phenomenology of nurse's knowing, they warn us: "Knowing a patient is a highly specific, situated knowledge . . . it would be a mistake to think that this discourse could be made completely formal, explicit, general, and objective, because it is the discourse of the particular so essential to clinical knowledge." As Hayes points out, when the "patients" are children with chronic conditions and their families, this task becomes most complex and perhaps most important.

As Hayes describes the body of literature related to families who have children with chronic conditions, she carefully weaves a tapestry about what we know and what we don't know. Much of what she describes is research that has been completed during my own lifetime as a nurse. As such, her words trace my professional life of understanding. As a young student I was taught that all patients and families eventually succumb to their vulnerabilities. Imagine my surprise when I began to hear the stories from families and children. I began to learn about the meaning that they ascribed to their situations, how they managed, and what they thought were the consequences for their lives (Deatrick & Knafl, 1990). I heard many different kinds of stories about their struggles within the family, as well as with illness, themselves, health professionals, and society that I did not see reflected in our literature. Since that time, I have seen the evolution of a much more balanced approach to describing their situations.

Certain children, parents, and families were especially important to my own learning. I learned from the father of a 12-year-old female with severe limb deformities that parents who are most successful at normalizing their situations often get accused of denying their children's physical differences. I learned from the parents of a school-aged female with neurofibromatosis that it is impossible and perhaps ill advised for some families to try to normalize everyday life. I learned from the parents of a 14-year-old male adolescent with developmental problems that we have a lot to learn about how we approach children, adolescents, and their families about health care decisions. I learned from many families how much effort it takes to successfully work with health care providers. I learned from hundreds of families about their tremendous ingenuity.

Throughout my years as an academic I have endeavored to translate my passion about families' experiences with childhood chronic conditions to the budding nurse, the accomplished specialist, and the career scientist in training. I believe that all share one common denominator in their learning needs. As reaffirmed by Hayes, theoretical notions about the family and childhood chronic conditions will have much to do with what is discovered about the families. Caretakers need to recognize their beliefs before they can refine them and use them to everyone's advantage.

A pediatric advanced practice nursing student commented about a clinical learning experience in her master's program that had helped her recognize some of her constraining beliefs about families (Wright, Watson, & Bell, 1996). Near the completion of her masters program she wrote the following note about a home visit:

> This family invited me, a stranger, into their home and shared some very painful and private information. There were times when all three of us had tears in our eyes. They thanked me for listening, they just kept talking. It was not what I expected. I did not come prepared with Kleenex, I did not come prepared to feel so connected to these people. I came prepared with a script, but a script was not necessary. I feel honored to have met them, I feel honored to have heard their story.

The responsibility inherent in the privilege of hearing family stories as a researcher is enormous. The newest breed of nurse scientists is now being prepared to shoulder those responsibilities. They are prepared to design not only theory-testing, but also, theory-building research. With required content in not only quantitative, but also qualitative methods, they have beginning skills to answer research questions that require more complex approaches. They are also being tutored by family scientists who have long grappled with the challenges of designing research of families (Feetham, 1991). Feetham (1991) suggests that a conceptual or theoretical framework, a conceptualization of the family, relevance for our understanding of family functioning and structure, and relevance to nursing practice are the hallmarks of both family-related research and research of families. While family-related research examines the responses of individual family members and/or concepts related to families or family members, research of families reflects the family as the unit or system in conceptualization, measurement, and analysis. In addition, the research adds knowledge to understanding family systems. These guidelines do not imply that either family-related or research of families is better, rather they provide a framework for enabling decisions about the design and conduct of research.

These guidelines have enabled me to address some of the complexities that Hayes directs us to consider. For instance, most recently, colleagues and I completed a study concerning mothers with relapsing remitting multiple sclerosis and their children (Deatrick, Brennan, & Cameron, in press). We conceptualized the family and their situation using Rolland's Family Systems-Illness Model (1994). This Model allowed us to consider family functioning, characteristics of the mother's illness situation, and the developmental life cycles of family members and the family itself. We were able to make decisions about these concepts and processes based on existing research and clinical knowledge, as well as on the resources available for the project. A family-related project was designed, using dyadic (mother-child) quantitative and qualitative data. Family functioning was represented by an instrument measuring maternal physical affection and by perceptions shared in an interview. Illness characteristics were represented by the mother's functional status, fatigue and symptom exacerbation. The children's development was represented by age and gender. The qualitative data were used to illustrate the quantitative results. Working closely with the editor of the journal that accepted the manuscript, we were able to clearly present the results of the study and their relevance for our knowledge of the functioning of family members, a family unit dyad, and nursing practice. Thus, the results of the study and the model for presenting them are both being disseminated.

In order to design and implement cutting-edge studies, both novice and experienced scientists need tremendous support. As Hayes points out, it may seem logical to carefully explicate one's theoretical perspective, use triangulated methods, use the family as the unit of data collection and/or analysis, and implement the findings for the family as a whole. Our present literature, however, provides few comprehensive guides and examples for these critical skills. Our institutional review boards, hospital research committees, faculties, grant reviewers, and journal reviewers have had little preparation in these areas. In addition, required formats may not be conducive to use of these cutting-edge approaches. Certainly review criteria may not favor those proposals that include complex procedures that require lengthy and difficult explanations.

In my own experience as a researcher most skilled in qualitative research of families, faculty and students make a tremendous number of requests for consultation. Such requests are not only personally gratifying but are also an indication that scientists are concerned and interested in answering the important mandates set forth by Hayes. We must all respond to her call.

REFERENCES

Deatrick, J., Brennan, D., & Cameron, M. E. (in press). Mothers with multiple sclerosis and their children: Effects of fatigue and exacerbations on maternal support. *Nursing Research.*

Deatrick, J., & Knafl, K. (1990). Understanding family response to childhood chronic conditions. *Journal of Family Nursing,* 5(1), 2–3.

Feetham, S. (1991). Conceptual and methodological issues in research of families. In A. Whall, & J. Fawcett (Eds.), *Family theory development in nursing: State of the science and art* (pp. 55–68). Philadelphia, PA: F.A. Davis.

Rolland, J. (1994). *Families, illness, and disability: An integrative treatment model.* New York: Basic Books.

Tanner, C., A., Benner, T., Chesla, C., & Gordon, D. (1996). The phenomenology of knowing the patient. In S. Gordon, P. Benner, N. Noddings (Eds.), *Caregiving: Readings in knowledge practice, ethics, and politics* (pp. 203–219). Philadelphia, PA: University of Pennsylvania Press.

Wright, L. M., Watson, W. L., & Bell, J. M. (1996). *Beliefs: The heart of healing in families and illness.* New York: Basic Books.

Chapter 6

Toward a Practice Theory of Caring for Patients with Chronic Skin Disease

Marit Kirkevold

OVERVIEW

The purpose of this study was to provide a description and interpretation of the practical knowledge embedded in the practice of a group of experienced nurses caring for patients suffering from chronic skin disease. A practice theory was uncovered encompassing the nurses' underlying "model" of persons living with chronic skin disease, the values/goals for their care, action strategies utilized to realize the values, and the context framing their understanding and practice. The practice theory is proposed as a useful tool to systematize, communicate, reflect upon, refine and extend the clinical practice of experienced nurses caring for this group of patients. The theory is also proposed as an example of how practical knowledge in other specialty areas may be systematized in order to communicate that knowledge efficiently. A scholarly discussion is needed about how best to communicate the invaluable resource of knowledge embedded in the practice of experienced nurses.

Note: Originally published in *Scholarly Inquiry for Nursing Practice: An International Journal*, Vol. 7, No. 1, 1997. New York: Springer Publishing Company.

INTRODUCTION

The purpose of this study was to identify and interpret the implicit practice theory of a group of experienced nurses providing care to persons with chronic skin disease. Chronic skin disease, such as psoriasis (PS) and atopic dermatitis (AD), is often considered to be mainly a "cosmetic problem." It may, however, lead to severe physical, psychosocial, and practical problems (Belk, 1983; Dunn, Cockerline, & Rice, 1988; Lombardo, Cave, & Bernadina, 1988; Updike, 1985). Recent research has found that patients suffering from chronic skin disease experience the disease as having a major impact on their daily lives (Ginsburg, 1989; Taylor & Buckwalter, 1988; Ramsay & O'Reagan, 1988; Updike, 1985). Despite these serious aspects, nursing care of patients with severe skin disease has received little attention, and there is almost no literature focusing on how nurses may assist this group of patients.

Nurses develop a wealth of knowledge as they care for patients over time (Benner, 1984; Benner & Wrubel, 1982; Ellis, 1969; Wiedenbach, 1970). So far, nurse researchers have not taken sufficient advantage of this resource. The provision of written accounts and interpretations of the knowledge guiding daily practice may facilitate reflection on this knowledge, assist in gaining new insights, and further the development of practice theories for nursing (Argyris, Putnam & Smith, 1985; Ellis, 1969; Juul Jensen, 1988; Kirkevold, 1989, 1990; Schön, 1983, 1987; Wiedenbach, 1970). Wiedenbach (1970) argues:

> Needed, I think, is understanding of the theory that underlies the nurse's way of nursing. This involves knowing what the nurse wanted to accomplish, how she went about accomplishing it, and in what context she did what she did" (p. 1058).

Practical knowledge has been conceptualized in different ways, but there seems to be an agreement that it encompasses essential assumptions, expectations, values, and norms integrated into practical decisions and actions (Argyris et al., 1985; Benner, 1983; Polanyi, 1962; Schön, 1983, 1987). Several authors have argued that practical knowledge may take the form of implicit theories embedded in practice (Argyris, Putnam, & Smith, 1985; Barnum, 1990; Schön, 1983, 1987; Wiedenbach, 1970). Practice theories make the actions of practitioners intelligible and plausible (Schön, 1987). For the purpose of this study, practice theory was conceptualized as shown in Table 6.1 (Juul Jensen, 1988; Schön, 1987; Wiedenbach, 1970).

The term "underlying model of phenomenon" is borrowed from Schön (1987). Schön (1983, 1987) and Argyris et al. (1985) have demonstrated how practitioners "see" situations differently depending on how they "frame the situation." Framing of a situation is based on the underlying model that practitioners hold of the phenomenon of concern. As there is no clear definition of the term, the following definition was adopted in this study: The "underlying model of the phenomenon" consists of nurses' assumptions and expectations of the essential characteristics of patients suffering from chronic skin disease.

Wiedenbach (1970) identified three ingredients in "the theory that underlies the nurse's way of nursing" (p. 1058): 1) the nurse's central purpose in nursing, 2) the prescription or general action that the nurse deems appropriate to fulfill the purpose, and 3) the context in which the nurse finds herself. This view of nurses' "practice theory" is in agreement with the Danish philosopher Juul Jensen (1988), who argues that

> the theoretical core of a discipline is its basic ideals (values). The actual action patterns and procedures must be understood in this light. The theoretical development within a discipline must start by determination of and reflection about the central ideals (p. 47–8).

In this study, basic undergirding values were defined as the values that could account for the way nurses structured their care, that is, the decisions and priorities they made in providing care to chronic skin patients. Strategies of action were defined as those nursing care actions that nurses performed in caring for chronically ill skin patients. Context was defined as the "background stage, or "world" which the nurses seemed to take into account in understanding patients' experiences and needs and in planning and providing care.

TABLE 6.1 Structure of Practice Theories

I. The underlying model of the phenomenon under consideration.
II. The basic undergirding values, pointing to the goals of the actions.
III. The strategies of action selected to reach the goals/realize the underlying values.
IV. The context/setting of the action.

For the purpose of this study, chronic skin disease was operationalized as psoriasis (PS) and atopic dermatitis (AD). These patients were admitted to a specialized hospital unit for treatment and care.

METHODS

Sample and setting

The sample consisted of 13 female registered nurses working in a specialized skin unit at an urban university hospital in Norway. They had worked an average of 7 years on the unit (ranging from 4 months to 20 years). Inclusion was based on the following rationale: All nurses were invited to participate in group interviews and to submit critical incidents on the assumption that practical knowledge is shared among a community of practitioners (Argyris et al., 1985; Biordi, 1984; Taylor, 1977). The eight most expert nurses (according to head nurse, supervisor, and peers) functioned as key informants; however, all nurses were observed while providing care. Participants signed consent forms after receiving information about what participation entailed. Anonymity and confidentiality were preserved by excluding names and other identifying data from the fieldnotes.

Data collection

The study used a triangulated research design in order to increase validity. Data collection consisted of a series of eight semistructured group interviews, the collection of 15 critical incidents, and participant observation of direct patient-nurse interactions, reports, and rounds during a period of nine months.

Interviews lasted an average of two hours and focused on eliciting the nurses' general and shared ideas about providing care to the selected patient population. Critical incidents focused on actual experiences with selected patients. The nurses were asked to describe in detailed narrative language at least one AD and one PS patient, the nursing care given, and the rationale for the care. The nurses were encouraged to reflect on the experience in terms of how they felt about the outcome and success of the nursing care provided. Selection of patients was based on the following criteria: (1) situation was typical in terms of providing nursing care to AD and/or PS patients or (2) situation was experienced as particularly successful or difficult (Benner, 1984).

Field observations sought to uncover implicit values and norms reflected in the way the nurses structured their nursing care. Observations encompassed group reports and direct patient-nurse interactions during morning and evening shifts, especially focusing on the morning and afternoon skin care sessions. In addition, physician rounds were included to observe how the nurses presented their interpretations of their patients' needs.

Data analysis

Data analysis focused on extracting the implicit practice theory guiding the nurses' practice. The analysis was guided by the model of practice theories elicited from the literature (Table 6.1).

The following procedure was used: Each critical incident was analyzed as an entity, identifying the underlying model of the phenomenon of chronic skin patients, the values/goals guiding the nurse's actions, action strategies used, and the context of the nursing care. The whole collection was then analyzed for recurring themes. The same procedure was carried out with the eight group interviews. These were compared with the themes uncovered in the critical incidents. The fieldnotes were analyzed in order to modify, refine, and verify the emerging practice theory. The results of the initial data analysis were presented to the participating nurses, who provided support for the findings and additional information that was used to refine the practice theory.

RESULTS

Each of the structural components of the practice theory is summarized in Figure 1 and delineated in the following sections.

The Nurses' Underlying "Model" of the Phenomenon of Chronic Skin Patients

The underlying "model" of the phenomenon of patients with chronic skin disease had three dimensions: (1) The relevant characteristic symptoms, causes, consequences, treatment and trajectory of the disease; including the characteristic appearance of the disease in its different stages and variations; (2) an understanding of what it means to live with chronic skin disease: and (3) assumptions and expectations about common responses to this situation. The model was an important basis for the rest of the practice theory, as it provided rationale for the values and goals to pursue and gave direction toward appropriate action strategies. The components of the "model" are summarized in the upper component of Figure 6.1.

Essential characteristics of PS & AD

The nurses considered the two diseases to share certain characteristics, but to differ in other respects. They underlined the following similarities: Both chronic diseases were characterized by (a) recurring flare-ups that required certain preventive, limiting actions, (b) a strong relationship between "stress" (particularly emotional burdens) and worsening of the disease, (c) being highly visible, and (d) being uncontrollable and unpredictable. The nurses differentiated the two diseases in terms of illness trajectory, degree of uncontrollability and unpredictability, and cardinal symptom (Table 6.2).

PS was assumed to be highly uncontrollable, because the only factor that was clearly known to influence the disease was stress, and total control of stress was considered almost impossible. Limited amounts of stress could be enough to precipitate a new eruption, setting off a vicious stress-worsening cycle. Explains one of the nurses:

> What is difficult about it, is that psychological stress exacerbates the rash. Rash, which is developing, does not stop, because the patients are psychologically influenced by it. The fact that they are sad about it, keeps it going. If they had been a little more optimistic, if they had been able to forget about it a little, so that they could get in better shape psychologically, then the rash would follow.

AD, although also clearly assumed to be influenced by stress, was seen as more controllable in that it could be associated with specific allergens or irritants that could be removed or avoided. It was also assumed that conscientious care to prevent dry skin could, to a certain degree, prevent an outbreak of the disease.

The burdens of living with the disease

The nurses recounted several ways in which they considered chronic skin disease to impact on the lives of their patients. They underlined

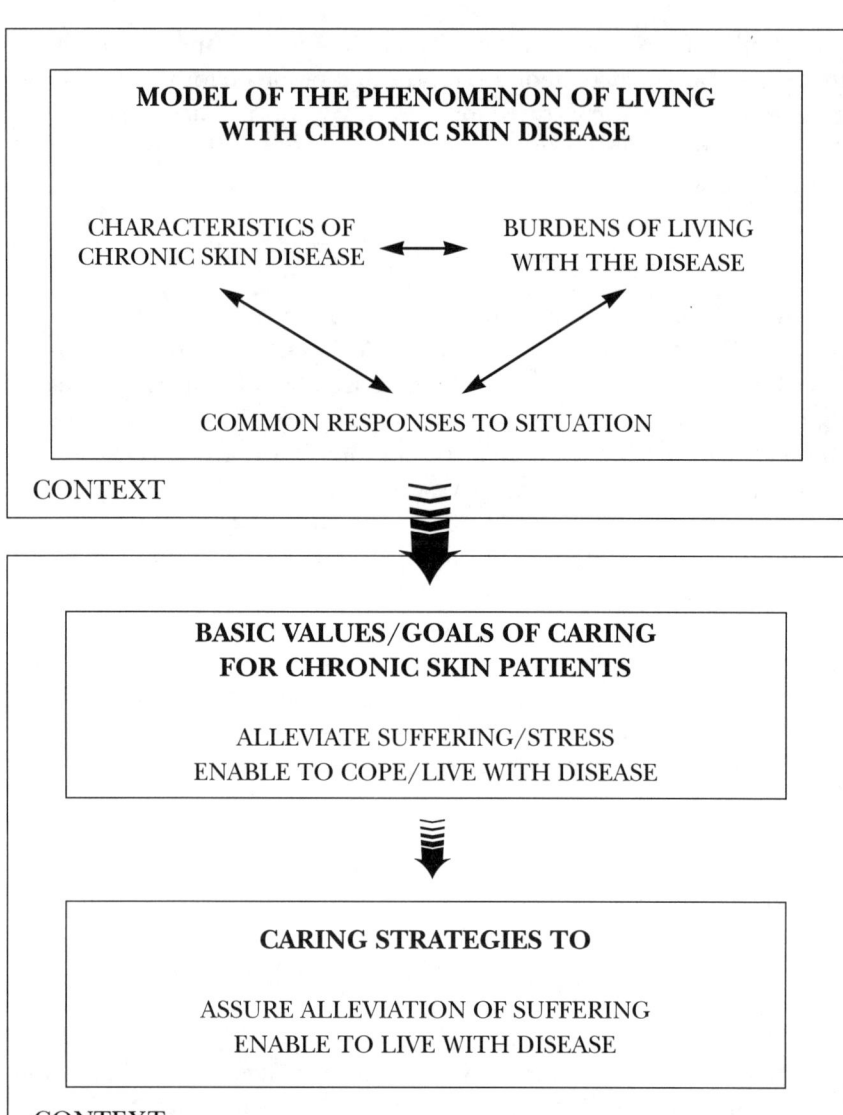

FIGURE 6.1 Components of the Nursing Practice Theory.

TABLE 6.2 The Nurses' Practice Theory: Differentiated Characteristics of PS & AD

Psoriasis	Atopic Dermatitis
Illness Trajectory:	

Psoriasis trajectory: young adulthood → (gradual worsening w/each eruption) / (limited stable) / (sudden exacerbation) → adulthood/old age

Atopic Dermatitis trajectory: children → (free) → puberty → (free) → young adulthood (pregnancy, etc.) → (free) → adulthood (specific allergies)

Psoriasis	Atopic Dermatitis
Degree of Uncontrollability:	
Very difficult to control, must control stress to control disease	More controllable *if* a) can identify & eliminate allergens b) take special care of skin
Degree of Predictability:	
Highly unpredictable, eruptions may occur at any time.	May predict to certain extent, according to usual trajectory & allergens/irritants
Symptoms:	
Flaking	Itching
Character of Eruption:	
Gradual development	Abrupt (in few hours)

that one frequently unappreciated aspect of living with chronic skin disease was the time associated with managing the disease. According to the nurses, preventive measures and required treatment, including different baths, liniments and topical applications, could take up to 2 or 3 hours daily. The nurses realized that the amount of time required to carry out the necessary regimen as well as its interference with other activities was frequently experienced as a great burden. The following quote from one of the interviews attests to this:

> It is important for us to see the whole picture of the person—see how much the psychological aspects mean. The disease impacts much more on the daily life than one would expect, for example, if you are to thoroughly apply liniments twice a day. And in terms of work, too, you have to get up very early to apply liniments etc., for an hour or so before even getting off. And, depending on the kind of work you have, in some positions involving representing tasks, this may become difficult because of eczema or bandages.

The disease gave rise to substantial demands in terms of self-control, self-monitoring, self-treatment, and stress-management, requiring that the affected person constantly monitor his or her condition and take appropriate measures to adjust the treatment regimen according to the condition. Also, the disease required self-control in terms of avoiding stressful situations, managing the stress response in such situations, as well as avoiding factors known to precipitate or worsen the condition. The nurses underlined that this could be experienced as an overwhelming burden at times because of its never ending character. In responding to the general, opening question in the first group interview about the characteristics of chronic skin disease, this was the theme that the nurses brought up.

Another serious impact, according to the nurses, was the feeling of stigma frequently experienced by affected persons. They underlined that both PS and AD could contribute to feelings of personal or social unacceptability in the person's relationships with family, friends, and colleagues. The nurses expected problematic relations whith spouse and boss to be a frequent consequence of the disease and assumed them to be closely related to ignorance and nonacceptance of the disease and its treatment by family and/or colleagues. The following fieldnote from an observation of a morning skin care session of an elderly professional woman illustrates the issue:

During the skin care session, the patient expressed that she had no illusions about getting cured. She should be happy as long as she could keep the itching and rash under control. The patient also said that she found it difficult to live with the eczema. She mentioned the characteristic smell associated with running sores, saying: "It is terrible to go around worrying about smelling badly. When I get the time, I will write a book about the inner life of the soul of eczema patients." She continued by saying that the worst part was people feeling sorry for her, people's curiousness, all the questions, and the foul smell.

Especially in acute stages, difficult or bothersome symptoms impacted greatly on the lives of patients. Frequently, they had to endure these for long periods of time. Both groups of patients had bothersome symptoms, varying from pain, soreness, and stiffness to itching, tiredness, and sleep disturbances. The two cardinal symptoms of scaling and itching had a profound, but very different effect on the patients. The itchiness associated with an outbreak of AD was seen as particularly bothersome because of its "maddening" continuous presence. The scaling of PS was frequently not as bothersome physically, but had an unesthetic character that underlined the stigma effect. The following fieldnote, from an observation of a morning skin care session, alludes to this:

> As the nurse applies the ointment, the patient initiates a conversation explaining that at home the skin care takes 4 hours a day, and that this is difficult to combine with working. The disease is also difficult because of his job. Being a salesman, it feels uncomfortable with all the flakes that he sheds wherever he stands. Says he: "Just lifting my arms, the flakes drizzle out of my shirtsleeves. The rash on the hands, too, is problematic, because you have to look okay as a salesman."

In accordance with the above quote, other assumed consequences of severe chronic skin disease were difficult or increased the challenge in carrying out other roles, notably the work-role, because of allergies towards allergens in the work environment, the time required for disease management, work-related stress, and frequent sick-leaves or hospitalizations due to the disease.

Common responses to the disease and its impact

According to the nurses, the impact outlined above led to certain common responses among this group of patients. The nurses argued that many of their patients were highly conscious of the presence of their disease and the reactions it caused in others. Explained one of the nurses:

> Psoriasis and dermatitis patients are very observant when they meet people for the first time (thinking): "Where do they look? Do they look at my flakes, my red spots, my hands?" Automatically, they watch where the person's eyes go. And their weak spots are focused upon every time. This feeling of not being as "good looking" as many others is a big psychological burden for many of our patients.

The nurses reported that the patients frequently responded to their disease by either covering the skin lesions by wearing long-sleeved clothes, turtlenecks, and trousers, or else isolating themselves from social situations involving exposure to the disease. These concealment measures were used to avoid the painful feelings associated with experienced or anticipated adverse reactions from others.

Another frequent response that the nurses expected to see was the boycotting of treatment or preventive measures necessary to keep the disease under control. The nurses reported that a large number of patients admitted to the unit had stopped caring for their skin in the months or weeks prior to the hospitalization, because they could not "take it" anymore. Returning to the situation of the salesman recounted above, the fieldnotes indicate that the patient continued the conversation by explaining that before being admitted, he had stopped applying the lotions and ointments, because "you just can't bear it anymore after a while." The nurses expressed an understanding of this response, but also saw it as a major challenge toward which they needed to direct their attention.

Basic Values/Goals in the Nursing Care of Chronic Skin Patients

Two basic values seemed to undergird the nurses' care of chronic skin patients. These were: 1) *alleviating* the patient of the stress/burdens associated with the disease, and 2) *enabling* the patient to manage the disease and its impact.

Based on their understanding of the impact of the disease on the daily life of chronic skin patients, nurses assumed that patients' experience of burden could be overwhelming at times, leading them to relinquish their frequently well-established and carefully implemented skin maintenance routine. This, together with the assumption of frequent lack of understanding and support in the patient's home milieu, led nurses to temporarily take over responsibility for alleviating the bothersome symptoms and managing the disease in order to help patients regain the necessary strength to continue this unending task. The following quote from one of the group interviews attests to this:

> We have patients who say that the disease causes family problems, because the partner can't accept the rash and flakes. Then it is good for them to come in here and we touch them and consider the flakes a natural part. . . . Therefore, patients frequently apply to get admitted when they have bad periods, because they just have to get away from it all until it gets a little better.

The principle of enabling, may be considered the exact opposite in that this principle emphasized the importance of assisting the patient to gain or regain control and responsibility for managing the disease and the associated life-situation. This principle emphasized the patient's own actions and underlined the importance of helping the patient to see that the disease could, in fact, be manageable and bearable. One of the nurses put is thus:

> We shall try to make the treatments a little more acceptable—show them that they are possible to implement without being a huge burden. . . . Our goal is teaching and treatments combined.

Action Strategies to Realize Basic Values/Goals of Care

The two principles are clearly related to action strategies utilized by the nurses.

Action Strategies to Alleviate Stress/Burdens

Several action strategies were used to realize the principle of alleviating the patient of the burdens associated with living with severe chronic skin disease. Some of these were general for all patients; others were more closely related to the particular characteristics and demands of the disease.

One general nursing strategy that nurses realized to be an effective, but more coincidental than planned intervention, was the creation of an environment that contributed to removing many of the burdens associated with the disease. As one of them explained:

> All the time we hear patients say: As soon as I learned that I was being admitted, I started getting better! Something happens to them then. (They seem to think:) Oh, how great. Now I don't have to stress so much anymore! Now I'll get in there, where people accept that this is how I am. This is a clear signal that where they presently are, they are not being accepted.

The environment that was created was characterized by (1) having only severely affected skin patients, (2) relatively long hospital stays (2–4 weeks) and (3) many patients who were familiar with the unit because of frequent readmissions. These characteristics led to an environment where having a skin disease was a shared experience and where an understanding of "what living with a chronic skin disease means" was present among fellow patients and health professionals. This shared understanding alleviated the patient of constantly having to explain and inform about his condition. The nurses and fellow patients "bore witness" (Benner & Wrubel, 1989) in the sense that they recognized and legitimized the patients' suffering as "real" and truly burdensome. The importance of this was supported by the frequent report of unacceptability and lack of understanding in the patients' home milieu. In one of the nurses' words:

> Here, they have no problems being accepted, because they have patients all around who have skin diseases. And we (the nurses) are used to seeing skin disease and do not react in the way that people do outside the hospital. . . . But they are only here a fraction of the year (or less). So it is what their situation is like outside that really matters.

The principle of alleviating burdens also gave rise to nursing strategies directed toward individual patients. One prominent example involved acutely affected AD patients suffering from unbearable itching. These patients were frequently admitted to the hospital in a desolate condition after weeks almost without sleep and their skin totally covered with a red, swollen rash, scratched until bleeding. Upon arrival, they were "gently" put to bed, offered itch-reducing baths and medications, and offered complete care by the nurses. The nurses as well as several patients and physicians commented on the abrupt improvement seen after only a day or two with this complete care. The nurses assumed that a plausible explanation was the complete alleviation of any responsibility for the management of the disease as well as the help received to control the bothersome symptoms. A quote from an interview testifies to this:

> Obviously, it is a big difference treating their "active" psoriasis attack at home and being here. Here, someone is taking over the responsibility for the treatments, and they are followed up upon daily. At home, they have to decide for themselves (thinking:) 'I wonder if I should use this ointment or that? For how long?' And so on. When they are admitted here, they totally relax, because they no longer have to decide everything for themselves.

Action Strategies to Enable Patients to Manage the Situation

Even more prominent in the nurses' practice theory was the principle of enabling the patient to deal with his or her disease and its impact on life. This was seen as an essential responsibility of the nurses, because of the chronic nature of the disease and because preventive care could limit the extent or frequency of the eruptions. One of their most important tasks, according to the nurses, was to help the patient realize that the disease was chronic and that it would not disappear by itself. Rather the patient would have to actively manage the disease in order to minimize its negative impact on his or her life. This was an especially challenging task in relation to young patients. The enabling principle was closely associated with the action strategies summarized in Table 6.3.

Teaching the patient to "read" and interpret the signs and symptoms of the disease were seen as essential tasks, because an adequate response at the appropriate time could limit the development of an outbreak of the disease. Teaching the skills necessary to "read" and interpret the disease was done during the daily interactions between the patient and nurse. The following fieldnote is from the daily morning bath of a young PS patient:

During the skin-care session, the nurse discussed and illustrated to the patient how to differentiate between rashes that required different kinds of treatment. The nurse pointed out areas of rash that required a tar-ointment (elevated rash), rash that required steroid application (flat rash); and rash that no longer required either, but only needed a moisturizer (healed, fading rash). She also had the patient touch the different rash areas in order to learn to "feel" as well as "see" the difference between the different types of rash.

The patients not only needed to learn to interpret their disease and its symptoms, but they also had to learn to initiate treatment measures at home. Nurses took care to teach the patients about what to do once different signs or symptoms were identified and interpreted. The relationship between interpreting the symptoms and the decision about what to do about them is evident in the fieldnote above. Another situation, involving an elderly AD patient, illustrates clearly how the nurses tried to help their patients learn to interpret the signs and symptoms and teach them how and when to initiate the appropriate treatment:

During the morning bath the patient told the nurse that one of the worst things about dermatitis was the awful smell associated with the disease. The nurse responded by emphasizing that it was during periods with infected, suppurating rash that the smell occurred. She underlined that the important thing, therefore, was to prevent or control any infection before it got too bad and the patient developed a body-wide rash. She continued by describing different ways of treating suppurating sores. . . . She also asked what the patient usually did at home, . . . and supported the patient's approach as one acceptable alternative. Finally, she suggested that they sit down together before discharge and write up some alternatives that the patient could try at home should the situation arise.

One important nursing "task" was to help patients learn *how* to implement the necessary treatment measures. That the actual implementation of different treatment measures was not easy and self-evident is clearly demonstrated in the following fieldnote from the same nurse-patient interaction as above:

TABLE 6.3 Nurses' Assumptions About Important Aspects of the Enabling Principle

1. Teach the patient to "read" (recognize) the signs and symptoms of the disease in its different phases.
2. Teach the patient to interpret the signs and symptoms and to decide which measures need to be taken.
3. Teach the patient how to do the actual treatment techniques.
4. Teach the patient about the consequences of different actions (e.g., food selection, environment, sanitation, etc.).
5. Coach the patient to do the necessary actions:
   a. Let the patient practice the skills in the hospital.
   b. Emphasize how to reduce the required effort to bearable levels (demonstrating that the skin care can realistically be done).
   c. Emphasize the consequences of not doing the preventive care.
6. Help the patient to evaluate his life situation (life-style. work situation, etc., in relation to the disease and its management) and support the patient in necessary decision-making.
7. Support the patient in getting used to "exposing" (asserting) him/herself (avoid hiding the disease or isolate self).
8. Help the patient seek meaningful activities to broaden his/her perspective on life and avoid assuming disease unnecessarily restricts life.

> The patient mentioned the use of steroid liniments to the nurse. She told about the last time she was hospitalized; she was discharged with the prescription for a strong steroid cream to use at home. It had had so many warnings written on it, however, that she had not dared to use it: '(Seeing that), I figured it was better to live with the eczema, than die from all those complications.' She illustrated her difficulty understanding the guidelines by commenting on one of the warnings: 'Do not stop abruptly with the treatment!—What does not stopping abruptly mean?' she exclaimed, referring to an earlier experience with steroid tablets. At that time, the dosage had been gradually reduced until she took half a tablet a week. 'Does this mean that one is to apply the cream once a week or what?' she asked.

The interchange clearly underlines the importance of helping patients to implement treatment measures under guidance while in the hospital. The nurses realized this and emphasized the importance of including the patients in daily skin care. Gradually, depending on the patient's willingness and energy, the nurses coached the patient to participate, providing guidance when needed. Again, an interaction during a morning bath may illustrate. The situation involves a young PS patient admitted to the hospital for the first time:

> The nurse asked the patient to apply the cream on those areas that she could reach, whereas she would do the others. The patient expressed reluctance, pointing out that she easily got the cream outside the rash areas. The nurse maintained that it was important that the patient participate, as practicing the application herself would ensure that she would be able to do it properly at home. . . .
>
> As the nurse and patient applied the cream, the nurse emphasized the importance of not getting the strong ointment on healthy skin areas, pointing out a few "burnmarks" where this had accidently happened, and demonstrating a particular technique that would minimize the possibility of touching the normal skin area surrounding the psoriatic spots (circular movements toward the center of the spot, rather than back and forth rubs). . . .
>
> The nurse also underlined the importance of applying ointments and creams systematically, suggesting that the patient finish one area at a time, starting, for example, with one arm, then the other, one leg, then the other, and so on. 'That makes it easier to remember all the rash spots,' she explained. The suggestion came as a response to the patient's unsystematic approach, taking one spot here, one spot there, and being unable to identify which specific spots had been lubricated.

Teaching patients about the consequences of different actions was also seen as an essential task by the nurses. As noted in the preceding quote, the nurse points out to the patient the consequences ("burn marks") of using an inadequate technique in applying the strong liniments.

This nursing strategy also encompassed more general issues. Nurses put great emphasis on exploring with their patients how their job activities, environmental factors, and dietary habits influenced the disease and the ability to control or contain the frequency of outbreaks. The nurses were also aware of the impact of personal relationships and individual coping strategies on the trajectory of the disease, although they seemed more reluctant to bring up these issues, unless the patient specifically mentioned them. Discussing this observation with the nurses, one of them commented:

> I am a little concerned about meddling in things that are none of my business. If the patient is admitted for a skin problem, is it our business to try to find other (psychosocial) problems? I don't think that I would have liked that.

The comment set off a discussion among the nurses about how to balance respect for the patient's privacy with an interest in helping patients deal effectively with their situation and possible associated emotional or psychosocial problems. The nurses admitted to feeling much less equipped to deal with such problems than with the pure bodily skin problems.

Nurses also emphasized the importance of helping patients come to terms with the concealment measures extensively used by many patients. This was done by "making exposure" of the skin a natural thing on the unit. The nurses expressed this expectation by caring for the patients' skin in their rooms rather than in an isolated treatment room. Also, they signaled an attitude of naturalness in regard to skin afflictions and in the way they touched the patients' skin. The following quote from a group interview illustrates this:

> Many patients don't dare to take off their clothes . . . because they have not gotten used to having other people look at them. This is something we try to support them in here. Part of the treatment is to learn in social situations to get used to not being afraid of exposing the rash (thinking:) I have some rash, I know that I have it, and I know I can do something about it, too, but sometimes it shows.

Finally, the nurses' realization that the chronic skin disease could lead to isolation and an excessive focus on the disease and its effects on the person's life led them to express a responsibility for assisting patients to try to step outside self-imposed boundaries. This was attempted by helping the patients explore possible activities to engage in, including hobbies that would take their mind off the disease, as well as possible alternative educational or work-related activities. The nurses also discussed with patients whether participating in such activities together with another skin disease patient might relieve the feelings of being different, which was a frequent reason for self-imposed social isolation. Again, a quote from one nurse illustrates the point:

> We must see if we can motivate patients to reach out, not only sitting at the window to watch what is going on out there, because I think some patients find it difficult to get out among others, and then it becomes a habit. And if you are first into a habit, it is difficult to break out of it, unless there is someone with similar problems, so they can support each other.

The Context of the Nursing Care

It is evident in the nurses' actions and their underlying assumptions and norms in caring for chronic skin disease patients, that the context of the nurses' care was kept within the limits of the hospital setting. The nurses had few interactions with patients outside the hospital setting and had no systematic interaction with their family or friends or primary health care settings, offering specific programs for these patients. It is interesting to note, however, that in understanding the disease and its impact, the nurses relied on a much broader context, that of the daily, significant life of the person and his significant others (partners, colleagues, friends).

DISCUSSION

The findings of this study support the notion that clinical nurses base their practice on practical knowledge about the characteristics of specific diseases and their meanings and implications for patients, and that they hold nursing values, goals, and action strategies based on this understanding.

An essential component of the nurses' implicit practice theory, was their conceptions of the "lived experience of the chronic illness." Their understanding of how chronic disease impacted on patients is in agreement with several reports about living with chronic skin disease

(Ramsay & O'Reagan, 1988; Taylor & Buckwalter, 1988; Updike, 1985) and other chronic illnesses (Benner & Wrubel, 1989; Kleinman, 1981). The nurses linked this understanding to the development of the disease, in that when the lived experience of the disease became burdensome, the disease process worsened. The nurses saw it as a major task to assist the patients in dealing with their experiences of burden or stress associated with the characteristics and consequences of the disease.

A central assumption of this study was that providing a systematic description and interpretation of the nurses' implicit practice theory may assist in reflecting upon, extending or refining the theory and the subsequent practice. It is possible to point to several areas where nurses might consider reflecting upon their practice theory and its application. First, although the nurses realized that the principle of alleviating the burdens was an essential component of caring for severely affected patients, this principle and its associated action strategies were not acknowledged as "good nursing care" in the same way as the enabling strategies. The nurses reported frustrations about not being able to move to enabling strategies within a few days of admission and felt that it was more difficult to invoke the alleviating principle than the enabling principle in explaining or defending their care. Reflecting upon the two caring principles might help nurses appreciate their own insights and consider how best to balance the two principles. Second, the participating nurses used no group teaching and support strategies to realize their enabling principle, despite the fact that they realized that fellow patients represented an important source of support and that the psychosocial aspects of living with the diseases were profound. Research and clinical experience support the value of group support in addition to individual care (Cole, Roth & Sachs, 1988; Logan, 1988; Lombardo, Cave & Bernadina, 1988).

Finally, nurses might consider reflecting upon widening the context of their care to include the context they relied upon to understand patients and their experiences in the home milieu. A major assumption underlying their enabling principle was to prepare patients to minimize the interference of the disease in their lives. A wider context of care could lead to better collaboration with the outpatient clinic and primary care system or to include relatives more systematically in patient-care.

REFERENCES

Argyris, C., Putnam, R., & Smith, D. M. (1985). *Action science.* San Francisco, CA: Jossey-Bass.
Barnum, B. S. (1990). *Nursing theories.* (3rd. eds.). Philadelphia: Lippincott.
Belk, D. (1983). Psoriasis. *Nursing Times,* March 3rd, 49–53.
Benner, P. (1984). From novice to expert. Menlo Park, CA: Addison-Wesley.
Benner, P., & Wrubel, J. (1982). Skilled clinical knowledge: The value of perceptual awareness. *Nursing Educator, 3,* 11–17.
Benner, P., & Wrubel, J. (1989). *The primacy of caring.* Menlo Park, CA: Addison-Wesley.
Biordi, D. L. (1984). The working knowledge of staff nurses: Control of uncertainty. (Doctoral dissertation, Northwestern University, Evanston, Illinois). *Dissertation Abstracts International, 45,* 2275A.
Cole, W. C., Roth, H. L., & Sachs, L. B. (1988). Group psychotherapy as an aid in the medical treatment of eczema. *Journal of the American Academy of Dermatology, 18*(2), 286–91.
Dunn, M. L., Cockerline, E. B., & Rice, M. R. (1988). Treatment options for psoriasis. *American Journal of Nursing, 88,* 8, 1082–87.
Ellis, R. (1969). The practitioner as theorist. *American Journal of Nursing, 69,* 1434–1438.
Ginsburg, I. H. (1989). Feelings of stigmatization in patients with psoriasis. *Journal of American Academy of Dermatology, 20,* 1, 53–63.
Juul Jensen, U. (1988). En teori i hånden er bedre end ti i hovedet. (One theory in the hand is better than ten in the head). *Klinisk sygepleje, 4*(2), 46–48.
Kirkevold, M. (1989). På tide å oppvurdere den praktiske kunnskapen? (Time to upgrade the practical knowledge?) *Sykepleien, 77,* 2, 4–7, 18.
Kirkevold, M. (1990). Practical knowledge embedded in the nursing care provided to stroke patients. Publication series 3/1990, Institute of Nursing Science, University of Oslo.
Kleinman, A. (1981). Comments: On illness meanings and clinical interpretation: Not 'rational man,' but a rational approach to man the sufferer/man the healer. Culture, *Medicine and Psychiatry, 5,* 373–77.
Logan, R. A. (1988). Self help groups for patients with chronic skin diseases. *British Journal of Dermatology, 118,* 505–508.
Lombardo, B., Cave, L. A., & Bernadina, D. (1988). Group support for derm patients. *American Journal of Nursing, 88,* 1088–90.
Polanyi, M. (1962). *Personal knowledge.* Chicago: University of Chicago Press.
Ramsay, B. & O'Reagan, M. (1988). A survey of the social and psychological effects of psoriasis. *British Journal of Dermatology, 118,* 195–201.
Schön, D. A. (1983). *The reflective practitioner.* New York: Basic Books.
Schön, D. A. (1987). *Educating the reflective practitioner.* San Francisco: Jossey-Bass.
Taylor, C. (1977). Interpretation and the sciences of man. In F. Dallmayr & T. McCarthy (Eds.), *Understanding and Social Inquiry.* Notre Dame: University of Notre Dame Press.
Taylor, D. E. & Buckwalter, K. C. (1988). Coping with psoriasis and its consequences. *Archieves of Psychiatric Nursing, 1,* 40–47.

Updike, J. (1985). Personal history. At war with my skin. *The New Yorker*, Sept. 2, 39–40, 43–44, 46, 57.
Wiedenbach. E. (1970). Nurses' wisdom in nursing theory. *American Journal of Nursing*, 70, 5, 1057–62.

Response
Nancy E. White
Judith R. Richter

The description and interpretation by Kirkevold of the practice of caring for patients suffering from chronic skin disease represents an excellent example of theory developed from the practice of nursing and based on nurses embedded knowledge. Although this theory was proposed as a useful tool to extend the clinical practice of experienced nurses caring for patients with chronic skin disease, it certainly could also apply to other chronic conditions.

A historical perspective on the origins of practice theory is useful in appreciating Kirkevold's work. Nightingale (1969) asserted:

> So it is with medicine; the function of an organ becomes obstructed; medicine, so far as we know, assists nature to remove the obstruction, but does nothing more. And what nursing has to do in either case, is to put the patient in the best condition for nature to act upon him. Generally, just the contrary is done. You think fresh air, and quiet and cleanliness extravagant, perhaps dangerous, luxuries, which should be given to the patient only when quite convenient, and medicine the sine qua non, the panacea (p. 133).

The structure of practice theory described by Kirkevold represents a nursing perspective in understanding the phenomenon of chronic skin conditions. Application of this theory would enable the nurse to put the patient in the best condition for nature to act upon him or her.

Stevens (1979) defined theory as "a statement that purports to account for or characterize some phenomenon" (p.1). The components of Kirkevold's practice theory are diagrammed to characterize the model of the phenomenon of living with chronic skin disease, the basic values/goals of caring for chronic skin disease patients and caring strategies. This practice theory clearly exemplifies Stevens' definition.

When describing the "underlying model of phenomenon," Kirkevold referenced Schön (1983, 1987) and Argyris et al. (1985) who demonstrated how practitioners "see" situations differently depending on how they "frame the situation." While this aspect of framing a situation is certainly relevant to Kirkevold's description of her theory, it is important to recognize that there are also universal aspects to her practice theory. For example, nurses throughout the world may hold common assumptions and expectations of the essential characteristics of patients suffering from skin disease.

There have been extensive debates in nursing about the nature of practice theory. For example, Dickoff and James (1968) challenged nurses to invent practice theories and test them against reality. Their set-of-rules approach was criticized by Beckstrand (1980), as difficult to justify and use. She also questioned the value of "practice theory" in nursing. Collins and Fielder (1981) argued that there is a need for practice theory that will integrate knowledge utilized in the practice of nursing and the particular set of moral ideals characterized by nursing practice. In the 1990s, we have moved beyond arguments about the value of practice theory. In fact, the practice model presented by Kirkevold not only describes the characteristics of chronic skin conditions, but also identifies action strategies utilized by expert nurses.

Two important pieces of literature offer further insight into managing chronic conditions. First, the Trajectory Framework developed by Strauss and Associates (Corbin & Strauss, 1988, 1992) provides insights into the complexity of issues and the unending nature of problems facing clients and families of persons experiencing chronic illness. Second, the Psychosocial Typology of Chronic Illness Framework introduced by Rolland (1987) allows for the comparison of similar psychosocial issues between people with different chronic diseases and different issues for people experiencing the same disease.

The trajectory framework has been inductively derived from interviews with patients and family members experiencing a variety of chronic conditions. Corbin and Strauss (1992) propose that the framework is useful for developing models for nursing care. Trajectory denotes the illness course in a general sense, but there are other critical concepts within the trajectory that require consideration. Trajectory phasing, for example, examines the particular subphases within a trajectory in order to understand the possibility for fluctuations in the illness process despite an overall stability in course.

Kirkevold identifies the illness trajectory of atopic dermatitis to consist of periodic exacerbations followed by periods in which the individual is free from the disease. This trajectory clearly differs from that of psoriasis despite the classification of both diseases as "chronic skin diseases." Both diseases may demonstrate subphases such as acute (active illness or complications) or stable (illness symptoms controlled by regimen) however, requiring individual differences in the management plan. Kirkevold recognizes the need to understand illness trajectory as an important feature in developing a model for understanding the experience of living with chronic skin disease. Corbin and Strauss (1992), however, emphasize the need to understand all aspects of the illness trajectory, such as trajectory phasing and subphasing; trajectory management, trajectory scheme, conditions influencing management, trajectory management, biographical and everyday living impact; and reciprocal impact (p. 16).

Similarly, Rolland (1987) introduces the psychosocial typology of illness which permits grouping together different chronic diseases which have similar psychosocial demands. The typology conceptualizes the broad distinction of onset, course, outcome, and degree of incapacitation, each along a continuum. Consideration of the psychosocial illness experience rather than a purely biological perspective allows practitioners to begin to understand the impact of illness on the individual and the family system, both of which are essential to a successful management plan.

Chronic diseases consist of those that have either an acute onset, such as strokes, or gradual onset, such as Parkinson's disease. The course of chronic illness may be progressive (emphysema), constant (spinal cord injury), or relapsing/episodic (lupus). Outcome refers to the initial expectation of the degree to which the disease can shorten one's life span. AIDS is considered to be fatal, lumbosacral disc disease is nonfatal, and emphysema or Type I diabetes are associated with a shortened life span. Incapacitation considers the kind of impairment (cognitive, motor, or social stigma) associated with the disease, the extent of impairment (ranging from none to major), and the timing of the impairment. For example, the impairment of Alzheimer's disease is gradual but inescapable.

Applying this framework to the two skin diseases in Kirkevold's study provides some significant insights. The course of psoriasis may be progressive, constant or episodic, depending on which form of the disease is present. For those experiencing the more progressive form, the issues for patient and family center on a perpetually symptomatic family member whose disability and care needs can be expected to increase in a progressive fashion (Rolland, 1987). Respite from the symptoms and demands of the illness are minimal and place the individual and/or family at significant risk for caregiver exhaustion. A more constant and stable course is characterized by clear cut deficits or limitations that are fairly predictable over time. The reduced uncertainty in this situation enables the family to anticipate and plan for future care needs without disrupting family roles. Relapsing forms of psoriasis are characterized by sudden flareups alternating with more stable periods in which symptoms are absent. This form of the disease is particularly stressful to the family system because of the frequent crisis states caused by the exacerbations and the uncertainty of when it may occur.

Neither disease is fatal or expected to reduce life span. Therefore, anticipatory grief may not be a care issue for either set of patients. The two skin diseases represent a different form of incapacitation and onset which require different approaches to care issues. For example, the severe itching which occurs abruptly in atopic dermatitis represents a sensory form of incapacitation requiring rapid mobilization of management skills and resources for effective resolution. Although both diseases are highly visible, the scaling and flaking associated with psoriasis contributes to greater stigma and social isolation. It is important to recognize that these two examples of chronic skin diseases share important similarities with other categories of chronic diseases and have important differences between them which may require different nursing management plans.

There are several advantages to reviewing Kirkevold's work in the light of the two frameworks described here. First, we begin to categorize diseases in more meaningful ways in order to realize the importance of psychosocial issues attached to the chronic illness experience in addition to the biological needs experienced. Second, these frameworks provide a basis for generalizing and extending Kirkevold's findings and practice recommendations to the care of individuals experiencing a variety of chronic conditions. Coping with long-term disability, shifting roles and responsibilities within the family system, caregiver exhaustion, and living with the stigma of a skin disease become the more salient issues to guide nursing practice and the nursing process.

There are a number of recommendations for studies that would expand Kirkevold's work. This theory is an example of how practical knowledge in specialty areas may be organized in order to communicate it more efficiently. Research that would apply this practice theory to other chronic conditions would be a step toward determining the generalizability of the theory. For example, identifying nursing strategies applicable to a variety of chronic illnesses would facilitate the development of a practice theory for "chronicity."

Another possibility would be comparing this practice theory with other theories of chronic illness. Kirkevold's work exemplifies the theoretical perspective of Corbin and Strauss (1992) and Rolland (1987);

however, Kirkevold's development of action strategies clearly extends the theory into practice. A study that would evaluate the effectiveness of action strategies developed in this practice theory would be invaluable for practicing nurses. For example, alleviating the burdens of managing chronic illness could be compared over time with enabling strategies in a given group of patients to determine benefits to the client. The need for longitudinal studies is more apparent with chronic conditions than with most health care issues.

Kirkevold has identified as the basic values/goals of caring for chronic skin patients the alleviation of suffering/stress and enabling the individual to cope/live with disease. While these are appropriate and essential practice directives, it is important to recognize that patients who experience chronic illnesses do not live in isolation. Rather, they are part of a family system in which the successful management of the disease rests with the entire family rather than the individual. Complex treatment regimens, for example, require the assistance of a spouse or family member. In addition, family roles must often be negotiated and renegotiated in order to meet the changing demands of the illness. Our work with women experiencing diabetes indicated that perceived social support was a significant predictor of successful psychosocial adaptation to chronic illness (White, Richter, & Fry, 1992). Further, we found that poor health status was associated with a decreased perception of support, indicating the possible depletion of resources at times when they may be most critical. Thus, any practice theory associated with chronic illness would benefit from a "family as client" perspective in the development and implementation of care strategies.

REFERENCES

Beckstrand, J. (1980). A critique of several conceptions of practice theory in nursing. *Research in Nursing and Health, 3,* 69–79.

Corbin, J. M., & Strauss, A. L (1988). *Unending work and care.* San Francisco: Josey-Bass Publishers.

Corbin, J. M., & Strauss, A. L. (1992). A nursing model for chronic illness management based upon the trajectory framework. In P. Woog (Ed.). *The chronic illness trajectory framework.* New York: Springer Publishing Company.

Collins, R. J., & Fielder, C. (1981). Beckstrand's concept of practice theory: A critique. Research in *Nursing and Health, 4,* 317–321.

Dickoff, J., & James, P. (1968). A theory of theories: A position paper. *Nursing Research, 17*(5), 197–203.

Nightingale, F. (1969). *Notes on nursing; What it is and what it is not.* New York: Dover Publications, Inc.

Rolland, J. S. (1987). Chronic illness and the life cycle: A conceptual framework. *Family Process, 26,* 203–221.

Stevens, B. (1979). *Nursing Theory.* Boston: Little Brown.

White, N. E., Richter, J. R., & Fry, C. (1992). Coping, social support, and adaptation to chronic illness. *Western Journal of Nursing Research, 14*(2), 211–224.

Chapter 7

Coping Amid Uncertainty: An Illness Trajectory Perspective

Carolyn L. Wiener
Marylin J. Dodd

OVERVIEW

This chapter offers an alternative to the conventional social/psychological definition of "coping." Using a theoretical framework of "illness trajectory," the authors examine the uncertainty of temporality, body, and identity inherent in coping with cancer. Analysis then turns to the interaction among these uncertain conditions and the complex work processes described by people with cancer, as they tolerate, i.e., "cope with," the disease. Although presented separately for purposes of clarity, these processes and their related activities are experienced in varying combinations and with varying and fluctuating importance by each individual. Viewed comprehensively, however, they constitute the larger process of coping with cancer, with implications for other diseases as well.

INTRODUCTION

As defined by Benner and Wrubel (1989, p. 62; see also Pearlin, 1989), "Stress is the experience of the disruption of meanings, understanding

---

Note: Originally published in *Scharly Inquiry for Nursing Practice: An International Journal, Vol.* 7, No. 1 1993.

and smooth function. Coping is what one does about that disruption. Since the goal of coping is the restoration of meaning, coping is not a series of strategies that people choose from a list of unlimited options. Coping is always bounded by the meanings and issues inherent in what counts as stressful" (Benner & Wrubel, 1989, p. 408). An alternative perspective is that "coping, adjustment, and stress are terms that seem to us as either obscuring very complex biographical processes and work processes or as missing many of the interactional and sociological aspects of what is happening during downward trajectory phases" (Corbin & Strauss, 1988, p. 170). In this chapter, we offer a "trajectory perspective," with its emphasis on work processes and their intertwining with interactional and sociological processes, as a way to view coping with a chronic illness. ("Process" is used here not to imply stages but in the sense of change over time.)

Tolerating the uncertainty of living with a chronic illness has long been of interest to social scientists (Comaroff & Maguire, 1981; Davis, F., 1963; Davis,M., 1973; Fox, 1959; Schneider & Conrad, 1983; Wiener, 1975; Weitz, 1989). Studies of the uncertainty surrounding chronic illness cannot avoid the self-evident proposition that all life is uncertain—that living requires coming to terms with uncertainty in much the same manner as described by people who are chronically ill: by developing strategies, balancing options and making choices. Chronically ill people, however, are not only dealing with a universal aspect of the uncertain human condition, but dealing with it in exaggerated form and with severely limited options. Most important, the elements which comprise tolerating the uncertainty appear in different combinations, and uncertainty takes, on varying degrees of significance in different illnesses. Thus, these variables must be tested, lest uncertainty become a facile explanation for all problems inherent in coping with a disease.

Analysis of interviews with families of cancer patients provided such an opportunity. From the reading of these interviews, the most problematic facet of living with cancer emerged. Taken literally as "loss of control," as expressed by respondents, this source of distress could be dismissed as a false sense of certainty in a demonstrably uncertain world. Analyzed sociologically as tolerating the uncertainty, however, the dimensions of their loss of control, the effect it renders, and their responses to it are illuminated. What do they mean by loss of control? Why do they feel they have lost control? How do they deal with the loss? These are the questions addressed in this paper.

SOURCE OF DATA AND METHOD

This report is part of a larger study that used a prospective longitudinal design to sample 100 patients and their families at three time periods, in order to describe family coping and self-care during six months of the chemotherapy experience. Patients had a diagnosis of breast, lung, colo-rectal, gynecologic, or lymphoma cancer and were receiving chemotherapy either for initial treatment or disease recurrence. In order to be eligible for the study, patients had to designate at least one family member who was willing to participate. Family was defined as interacting persons related by ties of marriage, birth, adoption, or other strong social bonds (Department of Family Health Care Nursing, 1981).

In addition to the quantitative component of this study (Dodd, Thomas, & Dibble, 1991; Dodd, Dibble, & Thomas, 1992), a 14-item structured interview, the Problem Centered Family Coping Inventory (PCFCI) (Lewis, Wood & Ellison, 1989) was used at each data collection point, with all participating family members present. These family members remained consistent over time. All family PCFCI interviews were conducted in the family's home and by the same nurse-interviewer. Respondents were asked to "brainstorm" problems or concerns that had occurred for the family in the last month. Using a 6-point Likert scale, respondents were then asked to select the most important problem or challenges they as a family had to deal with; how much it distressed the family; and how satisfied they were with the way the problem/challenge was managed. Interviews were audiotaped and transcribed verbatim onto Ethnograph software. In addition, a nurse-recorder was present at each interview to write down key phrases as a back-up to the audiotape system. A 5-item questionnaire was completed independently by each interviewer and recorder, who reported his/her overall impression of the interview, as well as his/her assessment of the family's willingness to be open, how well the family was managing, and any environmental factors which may have influenced the family's responses. Although the rationale of interviewing at three time periods was to determine shifts in the problems, challenges and activities that occurred over time, major shifts were not discernable. The patients' physical cancer status and the social/psychological consequences of the illness and of treatment (analyzed in this paper) remained central at all three times.

This chapter stems from the discovery by the principal investigator and coauthor (MJD) that significant findings existed in the qualitative data gleaned from the PCFCI. She enlisted the assistance of the primary author (CLW) to plum the data for meanings and interpretations of respondents that would enrich the quantitative findings. The verbatim transcriptions of 100 family interviews (at three time periods) were scrutinized to that end. This provided a unique opportunity to partially adapt an established qualitative methodology, Grounded Theory (Corbin & Strauss, 1990; Glaser, 1978; Glaser & Strauss, 1967; Strauss, 1987; Strauss & Corbin, 1990) to secondary data.

Among the tenets of the Grounded Theory method is that data collection and analysis are interrelated processes. Sampling proceeds on theoretical grounds, in terms of concepts, their dimensions, and variations. Thus, pure Grounded Theory cannot proceed without analytical memos through which concepts are developed, related and tested as part of the research process, guiding the direction of continuing data collection. These requirements cannot be utilized when analyzing secondary data—especially data which have been restricted by structured interview schedules designed with a different goal in mind. Nevertheless, the coding paradigm of Grounded Theory proved to be adaptable to retrospective data and led to the emergence of the core social/psychological process of living with cancer reported by respondents in this study: tolerating the uncertainty that permeates the disease. The method also enhanced the discovery of the dimensions of that uncertainty and of the management processes people employ as they deal with the disease and its consequences. In that regard, this research collaboration is an experiment in re-examining existing data from a perspective that departs from the original intent of the research project and examining the internal consistency of a developed theoretical perspective, that of illness trajectory.

THEORETICAL PERSPECTIVE

A distinction central to this analysis is that drawn between a course of illness and an illness trajectory.[1] The latter is a term borrowed from the physical sciences, used here as a metaphor. In ordinary usage, it signifies the path of a projectile hurtling through space. Just as the speed and direction that launches a missile can be modified in flight by the

---

1. This description of illness trajectory appears in Wiener, C. L. and J. Kayser-Jones, "The uneasy fate of nursing home residents: An organizational-interaction perspective" *Sociology of Health and Illness* 12:84–104.

push and pull of extraneous forces, so can the "natural course" of a disease be altered by the interplay of medical, social, political, economic, biographical, and psychological forces. Trajectory refers not only to the physical unfolding of a disease, but to the *total organization of work done over the course of the disease*—together with the impact that the consequences of the disease and its work exert on the lives of the people involved, namely, patients, family, and health professionals. Included also, in turn, are the reciprocal consequences of this interaction for the work itself.

Stemming originally from the seminal work conducted in the 1960s, which examined the correlative effects of patients, staff and institutional structure on the management of terminal patients (Glaser & Strauss, 1965, 1968), the concept of an illness trajectory was reformulated and expanded through research among the chronically ill (Fagerhaugh & Strauss, 1977; Strauss et al., 1984). Subsequent research identified the types of work which comprise contemporary health care and, most important, highlighted the role of the patient as central worker in his or her own care (Fagerhaugh, Strauss, Suczek & Wiener, 1987; Strauss, Fagerhaugh, Suczek, & Wiener, 1985). "Illness trajectory" has, through these vehicles, come to refer to all of the related work in a course of illness as well as to the impact on the workers—with not only health professionals, but patients and their families (in contradiction to the folk understanding of work) considered as workers (Wiener, 1989). It relates also to the relationship among these workers that then further affects both the management of that course of illness, as well as the fate of the person who is ill.

The value of this theoretical framework is that it focuses on the social context for work, as well as on the social relationships affecting the work (Corbin & Strauss, 1988). Its value for this analysis lies in the understanding that "coping" entails interaction among all of the actors involved in a course of illness, as well as interaction with external micro- and macro-sociological conditions: coping thus is highly variable. Although all of the families in this study were embarked on uncertain trajectories, the degree of uncertainty was affected by: the phase at which the interviews were conducted, the nature of family support, the type of financial resources, the quality of assistance from health professionals, and the extent to which the respondent was experiencing an initial diagnosis or a recurrence. It is important to stress that the interviews are at best a snapshot of frozen time in highly changeable trajectories. Nevertheless, by providing insight into how people manage uncertainty, they offer evidence of the resourcefulness and courage required in the human drama, and they offer health professionals and social scientists an insight into the management processes.

BIOGRAPHIES AND ILLNESS TRAJECTORIES

The initial exploration of the intertwining of biographies and illness trajectories (Wiener, Strauss, Fagerhaugh, & Suczek, 1979), has been more finely honed through subsequent research among chronically ill persons and their spouses (Corbin & Strauss, 1988). Biography is defined as "life course" in the sense of life evolving around a continual stream of experiences resulting in a unique identity. Contrary to the popular misconception that a serious illness is so devastating as to wipe out all other concerns, Corbin and Strauss found (as have other investigators of chronic illness) that the couples they interviewed never spoke only of the illness. Illness was always placed in a biographical context—what had been going on before, what life was like in the past, what hopes and dreams were interrupted or changed.

Biography is understood to consist of "conceptions of self," a self-classification of who one is at a particular point in one's life's course. We form these conceptions as we integrate various aspects of our self into a more inclusive whole. For each aspect of self, various tasks must be performed. For instance, as a health professional, one aspect of oneself, one may assess, monitor, and advise patients, record data or counsel with fellow workers. As a mother, another aspect of oneself, one may give guidance, feed, clothe and nurture one's children. All of these tasks related to various aspects of oneself take place over biographical time, for they are part of one's past, present, and, hopefully, the future. Not only does one's self feel integrated when all of these aspects have been successfully coordinated, but continual performance of the tasks related to these aspects of self requires an appropriately functioning body.

These three interrelated elements—(a) conceptions of self, (b) that evolve over the course of biographical time and (c) arise directly or indirectly through the body—must work together to give structure and continuity to who one is at any point along the biographical time line. An illness throws into disequilibrium the fine adjustment of these three elements that ordinarily work together. As illuminated by the Corbin and Strauss research, when a chronic illness intrudes, it sharply separates the person of the present from the person of the past and affects or even shatters any images of the self held for the future. "Who I was in the past and hoped to be in the future are rendered discontinuous with who I am of the present. New conceptions of who and what I am—past, present, and future—must arise out of what remains" (Corbin & Strauss, 1988, p. 10).

For the cancer patients in this study, these three elements of temporality, body and identity were permeated with uncertainty. Although dependent upon one another, they will be discussed separately.

The Uncertain Temporality

Biological research has confirmed that the highly developed frontal lobe in humans explains their ability to plan for the future, a distinguishing mark from other species. Thus, our perceptions of the present are imbued with expectations of the future, and we regulate our behavior by internalizing memory (Restak, 1988). Relevant here is Mead's (1934) explanation that the future is part of the present insofar as it is considered when the individual makes a selection between lines of action: "Intelligence is essentially the ability to solve the problems of present behavior in terms of its possible future consequences as implicated on the basis of past experience—it involves both memory and foresight" (p.100). In our daily lives, we see what we expect to see and hear what we expect to hear. A familiar example is waking up in a dark hotel room and reaching for a nonexistent glass of water, based upon the memory of the one on the nightstand at home. Thus, there is an interaction, a negotiation, between our expectations and what is really happening (Gevins et al 1989).

One facet of "coping" is facing the disruption of this innate temporal process. This is the message communicated by the most common complaint of respondents in this study: "I feel so out of control." Temporal disjunction, described in the life-cycle literature as "off-timeness" (Neugarten, 1966), is also captured in the distress of the mother of a 20-year-old son with prostate cancer: "It interrupts the family's developmental cycle—children getting cancer and especially prostate cancer is not supposed to happen." Similarly, the anguished question of a 66-year-old man with colo-rectal cancer, "Why did it have to happen to me now, so late in life?" reflects a loss of taken-for-granted expectations that life is like a sonata with three prescribed movements and that we are its orchestrators.

Although loss of this temporal *predictability* is the most recurrent theme in the interviews, other dimensions of uncertainty are related to biographical temporality: *duration* (How long will the illness last? How long will the side effects of treatment last? How long will it be before I feel better?); *pace* (Will the treatment outpace the disease? How long do I have to live? How soon and at what pace will deterioration take place? How soon before a recurrence develops somewhere else in my body?); and, *frequency* (How often must I go for treatment? How frequently will discomfort like nausea be present?).

Time may be *stretched-out,* as for patients who are unhappy about having to curtail work due to fatigue and are impatient with long unstructured hours at home, or as it is for patients who are waiting for a medical report on their status. Time may also be *constricted,* as when the date for another treatment appears to roll around too soon or plans for the future are unmet. Some people cling desperately to old perceptions of *limitless* time, as for instance the father who said, "I can understand how she feels but I think it's just like going to a doctor for a cold—if the medication he gives you doesn't work, he's going to give you something else—it takes time." The meaning of all of these dimensions is in a constant state of flux as conditions affecting the disease or treatment or everyday life change.

The Uncertain Body

When a chronic illness intrudes, the resultant body failure has to do with (a) the body's ability to perform an activity; (b) the body's appearance, that is, not only the way one looks to oneself and others, but the appearance of actions, what one and others *think* of what one does; and (c) the body's physiological functioning (Corbin & Strauss, 1988). For the patients interviewed in this study, uncertainty not only pervades these three elements of body failure but the body's response to treatment as well.

A shaken faith in the taken-for-granted body emerged frequently in the interviews. Although divided here into present and future concerns for purposes of clarity, these dimensions co-mingle and fade in and out of the picture depending upon imminent conditions. One present concern is with interpretation of bodily signs, based upon comparisons with the past. The interviews are permeated with self-recriminatory "I-used-to" reviews. Yet, typical of the ambiguity surrounding reading body signs is the following comment by a respondent:

> I have finally learned at the age of 49 and a half that I cannot work. This problem and my other physical fatigue thing which should be over by now, or is this middle-age, or is this something else, or is this leftover chemo or whatever?

This confusion was followed a few minutes later with further doubt as to the origin of her fatigue, "Granted we've been out almost every night this week." One woman told of her indecision over reporting a redness in the area of her intravenous treatment and of ignoring it, adding wryly, "I'm still alive." Her sister reminded her that she was told later that it should have been reported. The patient complained, "I was concerned about what am I supposed to tell them at Stanford and what am I supposed to ignore, and what's being silly and what's not being silly." Often the uncertainty centered on a new bodily symptom, e.g., "You always worry it will turn into cancer—I'm getting paranoid about aches and pains." Nor does the completion of treatment bring a return to normal nonchalance over bodily signs. As expressed by one patient at the end of chemotherapy, "I can spend my life with, 'what is this pain? what does it mean?' But that is constantly with me." Members of one family, all present at the interview, kept admonishing the patient to write down all of her complaints over her treatments, her spouse saying, "She forgets everything now, a lot." Unspoken was the implication of the roots of her faulty memory: was it stress? the disease? the medication?

Another present concern has to do with *what is being done to the body by others*. Many respondents expressed fear over what was happening to their veins, one adding that her worry included possible loss of the use of her arm. These fears were often coupled with criticism of the way the body had been handled by health professionals or with the general resentment over the assault on the body, e.g., "That's what they've pretty well done to me, right, is take my body and wear it out." While paramount in these patients' minds, these accusations still contain an element of doubt as to cause and effect.

A third present concern is that *the body's resistance has been jeopardized*. Some patients are ever mindful of their own responsibility to lessen the intrusion of further complications on their already failed bodies by avoiding crowds or persons with infections. Although these precautions are to some degree a means for maintaining control over the body, they bear within them the seeds of uncertainty for they are difficult to maintain if one is to proceed with normal living.

Future time concerns of duration and pace, when translated into body-failure dimensions, center on concern over the *efficacy of treatment*, "What's going to happen if the pills and the shots aren't working?," *the risk inherent in treatment*, "The chemo is the scariest; it goes after the good guys as well as the bad guys," and *recurrence of the disease*, "Every once in a while, I get scared and think, 'what if I get it again?' since there's a slight chance of getting other types of cancer because of the chemo and the radiation."

It is important to stress that the uncertainty of all of these dimensions is heightened by a central property of the disease itself—the unreliability of symptoms for the self-assessment of a disease characterized as "the silent killer." Most often, people with cancer have learned from the initial diagnosis that while they were symptom free, the disease was insidiously progressing. This becomes the ultimate tyranny of the uncertainty of reading signs of body failure.

The Uncertain Identity

As explained above, identity—conceptions of self, arising directly or indirectly through the body, as they evolve over the course of biographical time—must be in accord for there to be substance and constancy to who one feels one "is." Thus, the skewed temporality and failed body which inundate the cancer patient also deliver a blow to the patient's conceptions of self, making him or her feel that, as one patient put it, "The world is unraveling." The woman previously described, who had difficulty distinguishing which symptoms were "silly" and which should be reported, gave other dramatic testimony to the effect of the illness on her identity:

> About a month or 3 weeks ago, I was really wondering what this cancer really is and what was going to happen. Was it really going to go away? Did I really have it? Just a whole realization that . . . gee, is it really there? I saw Dr. W and I said to him, 'I really don't feel like there's anything wrong with me.' And he said, 'You are really sick, you have a disease that may kill you.' He just hit me square between the eyes . . . it's like, intellectually I believed it was real but emotionally I thought this isn't for real, this is some funny kind of game.

Urged by her sister to tell the physician of her intolerable fatigue, the patient said, "For a life-long time I go to the doctor's office and say, 'I'm fine, I feel great.' I'm learning that's not a good way to be but it's very hard to overcome that pattern." Her sister, after expressing her own uncertainty in interpreting bodily signs and her frustration over the patient's stubborn adherence to a previous identity, joked, "I told her last night, 'It's okay, we'll put that on her tombstone: She wasn't a hypochondriac!'"

Charmaz (1987) has delineated a hierarchy to characterize the way that ill people, over time, choose different types of preferred identities. One of these is the "contingent personal identity," which she describes as one people aim for when they believe that their hopes, aspirations and plans are fragile and tentative. "These individuals have already scaled down their hopes because they define so much uncertainty" (Charmaz, 1987, p. 308). The patients in this study, however, caught during the process of treatment, do not portray a sense of having either scaled down their hopes or of having chosen a preferred identity. Rather, they have had the uncertain identity thrust upon them. Furthermore, the trajectory framework underscores that *all* is contingent, that among the chronically ill, the interplay between mind, body, work, and behavior in always temporary and fluctuating.

IDENTITY AND WORK PROCESSES

Illness-related, Everyday-life, and Biographical Work

The trajectory framework, by emphasizing the organization of work that includes all actors—patients, kin, and health professionals—sheds light on the effect of this work on identity. In this study, patients and their families were performing tasks related to the various aspects of their conceptions of self, all part of what Corbin and Strauss (1988) have identified as three lines of trajectory work. *Illness-related work* consists of regimen work, crisis prevention and handling, symptom management, and diagnostic related work. *Everyday-life work* encompasses the daily round of tasks that help keep a household going: housekeeping and repairing, occupational work, marital work, child rearing, recreation, and activities such as eating. Associated with each type of work is *biographical work*, i.e., interactions with spouse or significant other, children, friends, health professionals, and others, in the gathering and dispersing of information, expressions of concern, caring or anger, and the division of tasks.

The performance of any one of these types of work can affect the performance of the other two. In addition, unforeseen contingencies affect all three of them. "Coping" consists of juggling all of these types of work amid emerging contingencies, while keeping some balance between illness management, biography, and everyday life. Most important, the balance is one of relative equilibrium with the weight shifting more toward one type or the other, (depending upon the illness, biography or everyday-life circumstances that are in play) (Corbin & Strauss, 1988, p.125).

The balance may differ for various actors in the trajectory. One mother made a wise observation about her children's reaction to their brother's cancer: "I think one of the biggest stresses in families is when they feel they have to go through it together. People have to be allowed to process it in their own way." In another case, the patient was focused on treatment while her adult children, brought together to care for her, were dealing with the day-to-day integration of their preferences and family conflicts. Or the family's focus on illness-related work may threaten the patient's biographical work. One patient spoke at length of the abundance of attention he was receiving from his sister and her family, who had taken him in:

> I can't even go at night to get water. Look up, here she's coming with this silver pitcher wrapped with a towel with ice cubes.... I don't want them altering their lives because of me.

Said another, of his friend's solicitude, "Before she was a lovely lady. Now she's my mommy."

Sometimes, despite the constant demands of illness-related work, the scale was tipped in favor of everyday-life work. One man, for example, although dealing with a succession of therapy-related discomforts, was nonetheless deflected from concern over these by the needs of his 93-year-old mother, who was blind and failing mentally. The focus of a woman patient on her own illness shifted suddenly at the time of her third interview. Asked about the problems she had dealt with during the past month, she forgot about losing her eyebrows and eyelashes and "peripheral issues dealing with chemotherapy" until reminded of these by her husband. Instead, she talked of a friend with renal cancer who had taken a turn for the worse and whose children the respondent was trying to help. Quite often, illness-related work crowded out the other two lines of work, illustrated by the husband who said of the patient's impending series of radiation treatments, "The more medically involved she is, the more she has cancer, and the less medically involved she is, the healthier she is." The tension between the three lines of work and the resultant undermined identity was most evident among those whose deteriorated physical condition had interrupted the taken-for-granted occupational schedule.

Shifts in identity, expressed as temporary "giving up" of past conceptions of self, are a consequence of unequal balance of the three lines of work—for example, the mother who found she was too weak to attend her son's baseball games, who worried over having to relinquish the household chores and the care of the children to her husband. Another respondent, the former naval officer, who by his own testimony always expected everything done by his crew to be "perfect," lamented, "I'd rather do the whole job by myself so it's kind of hard for me to discover that I can't go out and wash my car." One friend said of the patient's extended family (after a catalogue of complaints about their changed interaction), "We want there to be times to just have fun—this has always been an important part of our family unit."

Ultimately, the illness experience is transforming. As sociologist Arthur Frank (1991) has written out of personal knowledge, it "leaves no aspect of life untouched . . . Your relationships, your work, your sense of who you are and who you might become, your sense of what life is and ought to be—these all change, and the change is terrifying" (p. 6).

Uncertainty Abatement Work

To reduce the terror, and maintain a semblance of control over their lives, respondents in this study engaged in a fourth type of work: activities adopted to lessen the impact of the uncertainty of time, body, and identity. What we have called uncertainty abatement work becomes a means of defining and redefining the illness and one's changed identity. These activities take on different meaning not only for each patient but for each family member depending on the circumstances and sources of stress of the moment. Highly changeable as to appropriateness, they nevertheless provide an insight into how people manage their lives as normally an possible in the face of a disease as uncertain as cancer. Although discussed separately here, they may be employed in varying combinations and configurations.

1. Pacing

Patients spoke of modifying, cutting back or cutting out certain activities, of resting before and after routine activities. This entailed getting others to understand, i.e., "when I say I don't want to go somewhere they think it's negative, but I'm learning my limits" as well as getting oneself to accept the changed identity, i.e., "I felt like I couldn't work physically but mentally I felt like I would be a quitter."

2. Becoming Professional Patients

Patients and their significant others became mini-experts, rattling off four-syllable drug names with ease, reporting on their "counts" to the last digit, and speaking of "pleural effusions" and "lesions." They said they had learned to ask a particular nurse to administer chemotherapy to avoid someone "fiddling with the vein." Some tried to maintain a balance between expertise and super-medicalization, as for instance the women with lymphoma who said, "I try to learn as much as I can without going overboard."

3. Seeking Reinforcing Comparisons

Patients and family members lessened their own anguish by finding "worse-case" comparisons among others, for example a friend who had eight hours of chemotherapy in the spine. One man recalled that "The guy that I had been watching for almost all of my chemotherapy, who was able to walk in, is no longer able to, and I thought to myself, 'you've got nothing to bitch about.'" A young woman who was experiencing problems with morale and temperament, placing an admitted strain on her marriage, said, "Lots of people split up. The beautician who fitted me for a wig told me, 'you're lucky your husband hasn't left you.'" Although reassuring, these comparisons obviously contain an element of dread, evoking mixed feelings in the patient.

4. Engaging in Reviews

Some of the reviews consisted of looking back on the onset of symptoms and giving meaning to them in light of present knowledge. In some cases, the review included self-blame, revealing how theories about the mind/body relationship have sometimes filtered down to the lay public in their crudest form. Thus did a women with recurrent breast cancer say, "If I were more relaxed the body would be more relaxed too. Stress caused this to come up again." Some reviews, far from being consoling, merely exacerbated the uncertainty. One spouse struggled with causation in her remarks to the patient: "The seizure perhaps was activated by your weakness, your state of physical condition from your chemo, the temperature of the day," adding to the interviewer, "I felt responsible for taking him out." Also emerging frequently from the data were treatment reviews which focused on anger with health professionals, most often for not being listened to or for the absence of sentimental work (Strauss, Fagerhaugh, Suczek & Wiener, 1982).

5. Setting Goals

Not everyone was as explicit as the woman who said, "I can keep stretching this out, control it by setting another goal. I'd like to hang on until the one daughter I have who is unmarried gets married. Every year it's a new bride, a new baby, a new christening." Other examples of goal setting, however, such as a return home after completion of the treatment course, a trip to Europe, resuming an education, recur in the data.

6. Covering Up

As already noted, there are numerous references to avoiding the hypochondriac label. Patients also spoke of not wanting to make others feel bad, not crying in front of others, "not being a baby." They had gotten messages that they have to cover up more for some people than for others. One young women said, "Word was out through the family grapevine that my Dad was really down. I'll stop telling people if I think it too painful for them." Another found it hard to tell her friends she had cancer: "I didn't want people to feel sorry or talk about me. To be a cancer patient is embarrassing and humiliating because of the stigma."

7. Finding a Safe Place to Let Down

Covering-up necessitates an outlet, a safe place to let down. The woman who was concerned about stigma was also having trouble sharing with her husband her distress over physical and mental changes. Discovering that "I don't get to weep with my husband," she said she went to the clinic to cry, finding it a "safe sanctuary" and adding, "I felt better to cry around people who knew about this than around people who do not know."

8. Choosing a Supportive Network

Patients and family members were selective about sharing information concerning the problems that had occurred during treatment. Said one, about her decision not to tell her family, "They could only offer negative support and I couldn't handle that right now." Patients found they had preferred tenders—a sister who gave more emotional support than a spouse, one friend preferred over another.

9. Taking Charge

The form this action takes is a defiance of the health professionals, an assertion of the right to refuse all or part of the prescribed treatment. One woman reported she had challenged the doctor's order that she go every week for a blood test: "I said, no, the veins I have I save for chemo—when it's time for my chemo then I'll go and get my blood test." Some patients weighed the benefits against the side effects and opted out of treatment altogether.

DISCUSSION

The people interviewed in this study showed remarkable fortitude and resilience, demonstrable of the observation attributed (possibly apocrophally) to Ernest Hemingway, "everyone is broken by life, but some people become stronger in the broken places." For health researchers, their stories offer an opportunity to test the validity of the illness trajectory framework in regard to cancer patients. Further research could enlarge the scope of this framework and its relationship to uncertainty by theoretical sampling under different conditions, for example, in another culture, or among patients with other chronic illnesses for whom uncertainty takes on varying degrees of significance.

For other health professionals, the insight provided by these interviews can be utilized to facilitate a less troubled trajectory course for some patients and their families. Not only is there a need for health professionals to understand the myriad dimensions of trajectory-related uncertainty connected with cancer—and the work processes that constitute "coping"—but they, too, must be clear about how cancer differs from and how it resembles the uncertainty of other chronic diseases. Cancer trajectories differ from those of rheumatoid arthritis, for instance, by being potentially fatal and because of the historical meanings attached to cancer over time, as curse, punishment and embarrassment (Sontag, 1978). At the same time, as suggested by the respondent quoted above, cancer shares with other fatal chronic illnesses the fallout from that segment of the self-help world which has bought into the belief that there is a relationship between our personality and the diseases we get. Ignatieff (1988), in a thoughtful review of a number of works which deal with this subject, praises Susan Sontag for underscoring the accusatory side of seeking to enlist the patient's will to resist disease. He suggests that there in an obvious affinity between a philosophy that says that patients can cure themselves and an American cultural credo that insists that the individual is master of his or her destiny. He warns, however, that:

> The moral approval that we vest in the idea of struggle may burden the suffering patient with expectations beyond his forces. As soon as we understand a patient's experience as a struggle, we can evaluate whether he is struggling hard enough, and we can begin to treat him as if we were coaches on some exhausted runner, shouting encouragements that ignore his diminishing resources (p. 32).

Ignatieff suggests that we need to learn an ethic of ironical struggle, one that appreciates that we go into the battle against illnesses as underdogs. Citing Montaigne's equanimity about his fatal kidney condition, he says the French writer took illness as his teacher, and in becoming its student, he became its master.

Chronic illness, as John Lennon said of "life," is what happens when you're busy making plans. The uncertainty surrounding a chronic illness like cancer is the uncertainty of life writ large. By listening to those who are tolerating this exaggerated uncertainty, we can learn much about the trajectory of living.

REFERENCES

Benner, P., & Wrubel, J. (1989). *The primacy of caring.* Menlo Park, CA: Addison-Wesley.

Charmaz, K. (1987). Struggling for a self: Identity levels of the chronically ill. In P. Conrad & J. Roth (Eds). *Research in the sociology of health care* (pp. 283–321). Greenwich, CT: JAI Press.

Comaroff, J. & Maguire, P. (1981). Ambiguity and the search for meaning:

Childhood leukemia in the modern clinical context. *Social Science and Medicine, 15B*, 115–23.
Corbin, J., & Strauss, A. (1988). *Unending work and care.* San Francisco: Jossey Bass.
Corbin, J., & Strauss, A. (1990). Grounded theory: Procedures, canons and evaluative criteria. *Qualitative Sociology, 13*, 3–21.
Davis, F. (1963). *Passage through crisis.* Indianapolis: Bobbs-Merrill.
Davis, M. (1973). *Living with multiple sclerosis.* Springfield, Il: Charles C. Thomas.
Department of Family Health Care Nursing, University of California, San Francisco. Definition of Family. Published in Mission statement, Fall, 1981.
Dodd, M., Dibble, S., & Thomas, M. (1992a). Outpatient chemotherapy: Patients' and family members' concerns and coping strategies. *Public Health Nursing, 1*, 37–44.
Dodd, Thomas, M., & Dibble, S. (1991b). Self care for patients experiencing cancer chemotherapy side effects: A concern for home care nurses. *Home Healthcare, 9*, 21–26.
Fagerhaugh, S., & Strauss, A. (1977). *Politics of pain management.* Menlo Park, CA: Addison-Wesley.
Fagerhaugh, S., Strauss, A., Suczek, B., & Wiener, C. (1987). *Hazards in hospital care.* San Francisco: Jossey Bass.
Fox, R. (1959). *Experiment perilous.* New York: The Free Press.
Frank, A. (1991). *At the will of the body.* Boston: Houghton Aldine.
Gevins, A., Morgan, N., Bressler, S., Cutello, B., White, R., Illes, J., Greer, D., Doyle, S., & Zeitlin, G. (1987). Human neuroelectre patterns predict performance accuracy, *Science, 235*, 550–585.
Glaser, B. (1978). *Theoretical sensitivity.* Mill Valley, CA: Sociology Press.
Glazer, B., & Strauss, A. (1965). *Awareness of dying.* Chicago: Aldine.
Glazer, B., & Strauss, A. (1967). *The discovery of grounded theory.* Chicago: Aldine.
Glazer, B., & Strauss, A. (1968). *Time for dying.* Chicago: Aldine.
Ignatieff, M. (1988). Modern dying. *The New Republic, 199*, 28–33.
Lewis, F., Wood, H., & Ellison, E., (1989). Family impact study: The impact of cancer on the family. Unpublished preliminary analysis report.
Mead, G. (1934). *Mind, self and society.* Chicago: University of Chicago Press.
Neugarten, B. (1968). Adult personality: Toward a psychology of the life cycle. In B. Neugarten (Ed.), *Middle age and aging* (pp. 137–47). Chicago: University of Chicago Press.
Pearlin, L. (1989). The sociological study of stress. *Journal of Health and Social Behavior, 30*, 241–56.
Restak, R. (1988). *The mind.* Toronto: Bantam Books.
Roth, J. 1963. *Timetables.* Indianapolis: Bobbs-Merrill.
Schneider, J., & Conrad, P. (1983). *Having epilepsy: The experience and control of illness.* Philadelphia: Temple University Press.
Sontag, S. (1978). *Illness as metaphor.* New York: Farrar, Straus & Giroux.
Strauss, A. (1987). *Qualitative analysis for social scientists.* Cambridge: Cambridge University Press.
Strauss, A., & Corbin, J. (1990). *Basics of qualitative research.* Newbury Park, CA: Sage.
Strauss, A., Corbin, J., Fagerhaugh, S., Glaser, B., Maines, D., Suczek, B., et al. (1984). *Chronic illness and the quality of life.* Second Edition. St. Louis: C.V. Mosby.

Strauss, A., Fagerhaugh, S., Suczek, B., & Wiener, C. (1982). Sentimental work in the technologized hospital. *Sociology of Health and Illness, 4,* 254–278.

Strauss, A., Fagerhaugh, S., Suczek, B. & Wiener, C. (1987). *Social organization of medical work.* Chicago: University of Chicago Press.

Weitz, R. (1989). Uncertainty and the lives of persons with AIDS. *Journal of Health and Social Behavior, 30,* 270–81.

Wiener, C. (1975). The burden of rheumatoid arthritis: Tolerating the uncertainty. *Social Science and Medicine, 9,* 97–104.

Wiener, C. (1989). Untrained, unpaid and unacknowledged: The patient as worker. *Arthritis Care and Research, 2,* 16–21.

Wiener, C., Strauss, A., Fagerhaugh, S., & Suczek, B. (1979). Trajectories, biographies and the evolving medical technology scene. *Sociology of Health and Illness 1,* 261–283.

Wiener, C., & Kayser-Jones, J. (1990). The uneasy fate of nursing home residents. *Sociology of Health and Illness 12,* 84–104.

Acknowledgements. This research was supported by a grant from the National Center for Nursing Research (RO1 NRO1441).

Response
Marilyn T. Oberst

Coping with chronic illness, particularly cancer, has been the subject of numerous studies by investigators from many disciplines. In the majority of such studies reported in the last few decades, investigators have attempted to identify the specific coping behaviors employed, usually selected from a long list of options, and to link them to outcomes. While much has been learned from this work about the nature of illness-related stress and how people manage it, there are problems with both the method and the assumptions that limit its clinical usefulness.

A major problem in the study of coping with illness, and one which Weiner and Dodd point out, is the implicit assumption in the "strategy list" approach to measuring coping that all options are possible for any individual, in any situation when, in fact, one's options may be severely limited. A second problem arises from the multiple and often competing demands of illness and the fact that standard coping measures, even when respondents are asked to specify a particular problem as their response context, probably reflect multiple contexts. Once these multiple contexts are acknowledged, it becomes clear that summary measures, averaged *across* these contexts, will obscure coping efforts, rather than illuminate them; the problem here is that the sum tells us less than would examination of the parts. A final problem relevant to Weiner and Dodd's work lies in the evolution of what Benner & Wrubel (1989, pp. 272–274) have described as a normative model in which coping behaviors have come to be labeled as either "good" or "bad," irrespective of context.

The research reported by Weiner and Dodd, grounded in the sociological perspective of trajectory, represents a less usual approach to the examination of coping with illness. The authors are to be congratulated for being willing to apply the analytic method of one research paradigm to data collected in another, despite the obvious limitations in sampling and data collection that they point out. Part of what made this a viable approach in this particular instance was the massive data set consisting of some 300 family interviews; although they do not say so, the sheer volume of data likely allowed them to sample these data in a way that at least partially resembles the theoretical sampling approach usually associated with grounded theory.

The authors indicate at the outset that loss of control was the greatest source of distress, and appear to equate loss of control with uncertainty.

Conceptually, I find this the most problematic aspect of the paper. That uncertainty should be a major theme for cancer patients is not surprising; it has been well documented in the literature (e.g., Mishel, 1988, 1990) and is a finding that makes sense at an intuitive level. Similarly, loss of control is cited frequently as a problem for ill persons. My difficulty is with the assumption that there is uncertainty imbedded in all levels and kinds of problems with control.

The reported data do not always clearly confirm the presumed control-uncertainty link. For instance, a patient is quoted as saying that health professionals had taken her body and worn it out; while certainly reflecting loss of control over her own body, there may not be sufficient evidence for concluding that this accusation contains "an element of doubt as to cause and effect." Similarly, a spouse's observation about his wife that "she forgets everything" is said to carry an implication of uncertainty about cause; again, although this is a plausible interpretation, there could be alternate interpretations.

I think it is useful to clarify which of the authors' conclusions confirm prior findings and which represent new insights. Interestingly, although problems with both control and uncertainty are readily apparent in the work of other grounded theorists who focus on chronic illness (e.g., Corbin & Strauss, 1988), neither construct has been previously suggested as a central theme. Thus, by placing the elements of biographical time, body, and identity in a overarching frame of uncertainty, Weiner and Dodd present a somewhat different grounded perspective on coping with chronic illness trajectories.

Weiner and Dodd briefly review the three lines of trajectory work previously identified by Corbin and Strauss (1988), and provide some evidence that each type of work—illness-related, everyday, and biographical work—was present in this sample. In addition, they report the presence of a fourth type of work that they label "uncertainty abatement work," and it is this interpretation that makes their work seem unique. Each of the eight coping activities subsumed under uncertainty abatement is said to be a means of maintaining some semblance of control and most, indeed, could be interpreted in that way. It is less clear, however, that this group of strategies represents a type of work that is distinctly different from the three lines of work previously identified; certainly all eight could be categorized as fitting within at least one of the existing categories using the original definitions of Corbin and Strauss.

Inherent in the label "uncertainty abatement work" is an underlying premise that uncertainty and/or lack of control is always negative, something that must be relieved in order to "reduce the terror." This premise may be incorrect. One issue is that some things may not be controllable or perceived to be controllable precisely because they *are* certain; impending death, for instance, is a certainty that is not in the individual's control. Similarly, uncertainty may, in some situations, be preferable to certainty and, as Mishel (1990) has suggested, persons may act to "maintain the illusion" of uncertainty. Brown and Powell-Cope (1991) offer poignant examples of AIDS family caregivers' experiences and suggest that, while uncertainty is a pervasive and common social-psychological problem they all face, acceptance of some uncertainties may be the most productive way of coping. Similarly, Mishel's (Mishel & Sorenson, 1991) findings suggest that the efficacy of mastery (i.e., control) in mediating the effects of uncertainty on emotional distress is situation-specific, and depends largely on how the uncertainty is interpreted by the individual.

The data presented by Wiener and Dodd offer interesting insights about how families with cancer cope during periods of active treatment and, to a lesser extent, the personal interpretive context that motivates various coping strategies. The potential dangers inherent in a pervasive need for control are apparent in some of these data, a fact the authors allude to several times. Perhaps the most critical need in future research is to begin to sort out the work involved in *tolerating* uncertainty from that intended to *abate* or lessen it and to determine if gaining control or mastery in one sphere of activity affects the tolerance of uncertainty in other spheres. Only then can we begin to think about developing interventions that are supportive of coping efforts.

REFERENCES

Benner, P., & Wrubel, J. (1989). *The primacy of caring: Stress and coping in health and illness.* Menlo Park, CA: Addison-Wesley.

Brown, M. A., & Powell-Cope, G. M. (1991). AIDS family caregiving: Transitions through uncertainty. *Nursing Research, 40,* 338–345.

Corbin, J. M., & Strauss, A. (1988). *Unending work and care: Managing chronic illness at home.* San Francisco: Jossey-Bass.

Mishel, M. H. (1988). Uncertainty in illness. *Image, 20,* 225–232.

Mishel, M. H. (1990). Reconceptualization of the uncertainty in illness theory. *Image, 22,* 256–262.

Mishel, M. H., & Sorenson, D. S. (1991). Uncertainty in gynecological cancer: A test of the mediating functions of mastery and coping. *Nursing Research, 40,* 167–171.

Chapter 8

Chronic Sorrow: A Lifespan Concept

Carolyn L. Lindgren
Mary L. Burke
Margaret A. Hainsworth
Georgene G. Eakes

OVERVIEW

Losses are an integral part of chronic illness and disability. The term chronic sorrow, has been used to describe the long-term periodic sadness the chronically ill and their caregivers experience in reaction to continual losses. In this conceptual analysis of chronic sorrow, identified critical attributes are: cyclic sadness over time in a situation with no predictable end; external and internal stimuli triggering the feelings of loss, disappointment, and fear; and, progression and intensification of the sadness or sorrow years after the initial disappointment or loss. Model, borderline, related, contrary, and illegitimate cases illustrate what the concept is and what it is not. The meaning of chronic sorrow is compared to the meaning of unresolvable grief and depression. Chronic sorrow in various stages of life is illustrated in descriptions of: the situation and feelings of parents of handicapped children; multiple sclerosis patients in the middle, productive years; and elderly caregivers of spouses with dementia. Implications for research include the need

Note: Originally published in *Scholarly Inquiry for Nursing Practice: An International Journal,* Vol. 6, No. 1, 1992. New York: Springer Publishing Company.

to study the concept in various populations to determine its prevalence and operation. Through research, the meaning of the concept can be further clarified. This is a beginning step toward developing nursing theory that will give direction for providing care to persons encountering sadness over long periods of time.

INTRODUCTION

Confrontation of loss is a continual experience for chronically ill or disabled persons and family members who care for them. They may experience significant psychological distress from the sense of loss, and this distress in turn may serve as an obstacle to well-being and a potential threat to health.

The label "chronic sorrow" has been used to represent the emotional pain associated with the losses and disappointments of long-term illness and disability. The term was originally used to describe the feelings of parents of disabled or retarded children. They reported experiencing a recurrent sense of loss or sadness triggered by events such as the child's inability to walk at a normal age or start school with the other children (Burke, 1989; Wikler, Wasow, & Hatfield, 1981). The expressions of persons in other chronic illness situations, however, suggest that chronic sorrow is not limited to parents of handicapped children. Adjustment to negative events and losses is an identified task in any illness or disability (Stone, 1979, p. 233). Specific knowledge is needed of what chronic sorrow is and how it operates in persons across the lifespan.

Clarifying and establishing the meaning of chronic sorrow is fundamental to using the concept for nursing theory development and research, and to its pragmatic application in clinical practice. This chapter, therefore, presents a classic analysis of the concept, following the steps described by Walker and Avant (1983). As a basis for formulating research problems to test the utility of the concept, the analysis concludes with a discussion of what is known and not known in chronic sorrow as it operates in the lives of persons across the lifespan and in a variety of situations (Walker & Avant, 1983).

Dictionary and thesaurus definitions of chronic sorrow provide a beginning sense of the scope and characteristics of the concept. Webster (1983) defines sorrow as mental suffering caused by loss or disappointment, and expressed as mourning or lamentation. Synonyms are grief, affliction, sadness, regret, and lamentation. According to Webster (1983), grief is intense emotional suffering caused by loss, misfortune, injury, or evils of any kind; thus, the terms grief and sorrow are comparable. Each of the other synonyms for sorrow depicts a particular aspect of sorrow. Affliction connotes a weight or burden, cross, load, oppression, encumbrance, albatross around one's neck, a millstone (Roget, 1977). From this perspective, sorrow may be viewed as a heaviness or weight which the person does not have the strength or resources to move or lift. Synonyms for sadness are heaviness, heavyheartedness, and pathos (Roget, 1977). Thus sadness describes the emotions of sorrow. Regret implies grief, sorriness, or repining because of the loss of what was, or what was expected and did not occur (Roget, 1977). Lamentation describes the processes of mourning, grieving, and sorrowing and implies particular behaviors or expressions seen in persons in sorrow (Roget, 1977). The grieving process is the changing emotional reactions over time (Osterweis, Solomon, & Green, 1984). The distress or mental suffering that is a part of sorrow is seen in synonyms such as fretting, eating one's heart out, agony, ache, and joylessness and depressing feelings.

The term chronic may be defined as that which is perpetual, habitual, constant, continuing a long time, or persistent. When the term chronic is attached to sorrow, the sadness, regret, affliction, and lamentation that are a part of sorrow seem more oppressive. This sadness does not abate. Analysis of the experiences of persons who have reported these feelings brings further understanding of the nature of chronic sorrow.

INITIAL DEVELOPMENT OF THE CONCEPT

The historical perspective of the concept illustrates its progressive development. Olshansky (1962) first used the term chronic sorrow to describe the suffering of parents caring for a mentally defective child. Olshansky described this phenomenon as a pervasive psychological reaction. He contended that all parents of mentally retarded children probably experienced it to some degree throughout their lives as a reaction to the loss of the expectations they had for the child and to the child's ever present dependency. Based on his clinical experience as a counselor to parents of handicapped children, he concluded that chronic sorrow was a natural response to a tragic situation.

Searl (1978), a parent of a retarded child and a psychologist, confirmed Olshansky's view of the long-term suffering of parents such as himself. Searl described chronic sorrow vividly as shock, guilt, and bitterness that never disappear from the parent's emotional life. He spoke out against the notion that parents ever fully resolve or adjust to these feelings.

In 1981, Wikler, Wasow, and Hatfield conducted the first study of chronic sorrow to explore the pattern of grief experienced by parents of retarded children. In their descriptive, survey study, a selection of linear graphs depicting patterns of grief over time were included in the study questionnaire to describe the course of the parent's grief. They found that both parents and social workers perceived the parent's grief patterns as continual ups and downs. Parents reported that the later developmental years of the child were as painful as, if not more painful than, the early years, supporting the presence of chronic sorrow in their lives. The significance of this study was its documentation of the periodicity and progressivity of chronic sorrow in parents of the mentally retarded.

In a follow-up study, Vines (1986) described the feelings of fear, sadness, guilt, nervousness, anger, and helplessness experienced by parents of mentally retarded and/or physically disabled adolescents. Vines' study also supported the periodicity of the parent's feelings. Parents reported a resurgence of these feelings at developmental milestones which the child could not pass. The feelings were stronger among parents of the mentally retarded than among parents of physically disabled children. Vines labeled the phenomenon "regrief" rather than chronic sorrow.

Chronic sorrow was also documented by Fraley (1986) in a sample of parents of premature infants. These parents experienced a resurgence of the sorrowful feelings initially experienced at birth whenever the child experienced a stressful event such as illness, surgery, identification of a new medical problem, delay in achievement of a developmental task, manifestation of behavioral problems or entry into day care. At these times, specific feelings included sadness, depression, helplessness, frustration, fear, self-blame, and emptiness.

Davis (1987) philosophically examined chronic sorrow as it relates to society's expectations for the expression of grief. She contends that when grief occurs, it is expected to operate within a certain time frame and conclude with resolution. Health would be the expected resolution of a situation involving ill health. Since that is not possible in chronic illness situations, those in such situations are expected to "bear up" and control their grief. Society does not tolerate the visibility of grief that is not resolvable. Davis argues for recognition of recurrent grief and interventions to help persons deal with the conflict between the afflicted's need to mourn and society's expectation that they will hide grief.

Damrosch and Perry (1989) documented chronic sorrow in parents of Down's syndrome children and compared the responses of mothers and fathers. They used an adapted form of the graphs developed by Wikler and others (1981) to allow subjects to indicate their patterns of sorrow. The mothers reported their patterns of sorrow as periodic occurrences with peaks and valleys. The fathers reported more gradual, steady recovery.

Using a structured questionnaire, Burke (1989) studied the occurrence of chronic sorrow, the milestones or events at which it recurred, and factors that were or were not helpful to mothers of school-age myelomeningocele children in coping with the sorrow. Chronic sorrow was operationalized as a description of sadness at the time of initial diagnosis and at least at one later recurrence of the same feeling. Using this definition, chronic sorrow was identified in 91% of the sample of 47 mothers. The sorrow recurred with management crises, the child's failure to reach developmental norms, unending caregiving, and other painful experiences. The mothers' strategies for coping with their feelings included: interpersonal contacts, that is, talking it out with others; cognitive-emotional strategies such as appraisal of the situation; and, action or doing something. Subjects reported that their coping was facilitated by support from family, community groups such as churches and service agencies, and by professional care providers.

CRITICAL ATTRIBUTES

The definition of chronic sorrow has evolved from a broad, simple description of psychological reaction to a tragic situation (Olshansky, 1962) to a more specific description of recurring, periodic sadness that is permanent and progressive (Burke, 1989; Damrosch & Perry, 1989; Wikler, Wasow, & Hatfield, 1981). The loss is continually redefined in new situations with new problems and acts as a stimulus for sadness. These characteristics were incorporated into the formal description of the critical attributes or underlying assumptions of chronic sorrow, listed in Table 8.1.

These descriptions of chronic sorrow indicate that the phenomenon is a form of grief. Grief occurs in waves, even in acute stages (Lindemann, 1944; Schneider, 1980). At a death, the family members cry, then rally to make arrangements. Talking to friends, viewing the deceased or being alone to gather thoughts often trigger new waves of overwhelming grief. Throughout the grief process, reminders or triggers of the loss bring new waves of sorrow. Senour (1981) labels these waves "islands of sorrow." In resolvable grief they abate in intensity with time as the person reinvests in life and detaches from that which was lost. In chronic sorrow, however, the "islands of sorrow" continually occur from new losses and from old losses that are continually brought to mind.

Resolvable grief and chronic sorrow are reactions to loss—resolvable grief to one identified perceived loss, chronic sorrow to numerous losses that are a part of chronic illness or disability. Grief is a healing process that allows one to separate from that which was lost and form new attachments in order to survive the loss (Engel, 1960; Senour, 1981). In a chronic situation, the grieving process is a normal reaction designed to accomplish the same purpose. Each episode of sorrow is a step toward surviving in spite of the losses. The increasing intensity of chronic sorrow is probably related to the buildup of the numerous losses that are a part of a disease or condition and to the impact such losses have on the person's total being. The degree of commitment, or involvement with that which was lost, affects the intensity of the loss and the time needed to resolve the loss (Heikkinen, 1979). If physical wholeness is lost, a sense of control over one's destiny is lost, increasing the intensity of the grief (Senour, 1981).

If the underlying cause of continual losses is a handicap inflicted upon one's child, dementia in one's spouse or a devastating disease

TABLE 8.1 Critical Attributes of Chronic Sorrow

1. There is a perception of sorrow or sadness over time in a situation that has no predictable end.

2. The sadness or sorrow is cyclic or recurrent.

3. The sorrow or sadness is triggered either internally or externally and brings to mind the person's losses, disappointments or fears.

4. The sadness or sorrow is progressive and can intensify even years after the inital sense of disappointment, loss or fear.

such as multiple sclerosis, grief operates throughout the course of those diseases/disabilities. Quint (1969) describes chronic disease as progressive, periodic, and permanent. Chronic sorrow, as a reaction to chronicity, reflects those characteristics and is also progressive, periodic, pervasive, and permanent.

CHRONIC SORROW AS OPPOSED TO PROLONGED GRIEF

Establishing the boundaries of chronic sorrow makes it possible to distinguish it from the related concept of prolonged grief. The major difference between the two is that prolonged grief is a long-term reaction to one loss, and chronic sorrow is the reaction to multiple losses over time. In prolonged grief, the grieving person's reinvestment in a new life is hindered, slowed, or pathologically altered. Resolution is not achieved. The literature on grief, especially since the work of Kübler-Ross (1969) and Engel (1960), includes the notion that sorrow or grief occurs in stages from shock, disbelief, denial, anger, and depressive feelings, to acceptance and adjustment or resolution (Bowlby, 1973; Kübler-Ross, 1969). Even if persons fluctuate between stages, it is understood that the final stage of the process will be reached; not to do so is considered unhealthy or pathological. Pathological or unresolvable grief is recognizable by abnormal behavior patterns such as a delay in the reaction to a loss, taking on the symptoms of the deceased person or lasting loss of social interaction patterns (Lindemann, 1944).

In contrast, chronic sorrow is a normal reaction even though resolution is not the goal of the process. The loss occurs in bits and pieces and is such a part of the person's life that to replace what is lost and reinvest is not possible. Parents of a handicapped child may have other normal children, but their normality will not abolish the pain and suffering the ill child endures, or alter the developmental milestones the ill child is not able to reach. The elderly wife caregiver sees the continual mental losses her husband with Alzheimer's experiences, yet she is unlikely to divorce him and replace him with another man. Each new mental loss requires her to have sorrow.

CHRONIC SORROW AS OPPOSED TO DEPRESSION

Another important distinction is that between chronic sorrow and depression. Depression is considered unhealthy grief in which a real or imagined loss is felt at an unconscious level (Schneider, 1980). Depression is defined as a clinical syndrome of lowered self-esteem, overwhelming feelings of helplessness, profound sadness, apathy, negativism, and guilt (Gordon, 1987; Loomis, 1988; Schneider, 1980). Specific behaviors of depression include tearfulness, brooding, inability to shift one's thoughts from the loss or situation, inability to concentrate on reading, writing or conversation, a slowing in physical activity, insomnia with early morning awakening, loss of appetite, oversensitivity to others, and expressions of guilt and failure (Burgess, 1990; Schneider, 1980). Clinical depression is categorized as bipolar disorder, depressed, and major depressive disorder (Loomis, 1988). Often, no specific precipitating loss can be identified as bringing on the depressive state, and the condition is not self-limiting (Burgess, 1990). Clearly this is not chronic sorrow.

In depression, the person experiences emptiness and reduced self-regard. In contrast, in grieving or sorrow, the emptiness or loss surrounds the person (Osterweis, Solomon, & Green, 1984). Further, depression is a nonfunctional state, while chronic sorrow does not significantly inhibit daily functioning. Depression is not a periodic, off-and-on sensation, but a disturbance in a person's mood. Mood is a prolonged emotion that pervades or colors the whole psychological state of the person (Burgess, 1990).

Unresolvable or pathological grief can take the form of depression. Kübler-Ross (1969) identified a temporary state of depressive feelings in explanation of the grief process. For some this depressive stage may become permanent. This is not chronic sorrow.

Depression is commonly found in the elderly (Burnside, 1988; Ebersole & Hess, 1981), who experience numerous and varied losses such as suffering a stroke, losing the ability to drive, or having friends die (Lindgren, 1990b). The depression of the elderly is not chronic sorrow, but grief is considered a common feature of old age (Comfort, 1978). Such grief could logically be experienced as resolvable grief in circumstances of one loss or as chronic sorrow with multiple losses. It is not known how the elderly may experience various combinations of resolvable grief states, chronic sorrow, and depression related to their losses.

THE RELATION OF CHRONIC SORROW TO DEPRESSION

Chronic sorrow is not depression, but the two concepts may be related. Chronic illness and disability require mourning of the loss of parts of the body, functions, and potentials (Stone, 1979). If a person does not acknowledge that such mourning is necessary, or is not allowed such activity, this may contribute to development of an overriding negative state such as depression. It is possible that persons in situations leading to chronic sorrow can move into a pathological grief state or a depressive state for a variety of reasons such as personality predisposition, physical illness, overwhelming stressors that they cannot cope with, or a combination of these factors. It is also conceivable that a person might be depressed and simultaneously experience chronic sorrow. Burke (1989) interviewed several mothers with obvious symptoms of depression who also experienced chronic sorrow.

MODEL CASE

The model case of chronic sorrow presented here contains all the critical attributes of the concept. Mr. Jackson (fictitious name) is a middle-aged father of a retarded daughter in her 20s. When she completed a state vocational program for the handicapped, he was asked to give a few remarks. (His remarks are excerpted from an actual speech heard in Wyandotte, MI, Anonymous, 1988.)

> When she was born, the doctor said she was severely retarded and the best thing to do was put her in an institution. My wife and I were devastated. We cried. Then we dried our tears, took her home and loved her the best we could. When she was two, she still could not walk. We cried, dried our tears, and practiced taking steps with her until she walked at three.
>
> When she was five, we tried to enroll her in kindergarten. The teacher said take her home, she will not learn 90% of what is taught. My wife and I went home and cried. The next day we returned to the school with our daughter. I told the teacher to teach our daughter the 10% she could learn.
>
> When she finished special education classes at 18, they said she couldn't graduate. We cried. Then we took her out to dinner to

celebrate her last day of school. Now she has finished five years here at the Center and brings home a check for her work in the bakery unit. We cry in our hearts because she will never be able to be totally on her own, but rejoice at how far she has come.

Mr. Jackson's grief was progressive over time, periodic, and triggered by realization of his daughter's limitations.

BORDERLINE CASE

An example of a borderline case contains some of the attributes of chronic sorrow but does not represent the concept because the sadness described is periodic but not progressive. Margaret is an 84-year-old widow who lives in an apartment near her son. Six years ago, her daughter died suddenly at age 45. On the dining room table, Margaret keeps an arrangement of silk flowers that her daughter rearranged just before her death. Margaret gets a feeling of sadness sometimes when she looks at the flowers or when someone asks about them. Margaret's experiences differ from chronic sorrow because they originate from one unchanging loss as opposed to numerous, continual losses over time.

RELATED CASE

The following related case describes what at first appears to be chronic sorrow, but upon inspection is clearly not chronic sorrow. That is to say, forms of depression often appear at first to be chronic sorrow, but in depression, overwhelming feelings of self-worthlessness and self-hate appear. For example, Jane is the mother of three children, who are of school-age. One child, Timmy, is having difficulty reading and is two grades behind his peers. Her husband is working at two jobs to try to make ends meet. Jane feels trapped. One day Timmy brings home a paper stating that he is not eligible to sign up for the school pep group because of his grades. Jane wakes up in the night with a feeling of oppression and sadness, which continues for weeks. She feels she has failed as a mother and wife. She is contemplating ending her own life. Her behavior and feelings are indicative of depression.

CONTRARY CASE

A contrary case describes feelings which are clearly not chronic sorrow. Betty's son has just left home to attend college. He is the last of her children to "leave the nest." For a week she experienced sadness as she went about her daily activity: walking by the basketball hoop nailed to the garage where he spent many happy hours; seeing the neighborhood pool where he learned to swim; looking at the picture on the end table of him with his prom date. She is experiencing a grief reaction to the change that has occurred in her life; however, it is not chronic sorrow.

ILLEGITIMATE CASE

The following illegitimate case is an example of the misuse of the term chronic sorrow or chronic grief. Peretz (1970) inappropriately used the term chronic grief as a synonym for a pathological grief state. Peretz (1970) described chronic grief as persistent mourning of a loss characterized by denial of the loss and evidenced by behavior such as leaving the room of the deceased untouched long after the death. In this description, the grief process is blocked or inhibited by the individual's refusal to acknowledge that a loss has occurred. Peretz (1970) states that this blocking is a defense against grief and is pathological, yet he labels it chronic grief. Denying loss is not a part of chronic sorrow or chronic grief, nor is chronic sorrow or chronic grief pathological.

ANTECEDENTS AND CONSEQUENCES

Chronic sorrow is not an isolated process in persons' lives but takes place in relation to other events and happenings. The antecedents or events that must occur prior to the onset of chronic sorrow are:

1. The person experiencing chronic sorrow must be involved in a trajectory of chronic illness or disability, either as the one afflicted or as a caregiver.
2. The trajectory has an identifiable beginning such as the birth of an ill baby or a diagnosis of a chronic illness such as multiple sclerosis or Alzheimer's disease.

The consequences or events that occur as a result of chronic sorrow are the following:

1. The person is able to move into other phases of the chronic illness situation, having grieved losses of the previous phase. This is more likely if comfort and support have been received.
2. A depressive state or abnormal grief reaction may occur; this is more likely if the supportive network is inadequate.

The antecedents and consequences provide the sequential context of chronic sorrow. In the discussion section, the relationship of time and chronic sorrow is further explored.

DISCUSSION: CHRONIC SORROW AND THE ILLNESS TRAJECTORY

The Illness Trajectory

Chronic sorrow and the concept of time are inseparable. Years of people's lives are involved in feelings of loss and those feelings are affected by the individual's stage of life. Patients and families have a view of, or perspective on, their chronic illness as a course or category over time. Corbin and Strauss (1983) labeled this the trajectory of illness. Dimond and Jones (1983) called it the career of illness. The illness trajectory is a history that includes the events leading up to the onset of the illness/handicap, what is happening now, and what may or may not happen in the future. The trajectory is essentially a mental reservoir of the feelings, and experiences of other people involved with the illness, and tasks associated with the illness/handicap over time. Individuals may become aware of different parts of their illness trajectory or career at different times. At times, reflection may make them aware of the entire time sequence of the illness/handicap. At other times, they may have a heightened awareness of particular feelings occurring at certain times along the trajectory, such as the times of developmental tasks that have not been accomplished. Inevitably the long-term nature of chronic illness and chronic sorrow involves the integration of developmental milestones and events into the meaning of and reactions to the illness.

Chronic sorrow can be conceptualized as a sense of sadness that occurs at periodic intervals across the entire trajectory or career of illness. Chronic illness trajectories or careers are often fatalistic in nature;

that is, they are outside one's control and require conformity to changing patterns of disease and disability (Dimond & Jones, 1983). The trajectory, however, is broken into smaller parts which are experientially manageable. Chronic sorrow is the reflection of the grief work done in the small segments of the trajectory in order to align one's self-concept with the new reality (Stone, 1979). Chronic sorrow within the illness/disability trajectory can be seen in the descriptions of persons in various parts of the lifespan.

Chronic Sorrow in the Young Family Trajectory

Much of the joy of parenthood is linked to the growth, learning, and new experiences of the child. Illness/disability squelches that joy. Parents of a child with muscular dystrophy describe their chronic sorrow within the trajectory of their child's illness, thus: ". . . A healthy baby, so perfect in every way. His first innocent smile . . . his first words . . . the joy of first steps . . . always falling and hurting himself . . . thinking his odd walk was just a passing phase . . . The horror of learning that Duchenne muscular dystrophy was taking over our little boy's body . . . His tears when he couldn't be outside . . . The day he went for his first physiotherapy session . . . the painful operation to stretch his Achilles tendons . . . the sadness of the birthday when we knew he would never walk . . . and the wheelchair that has become part of his life" (Muscular Dystrophy Group of Great Britain & Northern Ireland, 1988).

Patterns of sorrow within this view of trajectory have been depicted by parents of handicapped children. In the Wikler et al. (1981) research, the parents' up and down feelings over periods of time were depicted in their peak and valley drawings.

Chronic Sorrow in the Illness Trajectory of the Middle Years

The middle years are characterized by fulfilling, productive activities and enjoyment of independence as an adult. Establishing a residential base, raising a family, building a career and working toward self-actualization are common features of this phase of life. Diseases/disabilities such as multiple sclerosis, which strike at this point in life, bring many disappointments and shatter the dreams of the future.

Multiple sclerosis patients have been described by Hainsworth (1987) as refusing to look at pictures taken of themselves when they were well, or when they were functioning at a higher level. Their regrets would overwhelm them, so they choose to block out such triggers to sadness. They elected to perceive only the current, manageable parts of their trajectory.

Strong (1988), whose husband has multiple sclerosis, has written of the chronic emotions of the spouse caregiver. Feelings of sadness, guilt, being trapped, and loneliness, jealousy, and annoyance at having no promise of an endpoint plague the caregiving spouse throughout the period of the disability. Strong (1988) verbalized her grief: "To be married to someone ill and to watch a man or woman you love suffer means you mourn. You mourn the lost marriage, the lost family, the suffering of the mate, and your lost self—the one who could feel dependent, who could ask to be indulged, the lighthearted you . . . you mourn a lost or reduced sexuality" (pp. 101–102).

Chronic Sorrow within the Disability Illness Trajectory of the Later Years

The elderly suffer losses such as widowhood, relocation, ill health, and the death of friends, which may trigger chronic sorrow. The losses suffered are usually related and form a trajectory pattern. For instance, falling and breaking a hip may lead to a string of related losses—loss of independence, relocation, loss of familiar surroundings and friends, and loss of financial resources (Ebersole & Hess, 1981; Lindgren, 1990b).

Because of the fatalistic trajectory that many ill elderly and their caregivers are involved in, it seems likely that they experience chronic sorrow. Anecdotal statements from caregivers of dementia patients indicate that they experience ups and downs of sadness as caregivers (Lindgren, 1990a). One caregiver noted that when frustration and sadness welled up in her, she would go into the bedroom and cry, bawling God out for picking on her and her husband and not answering her prayers. Then she would regain her composure and continue her tasks. Another reported that she told herself to be strong when the low periods came. Another recounted the feelings of devastation she had when her confused husband could only laugh at her mastectomy scar, or could not summon help when she fell down the steps. Several caregivers said they took life one day at a time, and sometimes that included one sorrow at a time. It was too painful to perceive at one time all the sorrows they had or to contemplate all the sorrows of the future.

RESEARCH IMPLICATIONS

The concept of chronic sorrow is in the early stage of development and understanding. Establishment of the major boundaries of the concept's meaning provides a basis for further exploration of chronic sorrow through research. A methodical program of study of chronic sorrow logically begins with exploring the manifestations of chronic sorrow in persons with various types of chronic illnesses and in family caregivers of the chronically ill. Major research questions to be answered are:

1. Does chronic sorrow occur in a variety of populations across the lifespan (i.e., affected individuals with diverse chronic or life-threatening conditions, their caregivers)?
2. What are the characteristics of chronic sorrow in these populations?
3. How does the expression of chronic sorrow in these populations compare with the chronic sorrow experienced by parents of children with disabilities?
4. Is chronic sorrow an inherent phenomenon in chronic illness situations?

Relationships between chronic sorrow and other concepts need to be explored. The differences and similarities of chronic sorrow, resolvable grief, and depression need to be examined in a variety of populations. Do some populations experience chronic sorrow concurrent with depression or does chronic sorrow precede depression? How does the depression the elderly are known to experience relate to their experiences of chronic sorrow?

Chronic sorrow is considered to be progressive. What are the variables related to increased intensity of the emotion? Is increased intensity of chronic sorrow related to added losses or to a changed perspective of losses? Beginning evidence indicates that support from others helps those experiencing the pain of chronic loss. What type and degree of support are most beneficial to persons with chronic sorrow? Is social support inversely related to the intensity of the chronic sorrow?

Exploring the incidence and nature of chronic sorrow and its related variables is a step in building the conceptual framework of chronic sorrow and a more comprehensive understanding of the concept. The framework can then be a basis for developing nursing assessment and interventions to help the chronically ill and their families deal with their losses over long periods of time.

SUMMARY AND CONCLUSIONS

Chronic sorrow is an identifiable phenomenon in the lives of persons in chronic illness/disability situations. This concept analysis has identified the critical attributes of chronic sorrow as progressive cycles of sadness triggered by personal, family, and social losses occurring as a result of the illness or disability. Chronic sorrow is not depression or pathological grief, but a normal reaction to a complicated, difficult situation in life. The information on the boundaries of its meaning can be used to determine the role chronic sorrow plays in the lives of populations of chronically ill or disabled persons and their caregivers across the lifespan. Understanding what chronic sorrow is and how it operates in the lives of patients and their caregivers is fundamental for providing effective nursing care to these people.

REFERENCES

Anonymous. (1988). Excerpts of an unpublished speech at recognition ceremony at the Jo Brighton Vocational Center, Wyandotte, MI.

Bowlby, J. (1973). *Attachment and loss: Vol 2. Separation, anxiety and anger.* New York: Basic Books, Inc.

Burke, M. L (1989). Chronic sorrow in mothers of schoolage children with a myelomeningocele disability. (Doctoral dissertation, Boston University, 1989). *Dissertation Abstracts International, 50,* 233–234B. (University Microfilms No. 89–20, 093).

Burgess, A (1990). *Psychiatric nursing in the hospital and the community,* 5th edition, Norwalk, CN: Appleton & Lange.

Burnside, I. M. (1988). *Nursing and the aged: A self-care approach,* 3rd edition. New York: McGraw-Hill Book Company.

Comfort, A. (1978). *A good age.* New York: Simon and Schuster.

Corbin, J., & Strauss, A. (1983). *Unending work and care: Managing chronic illness at home.* San Francisco, CA: Jossey-Bass.

Damrosch, S. P., & Perry, L. A. (1989). Self-reported adjustment to chronic sorrow, and coping of parents of children with Down syndrome. *Nursing Research, 38,* 25–30.

Davis, B. H. (1987). Disability and grief. *Social Casework, 68,* 352–357.

Dimond, M., & Jones, S. L. (1983). *Chronic illness across the life span.* Norwalk, CT: Appleton-Century Crofts.

Ebersole, P., & Hess, P. (1981). *Toward health aging: Human needs and nursing response.* St Louis: C. V. Mosby.

Engel, G. L. (1960). Is grief a disease? A challenge for medical research. *Psychosomatic Medicine, 23*(1), 18–22.

Fraley, A. M. (1986). Chronic sorrow in parents of premature children. *Children's Health Care, 15*(2), 114–118.

Gordon, M. (1987). *Manual of nursing diagnosis: 1986–1987.* New York: McGraw-Hill.
Hainsworth, M. A. (1987). An ethnographic study of women with multiple sclerosis using a symbolic interactionist approach. (Doctoral dissertation, University of Connecticut, 1986). *Dissertation Abstracts International 48,* 850. (University Microfilms No. 87–09, 033).
Heikkinen, C. A (1979). Loss resolution for growth. *The Personnel and Guidance Journal,* (February), 327–331.
Kübler-Ross, E. (1969). *On death and dying.* New York: Macmillan Publishing Co.
Lindemann, E. (1944). Symptomatology and management of acute grief. *American Journal of Psychiatry, 101,* 141–148.
Lindgren, C. L (1990a). *Experiences and reactions of spouse caregivers of dementia patients.* Paper presented at the meeting of Midwest Nursing Research Society, Indianapolis, IN.
Lindgren, C. L. (1990b). Loss in the elderly: A nursing problem. *The Older Patient, 4*(3), 15–17.
Loomis, M. E. (1988). Clients with mood disorders. In H. S. Wilson, & C. R. Kniesel (Eds.), *Psychiatric nursing* (3rd ed.) (pp. 424–429). Menlo Park, CA: Addison-Wesley Publishing Co.
Olshansky, S. (1962). Chronic sorrow: A response to having a mentally defective child. *Social Casework, 43,* 191–193.
Osterweis, M., Solomon, F., & Green, M. (1984). *Bereavement: Reactions, consequences and care.* Washington, DC: National Academy Press.
Peretz, D. (1970). Reaction to loss. In B. Schoenberg, A. C. Carr, D. Peretz, & H. Kutscher (Eds.), *Loss and grief: Psychological management in medical practice* (pp. 20–35). New York: Columbia University Press.
Quint, J. C. (1969). Some thoughts on a theory of chronicity. In C. M. Norris (Ed.), *Proceedings of the first nursing theory conference* (pp. 58–67). Kansas City, KS: University of Kansas Medical Center, Department of Nursing Education.
Roget, P. (1977). *Roget's international thesaurus* (4th ed.). (Revised by Robert L. Chapman). New York: Thomas Y. Crowell, Publishers.
Schneider, J. M. (1980). Clinically significant differences between grief, pathological grief, and depression. *Patient Counselling and Health Education,* (4th quarter), 161–169.
Searl, S. J. (1978). Stages of parent reaction. *The Exceptional Parent, 8*(2), 127–129.
Senour, M. N. (1981). Project loss: Sensitizing ourselves to grief. *The Personnel and Guidance Journal,* (February), 389–392.
Stone, G. (1979). *Health psychology.* San Francisco: Jossey-Bass.
Strong, M. (1988). *Mainstay: For the well spouse of the chronically ill.* New York: Penguin Books.
The Muscular Dystrophy Group of Great Britain and Northern Ireland. (1988). *Muscular dystrophy: A time of hope. Muscular Dystrophy Group annual review.* London, England: Author.
Walker, L. O., & Avant, K. C. (1983). *Strategies for theory construction in nursing.* Norwalk, CT: Appleton-Century Crofts.
Webster's New Universal Unabridged Dictionary (2nd ed.). (1983). New York: Simon & Schuster.

Vines, D. W. (1986). Regrieving in parents of disabled adolescents. (Doctoral dissertation, Boston University, 1986). *Dissertation Abstracts International, 46,* 387A. (University Microfilms No. 86–01, 381).

Wikler, L. M., Wasow, M., & Hatfield, E. (1981). Chronic sorrow revisited: Parent vs. professional depiction of the adjustment of parents of mentally retarded children. *American Journal of Orthopsychiatry, 51*(1), 63–70.

Response
Ida M. Martinson

The concept of chronic sorrow as developed by Lindgren, Burke, Hainsworth, and Eakes is a very helpful and thought-provoking treatise that attempts to combine their research with portions of what is found in the bereavement literature. Reading their article I was reminded of a phone call from the mother of a severely retarded child who had read of my work with dying children. She said, "I am dealing with a living death." I made a home visit and spent an afternoon with this mother and her severely retarded child. I was deeply moved by her story and contacted the local public health nurse. I urged the nurse to make regular visits to the family to support this mother in her difficult parenting role. The continuing losses that this mother was experiencing in caring for her child served as a powerful example and helped in my own understanding of the pain that is involved in living with seriously handicapped children. Over the years, I have continued to think of this mother and the chronic sorrow she was experiencing.

I strongly support these authors in their hope to engage in further research to develop interventions in this area. I also urge them to develop intervention strategies sooner rather than later. Attempts at intervention will add to the development of the concept of chronic sorrow necessary for nurses' understanding of the vicissitudes and sorrows of life. Although there is a risk in undertaking clinical interventions, as there will probably never be enough research data to have a complete, rational basis for intervention, I believe that nursing interventions can be very powerful if they are sufficiently planned and documented. Refinement of the model can always occur after the interventions have demonstrated effectiveness. From my years of experience with families, the availability of a nurse on call 24 hours a day, 7 days a week is a very powerful intervention. Accessibility to nursing consultation needs to be increased for individuals involved in chronic sorrow. A hospice team could really demonstrate its usefulness in conditions such as severe mental retardation or progressive Alzheimer's disease. I urge this team of investigators to do a national clinical research study soon.

Throughout the article, I had difficulty with only one of the critical attributes, that of progression and intensification of sadness over time. First, I was disturbed that chronic sorrow as conceptualized by Burke was operationalized as a description of sadness at the time of initial diagnosis and a minimum of one later recurrence of the sad feeling. To define only two points of measurement of sadness as chronic sorrow does not seem adequate. I am sure that all parents, even those with healthy, normal children, have at least two points of sadness regarding their children.

Second, Lindgren, Burke, Hainsworth, and Eakes undoubtedly speak to the increasing intensity of chronic sorrow because of the buildup of the numerous losses that are a part of a disease or condition. Based on my clinical experience and research in the area, there may not always be an increasing intensity of chronic sorrow. Instead, I might define chronic sorrow as a relatively constant state of sadness with peaks and valleys. Included in situations that I would identify as producing chronic sorrow are those where there are continuing losses, such as in caring for a severely mentally retarded child or a progressive Alzheimer's patient. Although I support the definition of chronic sorrow as a reaction to other types of chronicity, reflecting those characteristics as well as being periodic, pervasive, and permanent, I have not found the progressive attribute to be of use. The example of Jackson did not indicate to me that his grief was progressive over time. The borderline case of Margaret is a response to a one-time loss rather than to a series of losses. A series of losses may not always be progressive in intensity. Indeed, as described in their summary and conclusions, the progressive cycles of sadness or chronic sorrow do imply increasing intensity.

The authors' discussion of islands of sorrow reminds me of the empty space phenomenon about which several of my colleagues have published. We have found that one can reinvest in life and yet not completely detach from that which was lost. In our study of the empty space phenomenon, we found parents who would have a sudden resurgence of grief at an intensity that surprised them. Grief is a process, not a state, and a process dealing with emotion would not be spread out evenly over time. This notion needs to be integrated into the model of chronic sorrow.

The authors describe a series of phases that people move through as they deal with chronic sorrow. I am not sure that I understand what the authors were concluding with regard to these phases. For example, I doubt whether someone in the position of caring for a severely mentally retarded child or a progressive Alzheimer's patient could ever work through the phases and no longer experience sorrow. Phases and stages such as those described by Lindemann, Engle, and Kübler-Ross tend not to emphasize the individual patterns of coping and integration that occur over time. The works of Demi, Sanders, and Bugen may help to clarify and strengthen the model of chronic sorrow.

Chronic sorrow is a normal reaction to a complicated, difficult situation in life. The concept of chronic sorrow and the beginning development of a model that combines the authors' research and the literature on bereavement is an important contribution toward understanding a phenomenon of interest to all nurses.

REFERENCES

Bugen, L. (1977). Human grief: A model for prediction and intervention. *American Journal of Orthopsychiatry, 47*(2), 196–206.

Demi, A. S. (1989). Death of a spouse. In R. Kalish (Ed.), *Midlife loss: Coping strategies* (pp. 218–248). Newbury Park, CA: Sage.

Snaders, C. M. (1989). *Grief: The mourning after.* New York: John Wiley & Sons, Inc.

Chapter 9

Operationalizing the Corbin and Strauss Trajectory Model for Elderly Clients with Chronic Illness

Linda A. Robinson
Catherine Bevil
Virginia Arcangelo
JoAnne Reifsnyder
Nancy Rothman
Suzanne Smeltzer

OVERVIEW

A research team of six nursing faculty at Thomas Jefferson University College of Allied Health Sciences collaborated to develop a research proposal to provide nursing care to a selected population of chronically ill elderly persons. The Corbin and Strauss Nursing Model for Chronic Illness Management (1991) was selected as the organizing framework to guide research and care delivery. While conceptual models offer direction for nursing practice, specific guidelines for

---

Note: Originally published in *Sholarly Inquiry for Nursing Practice: An International Journal,* Vol. 7, No. 4, 1993, New York: Springer Publishing Company.

providing care can only be identified when major concepts of the model are operationalized (Fawcett, 1989). This chapter describes the first step in operationalizing the Corbin and Strauss Trajectory Model undertaken by the research team which resulted in the development of eight "Phase-specific protocols." Two of the eight phase-specific protocols are presented.

INTRODUCTION

Conceptual models are developed to provide an organizing framework for nursing practice, education, and research. Such models are highly abstract and general. While conceptual models offer general guidelines for nursing practice, more specific guidelines must be developed through operationalizing major concepts of the model and theory testing (Fawcett, 1989). This chapter describes the process undertaken by a team of nursing faculty members at Thomas Jefferson University, Department of Nursing, to operationalize major concepts described in the Corbin and Strauss Nursing Model for Chronic Illness Management (1991). Concepts of the model are briefly described to illustrate the research team's interpretation of how this body of work can be used to guide care for a group of chronically ill elderly adults and to design nursing interventions for a nursing research project. For the sake of brevity, the nursing model cited above will be referred to hereafter as the "Corbin and Strauss Trajectory Model."

BACKGROUND OF THE PROJECT

In response to a call for research proposals focusing on care of the chronically ill elderly, six nursing faculty members formed a research group to develop such a proposal. The chronically ill elderly residing in low income subsidized housing were identified as the focus of the proposal. This focus was based on data obtained during a community health experience of baccalaureate nursing students who made home visits to fifty elderly persons whose residence fit this description and is located in Center City, Philadelphia. Under the direction of a faculty preceptor, the students identified unrecognized and untreated chronic illnesses, made referrals of chronically ill residents to collaborating physicians, provided health teaching and counseling, and assisted in coordination of services. The experience indicated that elderly residents in low income housing in this large metropolitan area had a number of significant chronic health care problems that required screening, case finding, monitoring, referral, and follow up. Further, the students' experience indicated that many of the problems could be appropriately addressed by nurses. The data obtained through students' experiences were consistent with the documented incidence of at least one chronic illness in 85% of individuals 65 years of age and older, and decreased functional ability secondary to chronic illness in 40% of older adults (Folden, 1989).

SELECTING AN ORGANIZING FRAMEWORK

An initial step in developing a research proposal to test nursing interventions directed toward the health care needs of this population was to review nursing models and frameworks that might address the needs of elderly clients with chronic illness residing in the community and guide the design of specific nursing interventions. Following review of several theoretical approaches, the Corbin and Strauss Trajectory Model was selected because it was designed to enhance the individual's management of the chronic illness course. The long term nature of chronic illness necessitates that most management of the illness course occurs outside formal health care facilities, that is, in people's homes, and involves making adjustments to facilitate everyday life activities (Corbin & Strauss, 1991). The research team believed that nursing interventions designed for this proposal and project should promote wellness and empower elderly residents to care for themselves more independently. This perspective was considered by the team to be inherent in every concept of the Corbin & Strauss Trajectory Model.

THE RESEARCH TEAM

Once the Corbin and Strauss Trajectory Model was agreed upon as the organizing framework for the research proposal, meetings of the research team were held weekly over the course of five months to discuss how the model could be utilized in the process of planning, providing, and evaluating nursing care to chronically ill elderly people. The research team consisted of five nurse educators and one nurse researcher who came together in the fall of 1991 to develop the research proposal to address the health care needs of the target population. Clinical expertise of the research team members included backgrounds in community health, hospice, adult health, and geriatric nursing. The nurse researcher on the team also had extensive experience working with specific chronically ill populations and prior familiarity with the Corbin and Strauss Trajectory Model.

In addition to documenting the need for nursing services within this chronically ill elderly population, the anecdotal data obtained from the previously described community-based experience of the nursing students and their instructor were used to examine the applicability of the concepts of the model in relation to actual clinical situations. Furthermore, anecdotal data were invaluable in the research team's preliminary discussions about ways to operationalize the Corbin Strauss Trajectory Model. These early discussions helped to familiarize the research team with the unique terminology used by Corbin and Strauss.

MAJOR CONCEPTS OF THE CORBIN AND STRAUSS TRAJECTORY MODEL

The Corbin and Strauss Trajectory Model is based on evolving concepts described by Strauss and associates since the 1960's. This model is a result of over 30 years of studying the challenges of chronic illness management across settings. Corbin, a nurse, and Strauss, a social scientist, have drawn from the accumulated body of interdisciplinary knowledge referred to as the "trajectory framework" to formulate a nursing model (Corbin & Strauss, 1991). Their recently published work has more clearly specified the usefulness of the trajectory framework to the discipline of nursing.

The Corbin and Strauss Trajectory Model provides description of the four central concepts of the metaparadigm of nursing identified by Fawcett (1989) as: person, environment, health, and nursing. The process of reasoning leading to the model's development has been inductive, formulating generalizations from specific experiences nurses shared about working with chronically ill people. While it is not the intention of the authors to comprehensively evaluate the Corbin and Strauss Trajectory Model, its usefulness in guiding research and care delivery will be explored.

The major concept of the model is *trajectory*, which represents the chronic illness course. "Trajectory" implies a multi-dimensional course or unfolding of a chronic illness which affects an individual and those around him or her in all aspects of life. Illness, characterized by symptoms, influences a person's life, and aspects of life influence a person's ability to manage their illness. This differs from the view that an illness course is uni-dimensional, that is, affects only the physiological state of the sick individual (Strauss, 1984). Despite such multidimensionality, the Corbin and Strauss Trajectory Model is based on the premise that a chronic illness course can be shaped and managed over time even if the course of the disease cannot be modified (Smeltzer, 1991). The goal of nursing within this model is to assist those afflicted to shape their illness course while maintaining quality of life. Nursing care, referred to as "supportive assistance," centers around health promotion and collaboration with the individual, family, or community, and self care or management of the chronic condition (Corbin & Strauss, 1991).

Trajectory phase, another key concept of the model, refers to the various stages a person with chronic illness experiences. "Phases are a reflection of the illness course as defined by the patient" (J. Corbin, personal communication, May 5, 1992). Applying this concept in one manner allows the nurse to identify where the ill person is in his or her trajectory at a given specific point. Another way of using the concept of phasing is to look at the broad experience of the trajectory and the many phases experienced by the ill person over time. Essential to understanding the implications of trajectory phasing is the idea that people with chronic illness have a past, present, and a future experience with their disease. This concept has vast implications for planning care. The focus of nursing care must be specific to the individual's current trajectory phase, while simultaneously incorporating experiences the individual has had in other phases and has yet to experience in subsequent trajectory phases. Eight phases of chronic illness trajectory were identified and defined by Corbin and Strauss (1991) and are presented in Table 9.1. There is an unpredictable nature to the chronic illness course making definite plans and certainties about life goals difficult or impossible for the ill person. Daily fluctuations with symptoms, or ability to carry out everyday life activities, may temporarily place a person in a subphase that lies somewhere along the continuum of phases.

Biography refers to one's personal identity which reflects past experiences and current circumstances. This can be of particular importance when working with the elderly because they present a lifetime of experience or "baggage," which may influence their willingness and/or ability to carry out management strategies (J. Corbin, personal communication, May 5, 1992).

Trajectory projection, described as the vision of the illness course, relates to the future outlook for the illness course. While ultimately there are no cures for chronic illnesses, sufferers of similar chronic disease states have varying experiences. A trajectory projection or future outlook is held by the patient and all those who interface with him or her. Trajectory projections may or may not differ between the nurse and the ill person. The Corbin and Strauss Trajectory Model suggests that the trajectory projections of the nurse and the ill individual influence/determine management options and choices (Corbin & Strauss, 1991).

The *trajector scheme* refers to the overall plan of care. *Trajectory management* refers to the process and response of such a plan on the illness course. Nursing actions within the plan of care fall under the general categories of direct care, patient teaching, counseling, monitoring, referral, and arrangement making. In order to shape the illness course, the nurse providing "supportive assistance" would work collaboratively with the ill person, his or her support system, and professionals from other disciplines to manipulate conditions that interfere with effective management. Chronic illnesses can and do present many challenges in daily living; therefore, nursing's role could hypothetically range from providing direct care to advocating for increased funding and resources for particular chronic illnesses.

Reciprocal impact is a concept described by Corbin and Strauss as a "consequence component" (1991, p.165). The difficulties people face when trying to manage their illness course are affected by the illness, their biography, and everyday life activities. To illustrate this concept, a COPD patient may choose to smoke as an outlet for stress. Despite the fact that smoking worsens the symptoms, the individual continues to smoke to achieve a secondary gain. While smoking is contraindicated from an illness perspective, the model avoids labeling this individual as "non-compliant." Instead the model allows individuals to actively make choices about how they wish to manage their illness course. Such choices are influenced by their biography and everyday life activities. With management choices come consequences with which both the individual and the nurse must deal. While a medical model of care would not integrate behavior that perpetuates illness, the Corbin and Strauss Trajectory Model emphasizes the need for interactive and col-

TABLE 9.1 Definitions of Phases

Phase	Definition
1. Pretrajectory	Before the illness course begins, the preventive phase, no signs or symptoms are present
2. Trajectory onset	Signs and symptoms are present, includes diagnostic period
3. Crisis	Life-threatening situation requiring emergency/critical care
4. Acute	Active illness or complications that require hospitalization for management
5. Stable	Illness course/symptoms controlled by regimen
6. Unstable	Illness course/symptoms not contolled by regimen but not requiring hospitalization
7. Downward	Progressive deterioration in physical/mental status characterized by increasing disability/symptoms
8. Dying	Immediate weeks, days, hours preceding death

Note. From "A Nursing Model for Chronic Illness Management Based upon the Trajectory Framework" by J. M. Corbin and A. Strauss, 1991, *Scholarly Inquiry for Nursing Practice: An International Journal*, 5, page 163. © 1991 Springer Publishing Company. Reprinted by permission.

laborative efforts between nurses and individuals when managing lifelong illness. The model approaches the individual as he or she chooses to live, not necessarily how the nurse would prefer him or her to live. The illness can never be viewed or managed apart from the context of biography and everyday life activities.

OPERATIONALIZING THE TRAJECTORY MODEL

The research team was interested in using the Corbin and Strauss Trajectory Model as a framework for evaluating strategies toward assisting elderly residents to manage their illness course(s). The abstract concepts of the model combined with complex social and psychological phenomena inherent in chronic illness management, however, presented problems in measurement with respect to designing a scientifically sound research proposal. Therefore, to apply the model within the context and rigors of a research proposal, the team first needed to operationalize abstract concepts in order to enhance measurement and control for varying interventions within a formal study.

The first concept of the model to be operationalized was trajectory phase. The eight phases described by Corbin and Strauss were assigned to research team members based on their clinical familiarity in caring for ill people within the respective phases. Each of the eight phases was then analyzed by the research team member in order to develop what became referred to as a "phase-specific protocol." These protocols were purposefully designed to be non-disease specific, with an aim to standardize care within phases, among a diverse population. Each protocol incorporated the major areas to be assessed with patients, as well as the categories of nursing care to be provided. Efforts were made to clearly differentiate between the various phases through their application to case studies in research team meetings; the process resulted in numerous revisions of the protocols. While the impetus to develop phase-specific protocols was to enhance measurement and control of nursing interventions in a research context, the team gained some unexpected insights about chronic illness through their development.

Throughout this process it became clear to the research team that chronic illness transcends care settings. Each of the team members was relatively comfortable with particular phases of care, but no one team member could confidently describe care across all phases. It was the broad range of clinical expertise among the research team that enabled the process of describing the comprehensive care required across care settings and illness phases. The rather poignant realization for the research team, however, was the fact that chronically ill people have to cope with their illness challenges during every phase and across all care settings. The experience of operationalizing the phases of the Corbin and Strauss Trajectory Model deepened the team's sensitivity to the struggle chronically ill people face. The process helped the team become more aware of how traditional nursing education and clinical experience foster specialty care and "tunnel-vision," which are inconsistent with the lifelong, unpredictable nature of chronic illness.

APPLICATION OF THE PHASE-SPECIFIC PROTOCOLS

Applying the phase-specific protocols involves a four-step process reflecting the nursing process components of assessment, planning, intervention, and evaluation. The first step in applying the phase-specific protocols necessitates *locating the client and family and settings goals.* Corbin and Strauss (1991) define locating by the nurse as "identifying the management problem and giving a basis for establishing the specific goals of intervention" (p. 168). Three areas to be assessed in the process of locating the client are biography, everyday life activities, and the illness. The research team examined these three areas of assessment and delineated how they would differ among the eight phases. For example, in the Stable Phase an assessment of the client's knowledge about, and previous experiences with, the illness is made. If, however, the client was in the stage of Trajectory Onset, where the chronic illness is newly diagnosed, it would be important to assess the client's knowledge of and experience with other people who may have had the illness. Locating the ill person in a particular phase is not done by the nurse in isolation, but rather is a collaborative and interactive process between the nurse and client. The following case study is presented to illustrate the process of applying the phase-specific protocol:

> Mrs. G. is a 69-year-old woman diagnosed with diabetes mellitus 5 years ago. Mrs. G. had been caring for her father up until 6 months ago when he died at home from complications of diabetes. Mrs. G. recently had noticed increased thirst and frequency of urination. After being evaluated by her family physician, her blood sugar was determined to be high and daily insulin injections were prescribed.

This client is located in the Unstable Phase, given the presence of symptoms (polyuria, polydipsia, increased blood glucose), and she agrees that her condition does not yet require hospitalization.

Once the process of locating is completed, the second step in applying the phase-specific protocol is that of collaborative goal setting between the nurse and the client. The Corbin and Strauss Trajectory Model emphasizes that the setting of goals is a mutual process and should be phase-specific.

> Mrs. G. and the nurse agree that the immediate goal needing to be addressed is that of achieving and maintaining normal, or near

> normal blood sugar levels. The nurse learns from Mrs. G. that she has no intention of giving herself insulin injections. Mrs. G. states that "it was the insulin that killed my father." While in order to achieve the goal of normalizing blood sugar levels, it would be necessary to teach Mrs. G. safe administration of insulin, she clearly is not willing to do so at this time. Her biography presents experiences that color her acceptance of this aspect of diabetic management. Together Mrs. G. and the nurse agree that for now the focus of management will not be placed on the insulin injections. Instead, Mrs. G. is willing to learn to modify her diet. The nurse will provide the insulin injections until she can counsel and educate Mrs. G. further on the purpose and effects of insulin.

The third step in applying the phase-specific protocol involves implementing the trajectory scheme or overall plan of care. In determining the trajectory scheme the nurse analyzes the conditions that interfere with the client managing his or her illness trajectory. In this case, Mrs. G.'s previous experiences with diabetic management as well as the recent loss of her father interfere with her ability to manage her illness course. The nurse then initiates a plan to manipulate the conditions through the six categories of nursing actions: direct care, patient teaching, counseling, monitoring, referral, and arrangement making. As with locating and goal setting, the trajectory scheme is phase-specific.

> The nurse may implement the trajectory scheme by administering insulin injections (direct care), instructing Mrs. G. about her diet (patient teaching), allowing Mrs. G. to ventilate her grief over the loss of her father (counseling), performing daily capillary blood sugar determinations (monitoring), recommending Mrs. G. attend a local diabetic support group (referring), and begin identifying a support person who may be willing to assume responsibility for the insulin injections (arrangement making).

The fourth and last step in applying the phase-specific protocol is that of evaluation.

> A neighbor has agreed to prepare pre-filled syringes for Mrs. G. on a weekly basis. After receiving insulin injections for 2 weeks Mrs. G. states she feels "more like her old self again." With con-

tinued support and instruction from the nurse she has agreed to begin to give herself her daily insulin injections.

It is critical for the nurse and the client to periodically analyze the trajectory scheme in the larger context of the illness trajectory and determine in what direction, if any, the client is heading. If the client is in the Stable Phase, is everything possible being done to prolong this phase? Or is the client on a downward spiral? If so, are there modifications that could be made in the trajectory scheme that would reverse, slow, or ease movement in that direction? Tables 9.2 and 9.3 present two phase-specific protocols for comparison.

DISCUSSION

In developing the protocols, the research team members shared a common tendency toward wanting to "do and know everything" within every phase. For example, in the area of assessment, it has been traditional in nursing to collect a comprehensive and standardized data base on everyone. The research team's interpretation of the Corbin and Strauss Trajectory Model challenges that tradition. The assessment and locating process will vary by phase. The components of assessment (biography, everyday life activities, and illness) remain the categories of inquiry, but the emphasis on each of these components differs among varying phases.

The same is true within the Trajectory Scheme. A client with minimal symptomatology who is effectively managing asthma in the Stable Phase through avoidance of respiratory irritants and correct use of inhalers may need little or no direct care from the nurse. Instead, this client may benefit from additional health teaching and periodic monitoring to prolong this phase, thus improving overall quality of life. In contrast, the same client in the acute phase of the illness trajectory, characterized by severe wheezing and rapid respiratory rate, may require a great deal of direct care (such as administration of intravenous bronchodilating agents) to manage symptomatology. There would be minimal emphasis on health teaching within this phase.

While collaboration with patients to set goals has been traditional within nursing, the Corbin and Strauss Trajectory Model challenges the nurse to do so in a manner that places the client in a position of equal authority with the nurse. This stimulated considerable discussion among the research team as it related to clients who lack knowledge and/or acceptance of their disease process. The team had great difficulty reconciling whether it should be the nurse or the client who directs goal setting, given specific, yet frequently encountered, situations. A scenario often discussed by the team was that of a moderately hypertensive client who is asymptomatic and denies having high blood pressure. The nurse might want to instruct the client in making a number of lifestyle adjustments, such as following a low sodium diet and an exercise regimen with the long-term goal of normalizing the client's blood pressure. Clearly the client who denies a blood pressure problem would lack the motivation to work toward such a goal. Yet the team agreed that the nurse's failing to address the high blood pressure would be irresponsible and dangerous for the client. After much team discussion and clarification with Dr. Corbin via telephone consultation (June 8, 1992), it was decided that the client's perception is always the most important in determining planning and goal setting; however, negotiation may play a role in the goal-setting process. In this scenario, the nurse would first address the problem by increasing the client's awareness of and knowledge about high blood pressure. Until the client perceived the high blood pressure to be a problem, there would be little value in setting up a plan the client would be unlikely to follow.

The operationalization of the concepts biography and trajectory projection for an elderly population has been very challenging. The idea of obtaining biographical information from elderly clients conjures up lengthy interviews which may not be realistic in many clinical settings. Team members with experience in geriatrics warned of a common hesitancy on the part of most older people to reveal sensitive aspects of their biographical profiles until a trusting relationship is formed between the nurse and the client. Such a relationship cannot be established within a short time frame. It cannot, then, be expected that biographical information will be obtained in one or even several interviews. Time limits should be placed on discussions geared to elicit biographical information, but the client should be able to share experiences about any aspect of life no matter how unrelated to the chronic illness it seems to be (J. Corbin, personal communication, May 5, 1992).

It was fairly easy for the research team to imagine how trajectory projection could positively or negatively affect a client's willingness and/or motivation to carry out a trajectory scheme. For example, clients diagnosed with cancer who believe that there is little chance of survival may be less willing to consume a highly nutritious diet than a client with can-

TABLE 9.2 Pretrajectory Phase (Before the illness course begins, the preventive phase, no signs or symptoms present)

Locating the Client

Biography
1. Resident's risk factors from family history
2. Resident's risk factors relative to age and the aging process
3. Behaviors and factors from past life that serve as risk factors now
4. Resident's attitudes toward health and illness behaviors

Everyday Life Activities
1. Patterns that promote health and/or prevent illness
2. Patterns that place the resident at risk for illness

Illness
1. Not applicable

Trajectory Management Scheme
1. Current health management practices

Trajectory Projection
1. Meaning of current health status for this resident

Establish Management Goals

Trajectory Scheme

Direct Care
Patient Teaching
1. Develop education program with resident regarding healthy lifestyle (exercise, diet, smoking cessation, stress reduction, etc.)

Counseling
1. Provide counseling regarding at-risk health problems

Monitoring
1. Collaborate with resident to develop means of self-monitoring for at-risk health problems (i.e., symptomatology warning signs)

Arrangement Making
1. Collaborate with resident to identify primary health care provider

Evaluation of Trajectory Scheme

TABLE 9.3 Unstable Phase (Illness course/symptoms not controlled by regimen but not requiring hospitalization)

Locating the Client

Biography
1. Recent life changes, stresses, losses, etc., that may have had an impact on the illness course
2. Resident's knowledge of previous experiences with this illness
3. Resident's previous behaviors and responses to this illness
4. Resident's knowledge about, attitudes toward, compliance with, and abilities pertinent to current management scheme
5. Interaction of resident's age and history on current illness

Everyday Life Activities
1. Ability to carry out everyday life activities including ADLs and IADLs
2. Arrangements and adaptations made to allow resident to carry out everyday activities including ADLs and IADLs
3. Impact of current management scheme on everyday life activities

Illness
1. Identify changes in resident's symptoms and conduct a targeted assessment of them.
2. Identify other factors related to age, disease implication and secondary illnesses that are contributing to instability.

Trajectory Management Scheme
1. Review total plan of care for adequacy/effectiveness.
2. Examine conditions (technology, resources, experiences, motivation, setting, lifestyle, interactions/relationships and larger environment) for factors that inhibit/promote illness management.

Trajectory Projection
1. Meaning of this illness and this phase for this resident

Establish Management Goals

Trajectory Scheme

Direct Care
1. Provide direct care to manage unstable symptoms (i.e., energy conservation techniques for chronic dyspnea, preventive pulmonary strategies for respiratory symptoms, Kegel exercises

The Corbin and Strauss Trajectory Model for Elderly Clients 237

for incontinence.

TABLE 9.3 *(continued)*

   2. Change former plan of care in collaboration with resident to address new symptomatology.

Patient Teaching
   1. Educate resident about new changes in management regime and prevention of superimposed and/or secondary health problems (i.e., immunizations, avoiding infections).

Counseling
   1. Counsel resident to continue to develop a realistic, current, and future trajectory projection.
   2. Provide emotional support and facilitate adjustment to unpredictable nature of this phase.

Monitoring
   1. In collaboration with resident, revise strategies for self-monitoring of symptoms
   2. Review monitoring strategies utilized in past phases to ascertain if current phase was predicted.

Arrangement Making
   1. Identify appropriate collaborative services and assist resident in initiating those services (i.e., referral to home care or to physician for medical managment).

Evaluation of Progress Toward Management Goals

---

cer who believes that remission is at hand. Similarly, the nurse providing care for these respective clients might positively or negatively affect the trajectory scheme by choosing or not choosing to instruct about the benefits of good nutrition. The challenge for the research team was in operationalizing the critical, yet somewhat subjective and esoteric concept of trajectory projection. The research team discussed posing questions such as: "How much control do you believe you have over your health?" and "Do you believe you will feel better, worse, or the same, 5 years from now?" It would be useful for nurses to ask themselves the same questions about the client and to repeat the questions periodically throughout the trajectory scheme or plan of care.

While the impetus to develop phase-specific protocols was to enhance measurement and control of nursing interventions in a research context, there are a number of potential clinical advantages to be gained through their application. The protocols would serve as guides or cues toward focusing and differentiating clinical efforts between phases rather than approaching chronic illness care as the same for all clients in any stage of the disease process. The protocols would assist in providing more uniform and coordinated care by different providers and minimize frustration experienced by elderly patients who may see numerous health care providers with every encounter. The protocols would also ease the transition between care settings if adopted by nurses across settings. The phase-specific protocols might also be applied to contain costs by more accurately predicting needs, providing consistency of care, and establishing more realistic outcome measures and time frames reflective of the challenges of chronic illness.

Besides providing organization for thinking, observing, and interpreting data, Fawcett (1989) tells us conceptual models suggest when a problem is solved. This last aspect has special meaning for those working with chronic illness. Frustration and "burn-out" can occur when caring for the chronically ill. Sometimes the frustration stems from the lack of a cure for the illness, but often these feelings result from the long-term nature of chronic illness. The Corbin and Strauss Trajectory Model describes illness courses for which there are no cures. The model predicts there will be "ups and downs" along the trajectory, perhaps making set-backs seem less of a failure than an expected change (or progression) of the chronic illness course. Use of the model in clinical practice has the potential for reducing commonly experienced feelings of frustration and failure among health care providers who work with the chronically ill.

Summary

Development of the phase-specific protocols has been an important first step toward operationalizing the Corbin and Strauss Trajectory Model. Further application of the model and refinement and testing of the phase-specific protocols are needed to maximize their utility in nursing research and clinical practice.

The phase-specific protocols raise questions for further study. Do the protocols accurately describe the care that is needed in order to achieve the phase-specific goals? Can the protocols be useful in predicting care needs without being made specific to any particular chronic illness? For example, if an individual is suffering from heart disease, arthritis, and diabetes, will locating the person in one phase address care needs for all three conditions? These questions can only be answered through pilot testing of the protocols in a clinical setting.

While conceptual models are useful in education, practice, and research, they cannot be applied directly (Fawcett, 1989). Before applying conceptual models to nursing research it is imperative to clearly articulate how abstract concepts will be analyzed and evaluated within the study. This necessitates the preliminary step of operationalizing major concepts of the model. The process of operationalizing will continue to evolve to increasing levels of specificity in order for the model to become meaningful to practice. Operational definitions are an end point that enables precise analysis. By developing phase-specific protocols, the research team has begun the process of developing practical tools for nursing research and care delivery. The process of operationalizing the Corbin and Strauss Trajectory Model can help nurses grappling with similar challenges regardless of which conceptual model has been selected.

REFERENCES

Corbin, J. M., & Strauss, A. (1991). A nursing model for chronic illness management based upon the trajectory framework. *Scholarly Inquiry for Nursing Practice: An International Journal, 5*(3), 155–174.

Fawcett, J. (1989). *Analysis and evaluation of conceptual models of nursing* (2nd ed.). Philadelphia: F. A. Davis.

Folden, S. L. (1989). Caring for older homebound adults: A chronic illness perspective. *Journal Home Health Care Practice, 2*(1), 57–62.

Smeltzer, S. C. (1991). Use of the trajectory model of nursing in multiple sclerosis. *Scholarly Inquiry for Nursing Practice: An International Journal, 1*(3), 219–234.

Strauss, A. L., Corbin, J., Fagerhaugh, S., Glaser, B. G., Maines, D., Suczek, B., & Wiener, C. L. (1984). *Chronic illness and the quality of life* (2nd ed.). St. Louis: C. V. Mosby.

Strauss, A. L., & Glaser, B. G. (1975). Chronic illness and quality of life. St. Louis: C. V. Mosby.

Response

Juliet M. Corbin

When the article "A Nursing Model for Chronic Illness Management Based Upon the Trajectory Framework" was published (Corbin & Strauss 1991a, 1992), it was the hope of the authors that someone would perceive the potential of the model and take up the challenge to operationalize it. That is just what a team of nurse researchers from Thomas Jefferson University has done. Their process is described in the paper by Robinson and her coauthors.

Operationalizing an abstract model is not an easy task. One has to take a set of concepts, study them, discern their meaning, then devise a format for making the model usable, all the while staying true to the original intent. The eight "phase-specific protocols" developed by the researchers at Thomas Jefferson exemplify this process. This discussion will clarify and respond to some of the issues that were raised during the operationalizing process.

Someone asked at a recent meeting, why the term "trajectory"? Given the passage of time since the concept was first introduced (Glaser & Strauss, 1965), it is easier to discuss what the concept has currently become, than to explain where it came from. The aspect of trajectory that remains consistent throughout its developmental history is that the term was meant to refer to more than just an illness course.

Trajectory as Action

Action stands at the center of trajectory, action taken to manage illness within the context of actors' biographical and everyday living situations. Though fate, along with genetics and lifestyle, play a part in the development of chronic conditions, the meanings that persons give their illness, how they respond to the problems illness brings, plus the quality of their lives, are theirs to determine within limits imposed by personal and the larger political, social, and economic conditions.

Unlike the term acuity in reference to illness, which suggests short-term intervention, the notion of chronicity implies long-term management, an unfolding course of action that changes in response to changes in illness status. Since most of the work of managing illness goes on at "home," the responsibility for ongoing management rests mainly upon the shoulders of afflicted individuals and their families. Health professionals can play a supportive role in that management by providing persons with the information, technology, skills, and other resources that are necessary to carry out their trajectory work.

Assisting persons to manage at home, as well as caring for them during periods of hospitalization or when specialized care at home is necessary, opens the door to nursing because of the varied functions and roles encompassed within the profession. Nurses can move from hospital to home, can teach as well as provide direct service, and can care for individuals, families, and communities. Now, with the development of the "phase specific protocols," nurses have a tool to provide care tailored to the specific needs of the chronically ill and their families. Though it is possible to make the protocols more specific to each illness condition, this seems unnecessary unless a nurse works primarily with patients having one illness. Under these conditions, nurses can fit the protocols to their own practice. Keeping the protocols "generic" allows nurses to work with clients who have different illnesses and with those who have multiple chronic conditions.

Shaping Trajectory

Robinson and colleagues bring out the action aspect of trajectory with their emphasis on the "shaping" process. To clarify this term further, shaping was used in conjunction with trajectory to take the extreme form of fateful determinism out of illness. It denotes an "active agentry," or the interplay between fate and a person's ability to respond to conditions. Shaping in the actual management process takes the form of: preventing complications; carrying out regimens; handling disability by working out solutions to daily living problems; responding quickly to avert or handle a crisis; and carrying on with biography despite illness.

Trajectory Phasing

As expressed by Robinson and colleagues the notion of phasing is a very important one. Phasing gives management its preciseness. The phase-specific protocols included at the end of their paper make this very clear. It should be noted here that in the earlier article by Corbin and Strauss (1991a), the Comeback Phase (see Corbin & Strauss, 1988 & 1991b) was inadvertently omitted from the discussion on phases. This oversight probably explains why some authors who responded to the original article (Woog, 1991) had difficulty using the model to account for the "recovery" phenomenon seen with some chronic conditions. A protocol will have to be developed for this phase.

Biography

Since Robinson and colleagues use the term "baggage" in their discussion of biography, further clarification of the word seems called for to avoid any misunderstandings. As persons pass through life, they accumulate many experiences and develop both negative as well as positive habits that become part of their repertoire of behavior. These habits, along with a persons' desires, attitudes, and motives, influence their willingness to carry out regimens and the choices they ultimately make for managing both illness and life. As Robinson and her coauthors demonstrate with the case example, biographical knowledge can be very helpful in understanding patient behavior and in developing appropriate interventions.

Obtaining Biographical Information

Robinson and colleagues raise the issue that it might be difficult to obtain biographical information, especially from the elderly. To respond, some information is readily given, if *only* a nurse takes the time to ask. Other information, such as that which might be construed as discrediting to one's character, may be more difficult to elicit from a client. For instance, it is highly unlikely that in a first interview, a patient with COPD would readily admit to smoking. This type of information comes over time and with the development of trusting relationships. Since chronic conditions are long term and subject to periodic ups and downs, nurses are likely to encounter the same patients over again, as the chronically ill move between home and hospital, and in and out of clinics and/or doctors' offices. With repeated exposure comes the opportunity to establish trusting relationships and obtain information of a personal nature. Even the elderly are willing to give biographical information to nurses who are genuine and caring, who allow them the time to express their concerns, and who remain non-judgmental and accepting of clients' right to make choices.

Insights Gained

The most striking aspect of the operationalizing process, explained in by Robinson et al., is the insight the team from Thomas Jefferson gained as a result of their efforts. Most notable among the changes in their views of chronic illness are the following: (a) the "realization that chronically ill people have to cope with their illness challenges during every phase and across all care settings;" (b) the "deepened sensitivity to the struggle chronically ill people face;" (c) the increased awareness "of how traditional nursing education and clinical experience foster specialty care" and "tunnel vision," (d) the understanding that one nurse can't "do and know" everything about each phase; and (e) nurses can't force clients to make what they, as health professionals, view as the medically "correct choice."

Such changes come only when nurses are willing to "really" listen, thus are in touch with what the chronically ill are telling them. In essence, being sensitive is what the Trajectory Model is all about. By providing knowledge and understanding of what it means to be chronically ill, nurses will be encouraged to take the role of the other, to experience and feel what the chronically ill feel, while retaining enough professional distance to be effective practitioners. The issue is not whether nurses use this model or another, but that whatever model they choose, it brings them to a conscious awareness of the genuine problems faced by actual people living with chronic illness.

As Robinson and her colleagues state, work is still needed to operationalize the trajectory framework as a nursing model. Their eight "phase-specific protocols," however, are an important beginning. Even more relevant, in accepting the call to operationalize the Corbin and Strauss model, the team has undertaken an even greater challenge, that is, to provide nursing with the kinds of tools that it will need to meet the health care problems of the 21st century.

Chronic conditions are here to stay. With even greater life expectancy and technological developments, which will keep the chronically ill alive longer, radical changes are needed in the health care delivery system to accommodate and respond to the problems of chronic illness. Nurses can play a vital role in the development of new models of care. They can become central members of the caregiving team, because of their ability to provide quality and continuity of care, across cultures, age groups, and management settings—care that is both affordable and effectual. The paper by Robinson and colleagues illustrates what a group of highly motivated nurses with diverse clinical backgrounds can do to further that process.

REFERENCES

Corbin, J., & Strauss, A. (1988). *Unending work and care.* San Francisco: Jossey-Bass.
Corbin, J., & Strauss, A. (1991a). A nursing model for chronic illness management based upon the trajectory framework. *Scholarly Inquiry for Nursing Practice, 5*(3), 155–174.
Corbin, J., & Strauss, A. (1991b). Comeback: The process of overcoming disability. In G. Albretcht & J. Levy (Eds.), *Advances in medical sociology* (Vol. 1) (pp. 137–159). Greenwich, Connecticut: JAI Press.
Corbin, J., & Strauss, A. (1992). A nursing model for chronic illness management based upon the trajectory framework. In P. Woog (Ed.), *The chronic illness trajectory framework* (pp. 9–28). New York: Springer.
Glaser, B., & Strauss, A. (1965). *Awareness of dying.* Chicago: Aldine.
Woog, P. (Ed.). (1992). *The chronic illness trajectory framework.* New York: Springer.

Chapter 10

End-of-Life Family Decision-Making from Disclosure of HIV Through Bereavement

Barbara M. Stewart

OVERVIEW

End-of-life decision-making is conceptualized as the foreground against the background of a family, transitional model of illness with the human immunodeficiency virus (HIV). Both foreground and background represent new knowledge and theory development emerging from six research studies over a 7-year period. The research was phenomenological, longitudinal, ethnographic, descriptive, narrative, and grounded using the constant comparative method. In all, 100 families were studied in their home settings in the District of Columbia and 29 states across the United States. Throughout the transitional process from disclosure of HIV through bereavement, families engaged in end-of-life decision-making. Their decision-making style was primarily cognitive or primarily emotional or somewhere in between. Families using a cognitive style of decision-making were less disrupted and more able to surmount hurdles and move toward goals. Exemplars from 23 families illustrated family decision-making and components of the transitional, family model.

Note: Originally published in *Scholarly Inquiry for Nursing Practice: An International Journal*, Vol. 8, No. 4, 1994. New York: Springer Publishing Company.

INTRODUCTION

The human immunodeficiency virus (HIV) is the etiologic agent for a specific group of diseases or conditions known as acquired immunodeficiency syndrome (AIDS) and a pre-AIDS condition classified as AIDS-related complex (ARC) (Centers for Disease Control and Prevention, 1993). As Americans approach the 21st century, case fatality ratios as well as lack of prevention and cure distinguish HIV illness from most other end-stage illnesses. Moreover, HIV illness is unique because end-of-life family decision-making often occurs at the time of initial diagnosis of HIV seroconversion and disclosure within families.

In this chapter, end-of-life decision-making may be conceptualized as the foreground against the background of a family, transitional model of HIV illness. Both foreground and background represent new knowledge and theory development emerging from a series of research studies. Moreover, the substantive theory comprising the transitional model of HIV illness in the family supports prior findings with families facing cancer (Giacquinta, née Stewart, 1977).

Initially, the literature relevant to end-of-life family decision-making from disclosure of HIV through bereavement will be summarized. As part of the literature review, "family" will be defined and decision-making conceptualized as a major family coping strategy. Next I will chronicle my germane research studies from which the foreground and background emerged. The foreground and background model of HIV illness in the family will be briefly commented upon and then presented in table formats. By conceptually laying out the foreground and background, end-of-life family decision-making from disclosure of HIV through bereavement becomes clearer in the body of the article. Narrative exemplars from 23 families are provided to support family hurdles and goals of intervention within the model. Several of the same families will be portrayed in multiple phases of the transitional process. To protect the confidentiality of participants, names and identifying material have been changed in the exemplars.

Related Literature

Dating back to Freud's theory of individual developmental life stages, theorists have focused on intrastage individual or family behavior, and transitional theorists have described events and critical hurdles during or between transitions (Worthington, 1987). During end-of-life transitions, Kübler-Ross(1969) proposed a model of five stages through which dying persons proceed emotionally. Kavanaugh (1974) described a model of seven phases in an individual's bereavement process following a loved one's death. To identify concepts that emerged from families experiencing cancer, nursing research with observations in advanced nursing practice were combined (Giacquinta, née Stewart, 1977). A model of stages, phases, and hurdles was developed side by side with goals of nursing intervention to prevent or resolve crisis in living with cancer or restructuring in the living- dying interval, bereavement, and reestablishment.

Glaser and Strauss (1965) developed the concept of the dying trajectory, suggesting both a time-related and prognosis-related process. Clark, Curley, Hughes, and James (1988) identified objective and subjective factors influencing the dying trajectory of the AIDS patient. AIDS as a disease process is seen by Rolland (1984) as having transitional markers and phases. Disease transitional markers are characterized by prediagnosis symptoms, diagnosis of AIDS, initial adjustment, chronic long-haul, preterminal period, death, and mourning. The disease phases of AIDS are seen by Rolland as crisis, chronic, and terminal. According to him, the AIDS onset, course, incapacitation, and outcome contribute to family stress and crisis.

In the literature, families have been broadly defined by Walker (1991) as intimate networks that constitute the significant relationship contexts of persons with HIV infection, ARC, and AIDS. Thus, as defined in the literature and for the purpose of this article, families included homosexual or heterosexual couples, nuclear families, single-parent families, extended families or families of origin, and friendship networks of "buddies" or carepartners, or volunteers and friends who were providing care.

In traditional families, persons were joined together by bonds of marriage, blood, or adoption. Friedman (1986) provided definitions for various traditional family groups. The nuclear family was the family of marriage, parenthood, or procreation. The single-parent family was headed by one parent as a consequence of divorce, abandonment, or separation. Single-parent families included at least one child, who ranged in age from infant to adult. The family of origin was the family unit into which a person was born, and the extended family was made up of kin, such as grandparents, aunts, uncles, and cousins.

Families of choice were defined as variant forms of nonkin relationships, such as cohabitating couples, homosexual unions, and friendship networks providing care. "Variant" as a term avoided negative connotations and recognized the diversity of options available in society (Friedman, 1986).

After data collection and analysis were completed in a longitudinal series of research studies, I adapted family systems theory from the literature (Bowen, 1985; Guerin, 1976; Kerr & Bowen, 1988) and new theory and research in family stress (Burr & Klein, 1994) to theoretically advance understanding of family decision-making with the HIV virus stressor. As I see it, when HIV illness hits home, intense and dramatic family stress occurs. Stress signals that the family does not have the necessary coping strategies to handle the new stressor in ways that meet minimum standards in attaining individual and family goals (Burr & Klein, 1994). Coping strategies are used to help members manage, adapt, or deal with the family stress (Burr & Klein, 1994). A major coping strategy is family decision-making. It enables one or more family members to gain a sense of mastery or control, reducing stress in the living with an HIV stage and living-dying interval, and during bereavement.

Family decision-making has both cognitive and emotional aspects (Meyers, 1989; Wiens, 1993). Cognitive decision-making is rational and deliberative. Information is processed bit by bit; therefore, cognitive decision-making occurs over a period of time. In contrast, emotional decision-making is reactive. Responses occur or do not occur spontaneously, based on whether emotions are perceived or felt to be right or wrong, necessary or optional.

A family's cognitive strategies tend to change the least when stress occurs. The cognitive aspect of family decision-making, therefore, may be more insulated from stress than the emotional aspect (Burr & Klein, 1994). The family's emotional decision-making may be more volatile and the emotional climate of families with HIV illness may be described as a "roller coaster." Thus, under family stress, emotional decision-making may have the tendency to be disrupted the most readily and dramatically, while cognitive decision-making may have the least disruption or dramatic change.

Moreover, with or without stress, families may be differentiated along a continuum based on their capacity to distinguish between thoughts and feelings, and their ability to have thoughts rather than feelings guide their decision-making (Bower, 1985; Guerin, 1976; Kerr & Bowen, 1988). In turn, the degree to which families are able to distinguish between the cognitive and emotional aspects of their decision-making and are able to remain cognitive under stress may differentiate how successful they are in coping with the stress of the HIV life transitions.

Finally, three principles posed by Burr and Klein (1994) may direct thinking on how families may be helped to cope with stressful transitions: First, "if families focus on the unusual changes in their emotional systems during periods of family stress, then they will tend to cope more effectively" (p. 197). Second, if "they try to manage their negative emotions so they do not aggravate the stressful situation, it helps" (p. 198). Third, "positive feelings also help families cope with stressful situations" (p. 198).

Chronicle of Germane Research

My series of research studies is presented in Table 10.1. In November of 1986, I had unstructured conversations with gay and lesbian community leaders, AIDS crisis workers, clergy, and buddies or carepartners of AIDS patients. Several of these key informants provided entry to persons with AIDS (PWAs) and their families. By way of snowball sampling procedures (Polit & Hungler, 1978), nine families experiencing HIV illness were uncovered. With these families in their home settings, I conducted a phenomenological pilot study using the method developed by Colaizzi (1978).

One year later, I began a phenomenological study in the tristate New York area, using snowball sampling methods to obtain 15 families with a PWA. The nine pilot families were not included in the study. The purpose of the research was to describe family life with ARC and AIDS as family members experienced it. In accordance with the phenomenological method, presuppositions were bracketed (Oiler, 1982). Family members were asked "What is it like to have a family member with ARC or AIDS?" This initial open-ended question led to others. How do you interact with your loved one, once ARC or AIDS is disclosed? What are your resources? Has ARC or AIDS changed relationships in your family? How open is your family communication around lifestyle issues? How did you tell extended family and friends? What kind of social support, distance, or stigma did family and friends show? And, after the death of your PWA, how did your family grieve, use mourning rituals, and endure?

Because of the large number of families with HIV illness in the tristate area, it seemed that it would be easy to enlarge the number of families in the study. I couldn't have been more mistaken! Finding varied families was the greatest methodological problem. On average, four families were found each month through snowball sampling or by key informants. Because families were underground, I persisted with case finding beyond the usual number of subjects in a qualitative study. The sample grew from 15 to 59 families, not including the nine families used in the pilot study.

The 59 families were traditional and nontraditional with PWAs in all transmission categories of the disease. Exploratory interviews and then in-depth interviews were used in this phenomenological research project. Straightforward, processual, problem defining, comparative, triadic, sequential, and hypothetical questions (Fleuridas, Nelson, & Rosenthal, 1986; Palazzoli, Boscolo, Cecchin, & Prata, 1980; Penn, 1982) were used to fill openings provided by family members in individual and conjoint interviews. Parents, siblings, and then whole nuclear families were interviewed. These interviews lasted from 3 to 5 hours and all were audiotaped and transcribed verbatim. The seven steps outlined by Colaizzi were followed in the research process and audiotaped transcriptions were subjected to phenomenological analysis using his method (Colaizzi, 1978). From analysis of data, 3 categories, 10 themes, and 20 theme clusters emerged (see Table 10.2).

At the end of the first year in the field, methodological adjustments were made. I made the study longitudinal and gathered data from families at specific times. The periods of data collection were determined by the categories and themes. Significant themes occurred at the time of seroconversion, progression to ARC, when AIDS was diagnosed, during the chronic long haul, in the terminal period, and during bereavement. The process of fieldwork, methodological readjustments, and personal reactions were published after the first year in the field (Giacquinta, née Stewart, 1989).

After 15 months of the phenomenological study in which the analytic categories, themes, and theme clusters evolved, 20 of the 59 families provided direct access to witnessing their very private matters. Activities included sharing meals, driving and visiting extended family members' homes, admitting their loved ones to hospitals, visiting in hospitals, taking their loved ones home to die, waiting vigil at the bedside of dying PWAs, and planning or attending funerals, graveside anniversaries, or the Names Project quilt displays. The families who invited me to participate in their family life were well-functioning, as well as disorganized and chaotic. They lived in well-to-do neighborhoods and in impoverished communities hit hard by the AIDS epidemic.

With this subset of 20 out of the 59 families, the who, what, when, where, why, and how (Goetz & LeCompte, 1984) framework for partic-

TABLE 10.1 Germane Research

Time Design	Sample of 100 Families*	Phenomenon	Data Collection & Analysis	Method Reference
Pilot 11/86–10/87	Snowball 9 families	Experience of ARC/AIDS	Phenomenological	Colaizzi, 1978
Longitudinal 11/87–10/93	Snowball 59 families	Experience of HIV illness	Phenomenological	Colaizzi, 1978
Observation & interview 2/89–5/90	Critical case, 20 nested in 59 families	Experience of HIV illness	Ethnographic	Goetz & LeCompte, 1984; Bernard, 1988
Telephone interview 2-89–4-91	Same 59 families	Experience of HIV illness	Survey	Smith & Shamansky, 1983
Face-to-face interview 6-91–5-93	Critical case, 15 nested in 59 families	Experience of HIV illness	Life narratives	Riessman, 1993
Face-to-face Interview 6-93–8-93	Snowball theoretical & quota 41 families	Decision-making with HIV illness	Grounded theory	Glaser & Strauss, 1967

Note. *Total participants were 100 families, 59 in the tri-state area (samples of 20 and 15 were nested in these 59) and 41 were across the continental U.S., exclusive of the tri-state area. Distribution is found in Figure 10.1.

251

TABLE 10.2 A Transitional Model of HIV Illness in the Family

Categories Family Stage	Themes Family Phase	Theme-Clusters Family Hurdle	Theme-Clusters Family Goal
Living with HIV illness	Impact	Despair	Hope
	Disruption	Isolation	Cohesion
	Search for meaning	Vulnerability	Security
	Informing others	Retreat	Courage
	Engaging emotions	Helplessness	Problem-solving
The living-dying interval	Reorganization	Competition	Cooperation
	Framing memories	Anonymity	Identity
	Separation	Self-absorption	Intimacy
Bereavement	Mourning	Guilt	Relief
	Alignment of the social network	Alienation	Relatedness

ipant observation was applied. The method discussed by Bernard (1988) was also used. This ethnographic study enabled me to examine the themes and complex family processes and dynamics within the theme clusters of the phenomenological study. Twelve-hour periods of weekly intensive participant observation were spread out over several years. I recorded experiences as they were occurring or as soon as possible after they happened. Through dictation on the way home and transcription, I kept a separate personal field diary of my feelings and frame of mind during and immediately after each participant observation.

Within these field notes and diary were extensive side notes, identifying and labeling social relationships, activities, and behaviors. From participant observation, conversations, and interviews with families and key informants, I was able to validate interpretations and meanings. In most instances the key informants were part of the activities in which I was a participant observer. Therefore, this process of participation, observation, conversation, and interview with families and key informants enabled me to see if there were inconsistencies or contradictions between family accounts in the earlier interviews and what the key informants and I actually observed and experienced through participation and participant observation. Most important among these were the hurdles families faced and tracking how they were able to surmount them and achieve specific family goals. Coding and categorization of these data were checked with key informants. Analyses and interpretations were also referred back to them and checked with the 59 families in the sample.

Focus groups are an ideal way to determine if family members within a population of interest view a problem as do the investigators, share the same interpretation of the data, cross-validate research findings and theoretical notions, and find intervention goals consistent with their own needs and beliefs (Gross, Fogg, & Conrad, 1993). From November 1988 through May 1990, I co-led a weekly focus group of 11 HIV family members from the community. None of these members of the focus group was in the research sample. The members of the focus group, however, concurred with earlier data interpretations and communicated the necessity for mental health services that were consistent with the theory, data, and planned interventions in the evolving model.

As a way of further validating previous responses and quantifying patterns with numbers, I constructed a quantitative survey questionnaire. It contained 170 questions with fixed-choice answers obtained from interviewing the first 50 families in the phenomenological study. Between February 1989 through April 1991, the method outlined by Smith and Shamansky (1983) was used to collect data in a telephone, audiotaped survey with the 59 families.

In June 1991 through May 1993, I asked a different subset of 15 family members nested in the sample of 59 families to "tell the story" of their experiences with HIV illness and discovered an amazingly rich picture of the family's experience (Giacquinta, née Stewart, 1990). Riessman (1993) believes that the purpose of life narratives is "to see how respondents in interviews impose order on the flow of experience to make sense of events and actions in their lives" (p. 2). She notes that respondents often engage in storytelling when there has been a breach between ideal and real, or self and society. This life narrative study confirmed the order of themes and theme clusters that had evolved in the phenomenological and ethnographic studies.

Finally, in the last research study in this series, I engaged in face-to-face interviews with a snowball, theoretical, and quota sample of 41 families across the U.S. mainland. The purposes of this study were to describe the naturally occurring and unaided decision-making of families experiencing HIV illness and to develop empirical grounding for family decision-making with HIV illness. Audiotapes of the interviews were transcribed and the resulting data were sorted and coded according to the constant comparative method (Glaser & Strauss, 1967). Line-by-line analysis of the transcripts was used to look for indicators to describe the decision-making experiences of the subjects. Concepts were identified and named with a term that best described the data.

The inductive model that emerged from the above-mentioned six research studies was derived from multiple triangulation (Knafl & Breitmayer, 1989). Triangulation occurred across data sources (achieved by snowball, critical case, theoretical, and quota samples for the studies); data collection techniques (systemic questions, interviews, observations, a survey, and stories); time (over a 1- to 7-year period at times of comparable transitions); analytic techniques (qualitative and statistical); and subsystems of analysis (individuals, dyads or triads composed of parents, children, spouses, partners, lovers, grandparents, and families as a whole). In the combination of six research projects, 100 families were studied in their home settings in the District of Columbia and 29 states across the continental United States (see Figure 10.1). Characteristics of the participant families are shown in Table 10.3.

The Foreground: The Nature of Family Decision-Making

Throughout the transitional process from disclosure of HIV through bereavement, families engaged in end-of-life decision-making. The decision- making style of the family in transition may be plotted along a continuum from primarily cognitive under stress to primarily emotional under stress or somewhere in between. Families whose reactions to stress are mainly rational are cognitive decision-makers. These families deliberate and make decisions through various phases of family functioning. Their decision behavior and family change are stable. Their family climate is one in which stress is decreased. These families are less disrupted and more able to surmount hurdles and move toward goals.

On the other side of the continuum are the families whose reactions to stress are mainly reactive. These families are emotional decision-makers. They make decisions spontaneously. Their decision behavior and family change are volatile. Their family climate is one in which stress is increased. These families are more disrupted and fail to surmount the hurdles or move towards goals.

The data and description of the nature of families' experiences with HIV illness support the principles suggested by Burr and Klein (1994). If nurses and other health care professionals help families to recognize the difference between cognitive and emotional decision-making (see Table 10.4), and help them retain or regain a cognitive decision style, then

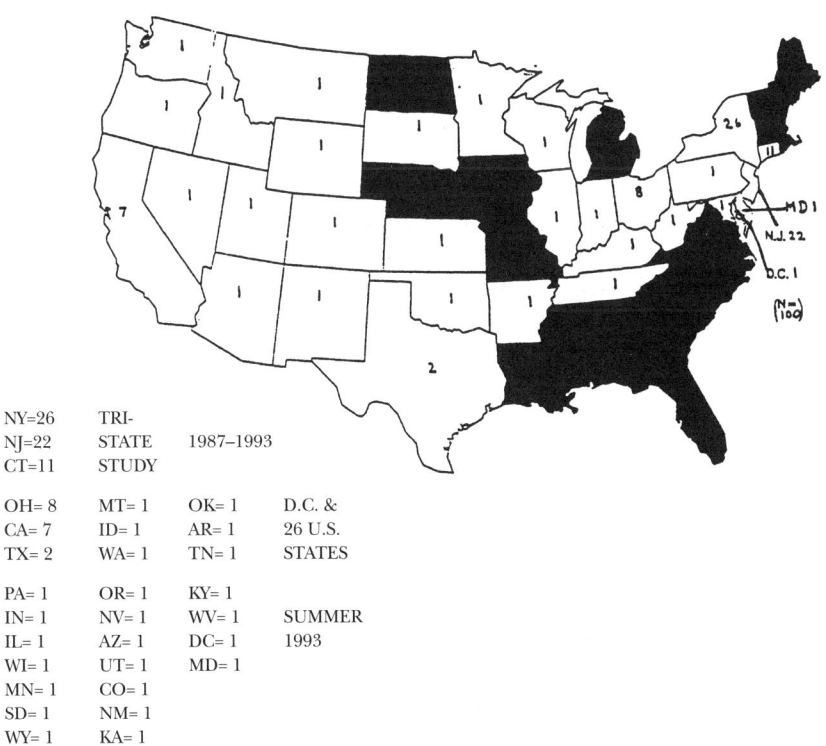

NY=26	TRI-		
NJ=22	STATE	1987–1993	
CT=11	STUDY		
OH= 8	MT= 1	OK= 1	D.C. &
CA= 7	ID= 1	AR= 1	26 U.S.
TX= 2	WA= 1	TN= 1	STATES
PA= 1	OR= 1	KY= 1	
IN= 1	NV= 1	WV= 1	SUMMER
IL= 1	AZ= 1	DC= 1	1993
WI= 1	UT= 1	MD= 1	
MN= 1	CO= 1		
SD= 1	NM= 1		
WY= 1	KA= 1		

FIGURE 10.1 Setting and sample for HIV studies.

families may cope more effectively. If the negative emotions inherent in the family hurdles are managed, the stressful situation will not be further aggravated. Finally, if nurses promote the positive characteristics inherent in family goals, then families may be further helped to cope with their experiences of HIV illness.

The Background: A Transitional Model of HIV Illness in the Family

It is hoped that presentation of a transitional model of HIV illness in the family may be utilized for identifying and meeting the needs of those in the epidemic of this generation. By way of this transitional model, nurses and other health professionals may obtain a theoretical basis for practice that is grounded in the lived experiences of families with HIV illness.

During the first stage, HIV-positive individuals or those with HIV illness received their diagnosis, but continued to carry out family roles. Within Stage I, a family may have undergone five phases: impact; disruption; search for meaning; informing others; and engaging emotions. Within each of these five phases are family hurdles, as well as family goals of intervention. In the body of this article, exemplars support these family hurdles and goals.

In Stage II, the living-dying interval, the PWA ceased to perform family roles and was cared for in a hospice, hospital, or home. Within this stage, the family may experience phases of reorganization, framing memories, and separation. Within the three family phases are family hurdles and family goals. Again, exemplars in the body of the article will illustrate these components of the model.

Stage III occurs with the death of the PWA. Mourning and alignment of the social network are the two family phases within this stage. Exemplars will convey the families' language within the hurdles of guilt and alienation and their experiences of trying to achieve the goals of relief and relatedness.

STAGE I: LIVING WITH HIV

Phase I: Impact

Impact occurs when family members learn that they have become HIV positive or when they are diagnosed with HIV illness. Shock and strain in this period can lead to emotional reactivity. Because hope cannot be

TABLE 10.3   Characteristics of 100 Participant Families

Race/Ethnicity	
White, not Hispanic	52%
Black, not Hispanic	38%
Hispanic	10%

Religious/Spiritual Preference	
Catholic	46%
Protestant	27%
Jewish	20%
Spiritual	5%
No Preference	2%

Reported Family Income Levels	
$1,000–$20,999	18%
$21,000–$40,999	17%
$41,000–$60,999	17%
$61,000–$80,999	19%
$81,000–$100,999	15%
$101,000–$200,999	8%
$201,000–$300,999	4%
$301,000–$400,999	2%

Risk Behavior/Exposure Category	HIV Study	U.S. Totals 9/93
Men who have sex with men	53%	55%
Injected drug use	26%	24%
Heterosexual	7%	7%
Men who have sex with men & injected drug use	6%	6%
Blood transfusion, blood components	4%	2%
Risk not identified	4%	5%
Hemophilia/coagulation disorder	0%	1%

Gender	
Female	23%
Male	77%

Type of Family	
Traditional	62%

TABLE 10.4 The Nature of Family Decision-Making

Family Decision Style	Reaction to Stress	Deliberation/ Change	Family Climate
Cognitive decision-making	Rational	Over time/ stable	Decreased stress
Emotional decision-making	Reactive	Spontaneous/ volatile	Increased stress

Family Decision Style	Family Disruption	Family Outcome
Cognitive decision-making	Less	Movement toward goals
Emotional decision-making	More	Unable to surmount hurdles

sustained without the support of significant others, it must be generated in the family (Giacquinta, née Stewart, 1977). When disclosures to families occur, in turn they experience impact. If families feel emotional despair, they make decisions emotionally, as though they have already received a notice of death. One female nurse, Judy, wrote this notation in her diary on the day she found out that she was HIV positive:

> To be told you have AIDS is a feeling only one who has experienced it can relate to. I don't think if God blessed me with 100 more years, I could describe the despair when I heard those words 'You have tested positive for the AIDS virus.' Having the virus and full-blown illness are two separate entities, but to the world there is no difference. I guess what's most frightening to me is that I myself cannot separate the two. I talk about it in terms of not actually being ill because of it, but I interpret it as a terminal state and see myself as a dying person. Getting a diagnosis of HIV was a hundred times worse than getting the diagnosis of cancer. I survived cancer, but this HIV is a fatal disease.

Because social support was necessary to foster hope and mediate coping with HIV infection, disclosure occurred within families. From almost immediately to several days before death, most HIV-positive individuals or those with HIV illness disclosed to their traditional families or families of choice. A newly wed wife who experienced an emotional impact from disclosure nevertheless responded cognitively to her husband by offering the possibility of hope. Her husband responded with emotional decision-making and despair:

> (Alice) My immediate reaction was Oh my God, despair. I had terrible fear of him dying. I wasn't afraid of catching it or if I had it. Those fears weren't real or there when we were told. I just said to Mike, 'Okay, we're in this together' and that's what I thought. I said, 'How can we survive this and beat the odds?'

> (Mike) Even though I had been completely drug free for 3 1/2 years, I said, 'We can't beat the odds. I'm going back to drugs. It doesn't matter because I'm going to die anyway.' It started through a prescription of 30 blue Valiums from a doctor, and 3 days later I was in the city with a needle in my arm. The Valium, for whatever reasons, makes you want to progress to the heroin and cocaine.

Although Mike made an emotional decision, Alice proceeded with cognitive decision-making. She said:

> For the first 9 or 10 months, all I did was research the disease. That's all I thought about. Sometimes he didn't want to hear it, but when he did, we'd have talks. I was doing all the research for him. I wanted him to get some hope. My purpose was to get him where I was, which was pretty peaceful, with the hope that everything was going to be all right.

Family members who were unable to find a shred of hope coped ineffectively. They could not retain a balance of cognition and emotion under stress. Rather than utilizing cognitive decision-making with their loved ones, such as finding information about the disease, they got stuck or engaged in emotional reactivity to stressors. This resulted in emotional imbalance for family members, who most often became angry. HIV- positive persons cognitively made decisions around arrangements for death, because they emotionally felt that there was no hope; and they were unable to reinforce family members who may have wanted to shift to a cognitive plan of action. One mother, Rosie, said:

I got in the car like you'd never believe. I drove like a maniac. I wanted to have a crash. I wanted to die. I felt the world came to an end. I was furious at the doctor for telling me while Carlos was in the room. If you're a doctor, I say, 'Use your mentality. Don't give a person a death sentence. Don't take away hope.' People always had called me 'Molly Brown.' You've heard of Molly Brown? I thought to myself, 'Molly Brown is sinking!'

My son was very sick and yet he had to make preparations immediately. We had to buy a cemetery plot. We had to make arrangements. We used to go to every cemetery. And, how much would it cost? It was gory and he was very morbid. Everything was dying, dying, dying. And I was very angry at Carlos because it was the first time I felt I failed. I couldn't get through to him. I kept saying 'Don't quit. I can't permit that. Okay now, let's fight it. You have a lot of fight in you. Come on now, let's fight it.'

Family members may have discovered their members' risk behaviors at the same time they learned of their HIV illnesses. Those members, who were reactive to these risk behaviors, made emotional decisions and had the most difficulty with cognitive decision-making. One brother, Marshall, confronted his brother and tried to coach him in dealing with their parents:

I went to my brother because it was very apparent that he was sick and he was gay. At first he denied both. Then he told me that he was bisexual. Then it was that he was bisexual with a preference for men. He was gradually moving over there and this was probably over a 6-month time period. It was probably when Jay had ARC that he told my mother about his gayness on the phone. I had urged him to tell both of them together because what happened was that my mother didn't tell my father for at least another year. My parents were really faced with a situation where they had never dealt with his lifestyle and then suddenly he was dying of AIDS. It was right after I'd come home for a weekend, probably 2 years into my knowing Jay was gay and 1 year into his being sick, and I vividly recall my mother saying to me, 'I don't understand, you knew that he was going to die, why did you let him?' It was as if I was in charge of the whole thing.

Family members may have blamed the individual with HIV illness. Caplan (1964) was the first to introduce the negative coping strategy called blaming. He proposed that blaming was a way of avoiding the truth and the problem. Although it may be an emotional decision-making strategy, it will make it harder for family members to emerge strengthened from crisis. Jay's father expressed the feelings of most others in the study:

> Why was he dying? He really did do it to himself. He could have lived to be in his 90s like his grandparents.

In despair, family members came to emotional conclusions that the family situations would have been worse if their loved ones were exposed to the HIV virus by other means. For instance, families having males who had sex with men as their risk behavior made emotional decisions that it would have been worse for the family if injecting drug use had been the risk behavior. Conversely, families whose members' risk behaviors were injecting drug use all agreed that the risk behavior category, men who have sex with men, would have been much worse for them to experience. These were decisions based on emotions. Family members used derogatory terms such as "junkies" or "fags" in describing people with risk behaviors. Sadly the stigma and ostracism expressed in over three fourths of the families mirrored the stigma and ostracism in society.

Only Mark's father, however, wished that another risk behavior had caused his son's illness. He said:

> I never knew Mark. If I said 'no,' Mark said 'yes.' If I said 'yes,' Mark said 'no.' All of his life, no matter what I said, he said the opposite. You know I always thought Mark was on a toboggan to kill himself. I blamed AIDS on his being gay. Taking drugs today is an accepted thing. Once you'd say he died of AIDS, people don't like that. I'd feel better if he did get it from the needle. People would accept it more. They will not accept the risk of being gay.

Interestingly, although all families were grappling with emotions, three fifths of the sample decided to cope by themselves, never knowing another family with HIV infection and never seeking individual counseling, psychotherapy, or community group services. They did not benefit from any services because they kept HIV illness a secret from the community. Even though individual and group support were sought by two fifths of the sample of families, they did not receive the hope for which they yearned. Hope would have enabled them to engage in cognitive decision-making.

Phase II: Disruption

Shock and despair in the first phase may have weakened family members' commitments to role obligations. Role dilemmas may occur. Time spent at hospitals may lead to role shifts. One mother who sought the services of a therapist cognitively decided to give up her work and daily routine because they interfered with the bond she wanted to create with her son. Mary Jane spoke of the closeness and cohesion that she and her son James were able to achieve:

> I made the decision that people don't always have the privilege of making. I chose to really get to know my son better in the 2 years that he had AIDS. Not that I didn't know him. I got to know his feelings, where he was coming from, and he got to know me, and how I felt. He told me things that I did as a mother that upset him, things I wasn't even aware of. We were able to talk about these things. To me this was a blessing. He could have died in a car crash and I would have never known how he felt about me. When he died there really wasn't much that we didn't know about each other. AIDS gave me more of an insight into what his feelings were about life in general and his philosophy of life and things like that. We were able to communicate together right up until his death.

Maria, a fiancée, made emotional and cognitive decisions in role changes and priorities:

> My life *had* to change. The first few months after Vinny's diagnosis of AIDS, he wouldn't touch me. He was afraid to touch me. He wouldn't hug me or kiss me and that hurt a lot. I still hugged and kissed him, but I no longer had the sensual feelings of being sexy or attractive or desired, none of that. That was the first confirmation that my life had changed. I wasn't a victim of AIDS. I just changed my roles and priorities. I abandoned my social life. There was nothing more that I could talk about with people. I abandoned my employment. I'm a godmother, and I haven't seen my

godchild in these 2 years that Vinny's been ill. I abandoned modern dancing, because when you're there, you have to be totally focused. I used to go twice a week. I went once after Vinny got sick, and it was disastrous! I had to leave, because I couldn't concentrate and let go. It was asking too much of myself. I abandoned planning for my future, travel, and vacations. I take 1 day at a time now. The more caregiving roles that I took on, the better it all worked. So my role changes and my priorities have been self-initiated at times.

Although disruptions were at times self-initiated and processed cognitively, Maria expressed the isolation that was insurmountable by some families:

I don't go out into the world now. The few times that I do, I feel plagued, too. Like there's something that has happened to me, that makes me different from everyone else, because my life is with a person with AIDS. When I am on the streets, nobody can see it on me, but I feel very much that I am this leper. I walk the streets, and I know I'm of this world, but not in this world.

Those who kept HIV illness and lifestyles a secret from their families remained isolated. Robert, who was bereaved over 5 years when interviewed, said that he wished his decision- making had been cognitive and his network cohesive:

I would have wanted more of a cohesive network supporting me. I wished my boss had said, 'Look, take the time you need, within reason.' José and I weren't totally abandoned like many are. He just didn't have family in this country, and my family wasn't very understanding. I wish I'd decided to be more outspoken with my family, saying 'Look mom, José is to me like your husband is to you. Dad, José is to me like mom is your wife. There's no piece of paper saying a, b, and c, but José means just as much to me as you two mean to each other. And if you can't give me some moral support and be kind, then don't do anything. Just let me alone and let me do it my way. If you can be more supportive that would be very nice. If not, I'll just wing it.' And knowing what I know now, with my boss, I would have probably said, 'I quit.' We'd live off whatever we could, but I'd be with José. Or I'd have taken a leave of absence or worked part-time if that could have been arranged. I wonder if there aren't a lot of other people out there who may be feeling the same way? I've never had anyone die on me. What do you do? I'm isolated from the rest of the world. Now, I'm a closeted widower.

Phase III: Search for Meaning

A search for meaning occurs because families try to acquire cognitive mastery over their emotions and family mortality. Family members who project blame to their loved ones for causing particular chronic or life-threatening illnesses, e.g., "he smoked too much" or "she never ate properly," have been found to reduce their emotional vulnerability, and increase their security that "out of the blue" this will never happen to another family member (Giacquinta, née Stewart, 1977, p. 1587). This phenomenon, however, exacts a severe emotional toll on the security of persons with HIV illness. Moreover, although blame may be projected to individuals because of "lifestyle" for instance, the search for meaning nonetheless brings a haunting, personal vulnerability to family members that *they* caused the illnesses. Jay's father shared the following:

> For our sake wouldn't it have been better if he was just walking the street and a stray bullet hit him, and that was the end of it. It's a tragedy and well, he didn't die of a communicable disease. I wouldn't blame myself. Now I feel I should have known all along. I don't know what I could have done. Maybe I could have been a more dominant parent and taken things into my own hands, and tried to straighten him out or something.

Jay's mother relayed her personal vulnerability and insecurity concerning her other two unmarried sons:

> Jay was a gifted child. He had an enormous IQ. He had the most wonderful SAT scores. He graduated with top honors. We were so proud. We were shocked. We used to think, where did we get this? He was unique and we just didn't know what the hell to do with him. To have a child like this, and to have him die at the age of 36, I decided it must be my fault. My guilt was that I wasn't intelligent enough or educated enough or knowledgeable enough to know how to handle this special human being.

> My husband and I are very grateful that we have two other sons. Without them, I think I would have gladly ended my life. If not for Richard and Ben, I would have gladly said, 'Goodbye world, I've had it!' The fact that our other two sons are not married bothers me very much. In fact, I was listening to somebody on the radio and I don't know how factual this is medically. He said that statistics have shown that if one member of a family is homosexual, it will carry to other siblings. I was having my breakfast, listening to the radio, drinking my coffee, and I got hysterical. I ran upstairs to my one son. He was getting dressed to go to work. Imagine the day he had! He said, 'Mom, don't worry, don't worry.' I was beside myself. I thought, 'Oh my God, no, not again.'

A mother whose HIV-positive son committed suicide said:

> I have feelings of guilt that maybe I gave birth to a child that ended up to be a homosexual. I have problems that I created it. See, it's my fault. This gayness caused his death.

Yet another mother who lost three sons to AIDS asked, "Do you think that my children are dying because God knows that I never wanted to be a mother?"

Emotional decision-making and reactive accusations by family members toward one another furthered the vulnerability of fragile family relationships. Rosie, who had been separated from her husband, could never forgive him or reconcile their marriage when her husband told her that their son's AIDS was her fault. She said:

> The father wasn't living with us at the time. I told him right away. When I told him he knelt down saying, 'Oh God, God, God, oh God.' But then he pointed at me and said, 'You, it's your fault!' And I said, 'Oh God, is it really my fault?' I never forgave him for that accusation.

One 80-year-old grandmother made the cognitive decision to experience her changing family rather than search for blame or a cause of the family's change. She said:

> My way of life is changing. When you're at your daughter's house and they have a happy birthday party to which 12 gays and their

partners have been invited, and I'm as natural as if they were my own blood relatives, I came home and I laughed my head off. What a changing world. I had such fun. That's how I feel about it!

Phase IV: Informing Others

Because of the stigma associated with HIV illness, persons often retreated from telling others inside and outside of the family. Judy lost her nursing job when she revealed her HIV seroconversion to her boss. Yet she received the courage from her priest in order to tell her children:

> Remembering the first thoughts after being told were those of rejection of my children, my friends, and ironically, even people I didn't know, the general population, came into mind. What would they think? This from a lady who never cared what insignificant others thought as long as I liked me. Maybe on another plane, I didn't like myself at that moment. Along with all of this, there's this nagging feeling to tell everyone who's ever touched my life. Why? Maybe to validate acceptance, testing true friends from strangers and most of all to seek the ultimate approval 'I'm okay, you're okay.' Then too, my feelings for family, friends, peers, and even enemies has always been upfront. To have lies goes against all I believe.
>
> When the priest came I said that I didn't know whether I should tell my children. I just couldn't stand losing them. If it came down to losing the rest of the world, I could take losing the rest of the world, but I couldn't take losing my children. I asked him, 'How do you live with telling your children?' The priest said, 'Count on that love from your children.'
>
> So I made the decision and called my daughter Nancy. I told her, 'I have something to tell you.' And I started to cry and she said, 'Mommy, my God, it's bad.' And I said, 'I'm sorry I have to tell you by phone, but if I don't tell you now, I don't know when I'll tell you or if I'll tell you. ' And I said, 'I had an AIDS test and it came back positive.'
>
> There was silence at first and then she cried. She said, 'Mom, I love you. And no matter what, you're my mother.' Her initial reaction was very courageous.

When I called my son Stan and he said, 'Oh my God, I drank from your glass and I ate from your dishes; Ma, can I get it?' I said, 'No Stan.' It was the most horrible feeling. It's like someone just cut out your heart. But I kind of expected it from Stan.

My daughter's reaction was nothing less than what I expected and hoped for. First, shock, but then her precious warmth, love, and ultimate loyalty were there as always. She makes being a mother easy. My son was unable to respond in the same way and it's strange, but he too reacted as I knew he would. Even in adversity, a mother knows her children.

Although Judy cognitively knew that her daughter would respond with courage and her son would retreat, she made the decision to tell both of them. The majority of family members, however, cognitively directed communication to only those whom they knew would give them courage, but in a third of these families there were surprises, resulting in emotional decision-making to cut off from family members who retreated:

Allen was coming home for Christmas, so I told my brother that Allen had just been diagnosed with AIDS. Now, my brother has come to my home every Christmas. We have always celebrated Christmas here, every year with the kids, his kids, my kids, and all my friends. And I wanted Allen to have a wonderful Christmas. He had just been through a lot and I had this big party planned. And my brother didn't come. He said he wasn't coming, nor his wife and kids. Then my brother did make one visit, before Allen went back to California, and that's when he had the talk with him that I hadn't known about because I wasn't here.

My brother gave Allen a lecture on God, and maybe if Allen didn't live his lifestyle, he wouldn't have AIDS. And Allen should change his ways and this kind of thing, which shocked me and made me really upset. My son felt terrible and so much hurt and anger with my brother that he never had anything to do with him again. And I've put space between my brother and me because of my love for my son and my hurt that my brother feels the way he does.

In this case, emotional decision-making by the brother, son, and mother resonated through the family. Emotional cutoffs occurred between the son and his uncle, and between the mother and her brother. There was multiple retreat in the family.

It was anticipated that retreat from family members might have occurred if particular members had been alive at the time of a loved one's disclosure of HIV infection. One grandmother stated:

> I was very delighted that my husband had died, because I don't think my husband would have accepted it—that Harry was gay. And AIDS and gayness kind of go together. I was glad that my husband was dead because I wouldn't have wanted him to hurt Harry's feelings. Neither would I have wanted to be torn between two sides.

Michelle, whose son Paul committed suicide when he learned that he was HIV positive, expressed this sentiment. "If my mother had been alive when Paul killed himself, my life would have been more hell than it is now, because it would have been 'poor her' instead of 'poor me.'"

Phase V: Engaging Emotions

From beginning to end, helplessness and ineffective coping were ever present in families with HIV illness. In all families there was a recursive emotional cycle, characterized by increasing helplessness, further retreat, vulnerability, isolation, and despair. Not one family found group support to enhance cognitive decision-making and coping with this resonating cycle. In fact, family members reported that attending community group sessions fostered great empathy for the helplessness of others, promoting further swells of their own helplessness.

Through examining family stress, Burr and Klein (1994) noted that "seeking community support has been a strategy that has been included in the literature since the beginnings of scholarly inquiry about family stress. Therefore, we expected it to be a very helpful set of strategies. Our data indicate that it is helpful to a majority but may not be as universally helpful as scholars have assumed" (p. 167).

If cognitive decision-making and problem-solving skills were taught to family members in community support sessions, they may have had greater ability to engage these skills and balance helplessness with cognitive problem-solving strategies for decreasing stress.

Emotions were volatile in families with HIV illness. When Ellen's son told her that he had AIDS, she projected her helplessness by blaming her son:

> I looked at him and I said, 'You bastard, you lousy rotten bastard, you're finally going to do it to me. You've been trying to do it to me as far back as I can remember, and you are going to kill me .And I went into the bathroom and I took a towel and I screamed. I didn't cry, I screamed. The despair came from my toes. And then later I went through the agonies of guilt. I decided that it wasn't right. Here he has got AIDS and he's going to die, and I'm calling him a bastard and worrying about myself going to die.

Sometimes emotions associated with AIDS led to family violence. A man named Essam spoke of his father's emotions:

> If my father could have killed my brother right then and there, he would have done it. My brother is an embarrassment to my father. My father is embarrassed because my brother is gay. My father is embarrassed because my brother has AIDS. When Hassim dies, my father has decided that he will not bury him in a cemetery around here. Even some doctor told my father that he could send my brother's remains to cemeteries upstate.

> My father *is* really sick in the head. Once or twice a week now, he goes through these rampages of abusing my mother and all of us and then blaming me for putting my brother in a hospital that's killing him.

Family helplessness and emotional decision-making went hand in hand. Some family members were unable to make a cognitive switch to problem-solving.

Family systems theory has offered an explanation for people who predominantly use emotion in their relationships with others. Guerin (1976), Bowen (1985), and Kerr and Bowen (1988) proposed that people with a higher level of differentiation, i.e., autonomy, were more able to retain cognitive functioning under stress. Conversely, persons with lower levels of differentiation, who were primarily relationship-oriented rather than self-oriented, processed events and situations affectively. In other words, those family members who were lower in their levels of autonomy and more relationship-oriented found the most difficulty in cognitive decision-making and problem-solving. With cluster stress and multiple intense stressful life events, however, even more highly differentiated family members may get engaged in emotional decision-making.

Multiple stressful life events have been found to precede or occur along with the AIDS crisis (Giacquinta, née Stewart, 1989). In one family with cluster stress, the father spoke of his inability to make cognitive decisions. Being primarily emotional in his decision-making process, he was unable to think of a way to respond to his son:

> What is most debilitating for me is that I have no solutions for any of Mark's problems. I don't have any control over any of what happens to Mark. My main problem has always been, 'Am I approaching this right for Mark's sake, not for my sake? Am I doing the right things? Am I acting right?' These are my main concerns. I've never been sure of how I should be responding. It is like you're walking on ice. I'll tell you right now, you don't know if you're doing right or you're doing wrong. I feel if I'm doing wrong, I'd rather play act it and do it right. I'd rather make one decision and know I was doing right by the boy.

STAGE II: THE LIVING-DYING INTERVAL

Phase VI: Reorganization

Reorganization of the family is needed to overcome role strain or to equalize tasks while a family member is very seriously ill with AIDS. Overfunctioning may lead to family conflict and competition. Cognitive decision-making may bring about a sense of cooperation among family members to ensure that family goals are met and overresponsibility by some members is relieved.

Jeff's mother Sharon, and her son's male partner, Dana, overcame competition for Jeff's love, and worked together cognitively as a cooperative team for about a year. The mother reported:

> When Jeff got AIDS real bad, I remember Dana coming in the hospital and asking, 'Would it be okay when Jeff gets out of the hospital if I come to visit you at home?' And I said, 'By all means you can come.' I valued the time I had left with Jeff. That's why I

made the decision to stop working so I could spend my time with Jeff, but Jeff doesn't know that. I didn't want him to feel that I stopped working, waiting for him to die. I stopped work so I could be here for his lunches and be available to him whenever. And I was making the time for me to help him.

Jeff's lover, Dana, and I worked together and decided who would do what. We worked it out so I take care of all of Jeff's medical forms, I help him take his medicines, and I take the car away from him when he's too weak. So I do all the driving for them. When Jeff was real bad one time, he wouldn't let me in the room. He'd only let Dana in. I decided to go into his room the next day and I cried and said, 'Don't shut me out because I'm hurting just as much as Dana is.' And after that Jeff didn't shut me out anymore. Not long after that, however, Dana took a new lover and walked out on Jeff.

Sharon relayed that she and her son's partner, Dana, both responded cognitively, when they worked together cooperatively and reorganized tasks so that neither was overburdened. Further, she stated that she and Dana made emotional decisions and became competitive when she said that she was hurting as much as Dana, and when Dana left to take a new lover because he was unable to share Jeff with Sharon.

Cooperation occurred rarely between a family of choice with HIV illness and all members of related extended families. Sara, a mother whose son was the partner of his significant other with AIDS, shared her story:

Christopher's parents were in the state of Idaho, my son David and Chris lived together in Texas, and my husband and I were residents of Connecticut. When Chris fell ill it was a natural thing that David would take care of him. I'm not sure if they ever discussed it. Probably there wasn't any decision made at all. They lived together, Chris took ill, and David cared for him. I think it was just such a natural thing, like between my husband and me. If he took ill I would take care of him. And, I think that's exactly how it was with David and Chris.

David had every Christmas with Chris's family. And even toward the very end they didn't think Chris would be well enough to travel the following year, so this would be his last Christmas, and next year Christmas, there were Chris and David back home again with Chris's parents! It was even in Chris' sister's eulogy that he just had such fight in him that each time he came home, they thought maybe this would be the last time he'd be able to make the trip, but turn around for his birthday or Christmas, he and David were there once again.

Chris surprised everyone, but he was so surrounded by love. David also had one of their best friends, a nurse, who was there for everything and she made it easier for David to take care of Christopher at home. They had an amazing network of friends. Everyone worked together. Chris's sister visited their home in Texas quite often. I went out for a week when Chris first took ill to help David take care of him. Before that my husband and I went out when Chris was still feeling fine. Then David gave a surprise party for Chris and I flew to Texas to surprise David. It was like a double surprise. David, the nurse, and one of Chris's best friends were constantly with him near the end, plus they had a handful of friends that stayed in their house so David was not alone if something happened during the night. Someone always made sure that he would always be there with David. David took the whole year off from his job and cared for Chris full-time that last year. Chris actually had AIDS for 5 years, but he traveled, did everything, and worked. And, David knew that whenever Chris wanted to go home and was able to make the trip, he'd find a way to get him there.

And David, of course, would always go with him. In fact, David wasn't home here with us for 5 years for Christmas because it was important for David to be with Chris and Chris's family. And we thought it was important for David to be with Chris and Chris's family. We knew this was where David wanted to be. We knew how much he loved Christopher. We've always given our sons' wishes a high priority. Our sons have their lives, we have ours, and whatever they want to do is fine with us, as long as they're happy. My husband and I have a very wonderful marriage. He's a wonderful man. If David had been ill with AIDS and Chris was his partner, my husband and I would still have let David and Chris be the decision-makers. I'd have to know from David that that was what he wanted. If David said, 'I want to stay in Texas and have Chris care for me,' then my husband and I would have no question that we'd support his decision. We'd just visit as often as they wanted.

There's a lot of sadness and pain with AIDS. But Chris was surrounded with love. His family was as loving as could be, and we were behind whatever our son wanted. We tried to give him all our support, and he's let us know we were there for him. He was very happy with our responses toward them and Chris's family.

Phase VII: Framing Memories

In this phase, slightly over two fifths of the families strengthened remembrances of their loved ones' lives and created additional memories for recollection after their deaths. Sharon made an emotional, reactive decision to go along with her son Jeff's wishes, because he had been jilted by his male partner. She made cognitive decisions, however, by learning to drive, mapping out a journey, and braving her husband's fury, so Jeff could shoot the rapids. She relayed the following:

> I thought of all the times when Jeff wanted us to do things with him and remembered how furious my husband always got. We had a camper and I didn't know how to drive it. And Jeff wanted to run the rapids in Wyoming in a kayak for 8 days. Since I've learned that my husband was always going to be mad anyway, I took the camper and drove Jeff all the way to Wyoming. Now I can say 'Thank God that I did that before Jeff died.' Those are my memories now. That's how I'll always see Jeff, so brave and strong.

In this case both cognitive and emotional decision-making established an identity for both mother and son, reflected in the metaphor of a mother and son's journey together and the son's courage to ride the swift currents and dangers of his life's path.

Families' memories may have been framed in special conversations with their loved ones. A father gave this account:

> I spent 3 days in New York at a convention. I took the opportunity because it was a good time for us to talk. I wanted to say a lot of things that I hadn't ever said to him. I told him how much I cared for him and loved him. Even though he drove me crazy, I never

stopped loving him. I wanted him to know that I finally accepted his way of life, because I never told him that in words. And I told him that I wished he'd shared his situation with me earlier so I could have been there for him longer. His keeping it a secret was a burden that he had to share alone and it really wasn't necessary. I wanted him to know he could have told me.

And I guess I said more in those 3 days than I would have said otherwise, because I felt that he was cheated because he feared my rejection. I also knew, perhaps not consciously, that I wouldn't have him much longer.

In Contrast, Jay's mother lamented that she never chose to have a conversation with her son:

Because we didn't talk about his dying, I keep thinking to myself, 'I just wish I had him back so that we could hug and kiss and say goodbye.' We never said goodbye. We faked the whole thing. We fooled each other. We fooled no one. I think I would have rather been able to say goodbye with a hug and our crying together. I don't know, maybe that would have been more devastating for me to live with. I just feel there was no ending, no finish. We played a game and lost. Yet, he never took the lead. I waited for him to say something. And, he never said, 'Ma, I'm dying.'

In another way, a traditional family together with a family of choice selected an activity that enabled their PWA's memory to live on through others in the future. Sara, her husband, David, Chris, and their network of loving friends created a living memorial by making a garden. Sara told of this decision:

Christopher had such love of a garden. All of us actually decided to make a garden in his name while he was still alive. It was made from all the donations from his friends. We chose to make it at an AIDS hospice in Houston. It was absolutely beautiful.

Three mothers individually decided to start community groups for others having HIV-infected family members. One mother described her decision-making:

I made a promise to Carl. We were in the hospital as we were for many, many days. He was in one of his more grouchy moods. He said, 'Mother, leave me alone. That's enough. Why don't you go out and do something to help people with AIDS?' My first reaction was 'What the hell do you think I'm doing? I'm here with you.' But I knew he was serious. Even though he was angry I said, 'I will, but please not now. Don't push me now.' Carl said, 'I think you should be out doing something for people with AIDS. In other words stop hovering over me. Leave me alone.' He just looked at me and I looked at him and said, 'I made you a promise.'

We never discussed it. But he set me up as he always did as a kid. He was the one who could put me in motion. Every once in a while now I talk to his picture, 'Alright, what are you going to do for me now? Now you got me in the middle of this.' I'm really not sorry I started it, because I get as much out of the AIDS group as everyone does, knowing that these people have someplace to go. As a group we were trying to find a name for the group. I was taking his initials. I had dictionaries out. We were working and working and there was nothing that we came up with that was appropriate. And then one group member, a sister of a young man who was carrying the virus, said, 'Why not call the group "The Promise"? You did make a promise to your son and that's why we're here.' And that was it. I went after all of my friends, the journalism majors, and my goddaughter, we got a blurb saying what "The Promise" was, and a community group to print it for us.

In this phase, the greatest fear of the two fifths of families who decided to accept and join with their PWAs were that memories would fade too soon. Anonymity was a severe threat for these families. On the other hand, for slightly less than one tenth of families who rejected their PWAs, memories couldn't fade soon enough and anonymity was a blessing. For about half of the families in between, the majority of members made cognitive decisions to engage a strategy called thought-stopping to block out recollections of their loved ones. Their emotional pain tied to remembering was too great.

Phase VIII: Separation

This eighth family phase coincided with the time when the PWA's consciousness diminished and awareness of the family faded. At this time family members experienced the loss and loneliness of separation from their loved one. Self-preoccupation with gearing up for the separation and getting through the loved one's death were paramount in this phase. Only a handful of families were able to achieve final family intimacy and complete all unfinished business.

Sharon shared her inability to remain cognitive under the emotional strain of her son Jeff's grief, goodbyes, and gifts:

> Jeff only said once that he was dying. He called us from the apartment and wanted us to come up. He had all of his worldly possessions in piles for each of us. And he stood there crying and sobbing as he explained to us that he was dying. He wanted us to have all of his things. We decided to tell him to put his things away for now. We specifically said that he wasn't going to die now.

> I wish I could remember those things that he separated. He had every closet and every drawer emptied in the apartment. You couldn't move in it with all the piles. And he had all of his papers out. He said that he wanted me there because he wanted to give me instructions on how to give all this stuff out. He told me all about his will. I kept saying to him, 'Oh Jeff, put that away. We don't need it.' Nobody else in the family said anything. I should have let him get it all out, but I kept hushing it. He was telling us all the things that a mother just does not want to hear.

A male partner, Robert, discovered that his lover José wrote a plea to finalize this period. Robert spoke of what decisions he would have made if he knew then what he currently knew:

> When they took José down to the intensive care unit, I found on the bedside table a piece of paper with some scribbling on it in Spanish. I looked at it and couldn't understand what it was, so I saved it. And to everyone who spoke Spanish I'd say, 'What is this?' I eventually found out what he wrote, just before they put him on the respirator. The words he wrote meant basically, 'What are we waiting for?' What he was trying to say was, 'What are we waiting

for, let's get this over with. Let's not do any of this stuff with the respirator.'

I should have stopped them putting him on the respirator because it didn't do a damn bit of good. All the tubes and all that crap. I couldn't talk to him and he was on morphine. I'd pull his eyelids open to look at him. I talked and talked to him and his eyes were closed all the time. He couldn't squeeze my hand—nothing. So I slept in the waiting room.

The nurse came in about two o'clock and told me to come in. They were pounding on José's chest, trying to resuscitate him. There were still vital signs, so I stood there and talked to him. The signs on the monitor started to level off and they took a hyperdermic end put it in. And I said, 'Don't do that please.' And the nurse said that he had to. The graph started popping up again. I leaned over and said, 'Go to sleep' and his heart stopped. And they turned off the respirator. That was it.

If I knew then, what I know today, I'd have kept the respirator away and all the gowns, masks, and everything else. I would have just loved to take off all that garb and gotten into the bed and held him in my arms and talked to him.

A mother who signed a Do Not Resuscitate form told of her personal conflict in making this decision:

He was dying and I was watching the breath stopping and starting and stopping and I could not cry. The doctor came to me and said, 'You have to sign a paper.' He said that the paper stated that no extra means would be taken to keep him alive. I remembered that my son had told the doctor first thing, 'I'm telling you in front of my lover and my mother, I don't want to be put on a respirator. If you know you have a medicine that's going to bring me back, fine, but no code.'

Signing was the time that was most difficult for me. Not knowing if it was really right. I was doing what my son wished, but I didn't know if it was really the right thing to do in the religious sense. My son's sister and his lover were very upset to find out that I had to sign that paper because they had already written and signed that they knew that this is what my son wanted. The doctor chose not to accept this, however. He said that the hospital said it wasn't good enough. I, as my son's closest relative, had to sign the form.

A woman named Donna, whose husband oriented himself to the gay lifestyle while they were married, divorced her husband. Yet, in her own words, she could not let him die alone (Giacquinta, née Stewart, 1990). She shared her decision-making dilemma. It vacillated between her own emotional self-absorption, the "truth," and the information and intimacy she wanted to convey to her ex-husband:

> I tried to hold him in my arms. At a moment like this, you don't have time to plan what to do. I said to myself, 'This is the last thing he's going to hear. Tell him that you love him. That is what he needs to know before he goes.' Then I corrected myself, 'I can't tell him I love him because I don't love him anymore.' But then I thought of a way around that, 'Tell him that you care a lot about him. Let him hear that.' But I realized, 'If I tell him that I care about him, he will know I'm saying that because I'm unable to say that I love him. You don't want him to know that.' It sounds crazy to have such a dilemma.

> But finally I said to him, 'Glen, it's Donna. I love you.' And I held him in my arms, repeating who I was, and that I loved him. And I was so glad he didn't have to die alone. Although afterwards, I felt guilty for telling him what he needed to hear at the moment of his death, rather than telling him the absolute truth.

Michelle's son Paul took the act of separation into his own hands by committing suicide. Michelle spoke about her son's decision and the self-absorption that she experienced. During separation, she continually reviewed her thoughts and feelings:

> Paul found my mother's bag of medicines in my drawer and decided to take all the Darvon. He wrote a note to me, the young man he was seeing, his roommates, my girlfriend whom he called 'auntie,' and one 'to whom it may concern' about what he wanted to be buried in. He'd already had something in him when he wrote because there were misspelled words. Maybe I wanted him to say

more to me. He didn't say that much. He said 'I hope you understand. I tried to be strong and I couldn't. I'll be with people who love me, nanny and Alfredo. Please have a mass said for Alfredo on November 19th.' And he said, 'Love you,' and signed it, 'Your Paul.'

I gave everyone Paul's notes, but they didn't say anything to me. It surprised me that he didn't write to his middle brother, because they had started to get very friendly. But I think he intended to write more and the pills got to him. They never told me how many Darvon he took, but I found out that he crushed the pills and put them in alcohol.

At the time of Paul's death, I thought it was unfair that they wouldn't let me see him. But if you remember, it was an extremely hot summer. Paul never liked air conditioning and it wasn't on in here for 2 days. And he was dead in the bathroom with no window open. They said there was a great deal of decomposure. And the policeman said, 'No mother should see her child like that.' I had a very hard time. I wanted to come in and see my son. But they wouldn't let me and when he got to the funeral parlor, I begged them to at least have a viewing and the medical examiner said, 'No, there was too much decomposure.' You have mixed feelings. I felt very robbed not to see him and hold him. And yet, at other times I say, because he was always so meticulous and wouldn't go out without a shower, if I saw him maybe looking so terrible, maybe I would never be able to get that out of my head. Which is worse, the reality or the fantasy? I don't know. When he was viewed it was a closed casket, and he wasn't in the casket. I didn't tell too many people that. I think that's the only way I got through it, knowing he really wasn't in that casket. They wouldn't allow him to be put in the casket because he could not be embalmed due to so much decomposure. So Paul was not in the casket. He was downstairs. When the service was over, he was put in the casket. I say that's how I got through the service.

A mother, Mary Jane, told of the intimacy that she achieved with her son Thomas right up until his death:

I was sitting next to Tommy and he was cold and taking these deep breaths. AU he had was his oxygen because the doctor had stopped the medication. It wasn't doing him any good and it was just prolonging the agony. And Tommy kept taking these deep breaths and his eyes were open. It was from about 12 o'clock at night until 3 in the morning, and I thought he was sleeping. But he must have been in a coma. I didn't know if he could hear. I don't know because I saw that struggle he was having to get air and I saw his eyes. But I made the decision to talk with him. I said, 'Tommy, please, in God's name stop fighting. Don't fight anymore, Tommy. Tommy, please let go.' And tears ran down his cheeks, like he couldn't respond to me orally or even physically. Or, it was just in the part of the dying process when he was losing the fluids from his body. I don't know, but tears ran down his cheeks. And then I said, 'You put up a great battle. You did so much and you helped so many people.' And I just turned my head a little and I turned back again and saw him take his last breath. And I thanked God. I couldn't watch him struggle like that. I was glad I was there because it made the dying real for me.

STAGE III: BEREAVEMENT

Phase IX: Mourning

Relief for family members occurred through mourning rituals. The Scattering of ashes and the Names Project quilt provided a mourning ritual for one fifth of the families. Robert shared his decision-making with his lover José and José's family:

> After José died, his family and me had decided that he was to be cremated. I brought the ashes home and put them on the fireplace. I had some people up and we just had wine and cheese and sat around and talked. The next morning I flew to José's homeland with his ashes. Before José had died, he spoke to me of his death and said, 'Baby, when I die, I want my body burned and you take my ashes back to my country and put me near my mother.' His mother was buried there and he wanted to be in the plot next to her. So I carried out his wishes. But because he was not buried here, I was alone with nothing but tears and constant sobbing. I really thought the only solution was suicide. On the fifth anniver-

sary of José's death, I thought to myself, 'God almighty am I going to make it?'

So I called a hotline and went down. It was there that I decided to make the quilt. I had written a poem shortly after José died and I had it laminated and tied to the quilt. I got a little bag, a thing that I made, with drawstrings. And it has some very special things in it that mean things to José and me. The quilt is a substitute for a grave because he's not buried here. I have one strip on the quilt that says, 'I loved you more than you knew and you loved me more than I deserved.'

In this Case, Robert gained some relief from his guilt by engaging in this very special mourning ritual.

Sara's nuclear and extended family, her son David, and his family of choice worked together and contributed to the Names Project quilt:

My husband and I made a panel for Christopher, which is part of the huge Names Project quilt. We went to Washington last year with it. It was very healing for us. My husband had taken me to all the stores for the fabric. He picked out the paints and flowers. He even ironed them on. We had gone shopping together. We picked out each other's flowers. And since we made it all flowers we asked everyone in our family to make a flower, because they had known of Christopher's love of a garden. And so we asked all of our family, my husband's family, and my side of the family. Everyone made a flower. Some of them crocheted them. My mother crocheted and my sister-in-law made one out of crewel. There were 18 flowers. Every person knew in the family and every person made a flower. We all put it together. And David made one for Christopher and one for each of his six very dear friends and we shipped it out.

And they put the eight panels together in one piece. They are all together. Our panel was next to the one David made for Christopher, and the six friends of David and Christopher are right there in the same piece.

Designing or selecting the inscription of a tombstone or carrying out the wishes of the deceased provided a mourning ritual for some. Several families did what they wanted, rather than what their loved ones had instructed them to do. For instance, while alive, one husband who was a church deacon refused to disclose his risk behavior to his wife, who consumed alcohol to cloud her suspicion of his bisexuality. She, however, seized control when it came to designing his tombstone:

> I was thinking about my husband's tombstone and said to myself, 'Well, you're not going to get your broken obelisk.' My husband wanted that on his tombstone because he wasn't completing his full potential. But we have symbol in the diocese. It's a special cross that had a double meaning. The bishop introduced my husband to the cross, saying that it was the cross with the shroud of Christ wrapped around it. But my husband knew it as the Greek wedding cross, which is the symbol of unending love. For many years my husband had it on all of his fishing lures, because fishing was his unending love. So rather than giving him the broken obelisk on his tombstone, I chose to symbolize our marriage by putting the Greek wedding cross on it. I explained to the bishop that this symbol was for married clergy.

Michelle spoke of the *inability to make decisions* in the mourning phase after her son committed suicide and she found his notes:

> My middle son tried to reach out. When I say reach out, he was here and he helped me with everything. I couldn't even write a check. I just signed my name. I couldn't write anything. I said, 'You know it's too bad when a crisis like this happens, that a person who isn't emotionally involved can't step in.' You don't know what you're doing. I mean I bought three graves. I put my ex-husband's name on the tombstone. You could have talked me into anything at that point. I didn't know what the hell I was doing. Does it now mean that I have to bury my ex-husband when he dies?

Mourning is as unique as the relationship that has been severed. Donna, ex-wife of Glen, and her four children discussed their decision-making in creating a mourning ritual (Giacquinta, née Stewart, 1990):

> Glen wanted to be cremated and he did not want any kind of a service. I realized after he died, the people who were living needed a sense of closure. In a sense, we evolved our own ritual to bring relief and closure. First, I talked to the kids about having a memorial ser-

vice and they did not want that. And we were thinking about what Daddy would want, that kind of thing. And I did not want the ashes to be around. I wanted something to happen to them.

Cape Cod was a very special place for all of us for different reasons. And so we decided that we would go to Cape Cod and go on a whaling boat. Even though it's against the law, when they got out to sea, we'd just put the ashes over. Then Glen Jr., who had such mixed feelings about his dad, decided that he wanted to make a boat for his dad, to put the ashes in. My son Glen has a way of incredibly dragging things out and never finishing things and the rest of us needed to finish it.

And Glen Jr. made this magnificent Viking boat. He carved it out of wood—maybe 3 or 4 feet long. He went and got a special piece of wood from a house that we had lived in. He went in the back yard of this house and cut down a tree that we had planted when they were little. He would have gotten arrested because someone else owns the house now. We made a sail and divided it into sections. Each one of us drew something on it that was kind of special. I told the kids, if they had anything special that they wanted to put in the boat, that they could—I mean besides the ashes. It was interesting how it evolved and turned into a ritual, even though it didn't start out that way.

I had taken my ex-husband's adopted mother's beautiful embroidery pillowcase and put the ashes in that. My older daughter put a picture of herself in. I put rose petals in the boat for a special reason. Sandy wrote him a goodbye letter and put it in. Then we brought the boat up to his favorite beach. I just wanted to float it. Glen Jr. said he didn't want it washing back on shore, so he soaked it with gasoline. He took it way out and set it afire. That was the finish we needed. It was kind of weird. I was thinking, 'Oh my God it's a pagan thing. I'll go to hell forever!' But it made me realize that you do need some formal kind of closure, and for us that did it.

Phase X: Alignment of the Social Network

This final family phase may occur after the completion of mourning. Family members bereaved from AIDS have a shadow grief that never leaves them. If family members become alienated from others, whether by making decisions to exclude or to distance themselves from stigma in society, this grief never leaves them. Grief cannot become less devastating following bereavement if it is unexpressed, unshared, and is not worked through in the presence of caring others.

The AIDS epidemic has created two kinds of families who have experienced HIV illness in the family. One group of families is completely disconnected and alienated. The other group is so related and connected to AIDS in the U.S. or to PWAs that every death is felt, experienced, and added to the "till." These family members suffer for every AIDS loss they learn about—past, present, and future.

In overcoming feelings of alienation, family members must relate to their changing identity. As families expand their social networks, they accept that death in the family was inevitable, but not insurmountable (Giacquinta, née Stewart, 1977).

Robert, who considered suicide on the fifth anniversary of José's death, spoke of needing relatedness:

> I didn't have anything to do with gay life. But when I called the hotline and went down, I started getting deeply involved, heavily involved, sleeping at the Center, and working on the newsletter. It was great. I made some friends. People paid attention to me. A couple of times I needed a shoulder and it was there.
>
> I asked myself, 'Should I get a Buddy? Really should I get a Buddy, or should I stop working with AIDS?' I made the decision to get a couple of buddies who had absolutely nobody at all. That just furthered my need to see somebody through to the end, the right way.

Metaphorically, Robert made the decision to complete the transitional process "the right way."

CONCLUSIONS

This chapter presents the view that end-of-life family decision-making occurs at the outset of HIV seroconversion and disclosure within families. Through qualitative and quantitative methods and exploratory research aimed at identification, description, and explanation-generation (Crabtree & Miller, 1992), a transitional model of HIV illness in the family is used to direct thinking about how families cope with stressful transitions and to further explicate for nursing practice the three principles posed by Burr and Klein (1994).

There is always difficulty in proposing a model that may be misunderstood as stereotyping and reducing the complexity and uniqueness of family life. Rather, it is hoped that this model, along with the conceptual ideas, adds new insights to the literature about end-of-life family decision-making, and provides further questions for subsequent nursing research.

Understanding the experience of living with HIV illness, the living-dying interval, and family bereavement are primary foci for nursing research. Larson and Ropka (1991) state "there is a continued gap in the research literature related to the care aspects of HIV infection. This gap needs to be filled by nursing investigation" (p. 4). Provision of a transition model may be valuable, according to Murphy (1990), because "to the extent that transitions are anticipatory, preparation for role change and prevention of negative effects can be instituted" (p. 344). Therefore, the model's usefulness may relate not only to scholarly inquiry, but also provide directions for nursing assessment, diagnosis, intervention, and evaluation of individuals and families as they attempt hurdles and progress through HIV illness.

REFERENCES

Bernard, H. (1988). *Research methods in cultural anthropology.* Newbury Park, CA: Sage Publications.
Bowen, M. (1985). *Family therapy in clinical practice.* New York: Jason Aronson.
Burr, W., Klein, S., & Associates. (1994). *Reexamining family stress: New theory and research.* Thousand Oaks, CA: Sage Publications.
Caplan, G. (1964). *Principles of preventive psychiatry.* New York: Basic Books.
Centers for Disease Control and Prevention. (1993). *HIV/AIDS surveillance report* (No. 2). Atlanta, GA: National Center for Infectious Diseases, Division of HIV/AIDS.
Clark, C., Curley, A., Hughes, A., & James, R. (1988). Hospice care: A model for caring for the person with AIDS. *Nursing Clinics of North America, 23,* 851–862.
Colaizzi, P. (1978). Psychological research as the phenomenologist views it. In B. Valde & M. King (Eds.), *Existential phenomenological alternatives for psychology* (pp. 48–71). New York: Oxford Press.
Crabtree, B., & Miller, W. (Eds.). (1992). *Doing qualitative research.* Newbury Park, CA: Sage Publications.

Fleuridas, C., Nelson, T., & Rosenthal, D. (1986). The evolution of circular questions: Training family therapists. *Journal of Marital and Family Therapy, 12,* 113–127.
Friedman, M. (1986). *Family nursing: Theory and assessment.* Norwalk, CT: Appleton-Century-Crofts.
Giacquinta (née Stewart), B. (1977). Helping families face the crisis of cancer. *American Journal of Nursing, 77,* 1585–1588.
Giacquinta (née Stewart), B. (1989). Researching the effects of AIDS on families. *American Journal of Hospice Care, 6*(3), 31–36.
Giacquinta (née Stewart), B. (1990). Psychosocial case report: Attachment responses in a family affected by AIDS. *AIDS Patient Care, 4*(2), 19–22.
Glaser, B., & Strauss, A. (1965). *Awareness of dying.* Chicago: Aldine Publishing Company.
Glaser, B., & Strauss, A. (1967). *The discovery of grounded theory: Strategies for qualitative research.* Chicago: Aldine Publishing Company.
Goetz, J., & LeCompte, M. (1984). *Ethnography and qualitative design in educational research.* New York: Academic Press.
Gross, D., Fogg, L., & Conrad, B. (1993). Designing interventions in psychosocial research. *Archives of Psychiatric Nursing, 7,* 259–264.
Guerin, P. (Ed.). (1976). *Family therapy: Theory and practice.* New York: Gardener Press.
Kavanaugh, R. (1974). *Facing death.* Baltimore, MD: Penguin Books.
Kerr, M., & Bowen, M. (1988). *Family evaluation: An approach based on Bowen theory.* New York: W. W. Norton & Company.
Knafl, K., & Breitmayer, B. (1989). Triangulation in qualitative research: Issues of conceptual clarity and purpose. In J. M. Morse (Ed.), *Qualitative nursing research: A contemporary dialogue* (pp. 209–220). Rockville, MD: Aspen.
Kübler-Ross, E. (1969). *On death and dying.* New York: Macmillan.
Larson, E., & Ropka, M. (1991). An update on nursing research and HIV infection. *Image: Journal of Nursing Scholarship, 22*(4), 4–12.
Meyers, D. (1989). *Self, society and personal choice.* New York: Columbia University Press.
Murphy, S. (1990). Human responses to transitions: A holistic nursing perspective. *Holistic Nursing Practice, 4*(3), 1–7.
Oiler, C. (1982). The phenomenological approach in nursing research. *Nursing Research, 31,* 178–181.
Palazzoli, S., Boscolo, L., Cecchin, G., & Prata, G. (1980). Hypothesizing-circularity-neutrality: Three guidelines for the conductor of the session. *Family Process, 19,* 3–12.
Penn, P. (1982). Circular questioning. *Family Process, 21,* 267–280.
Polit, D., & Hungler, B. (1978). *Nursing research: Principles and methods.* Philadelphia: J. B. Lippincott Company.
Riessman, C. (1993). *Narrative analysis.* Newbury Park, CA: Sage Publications.
Rolland, J. (1984). Toward a psychosocial typology of chronic and life-threatening illness. *Family Systems Medicine, 2,* 245–260.
Smith, D., & Shamansky, S. (1983). Determining the market for family nurse practitioner services: The Seattle experience. *Nursing Research, 32,* 301–305.

Walker, G. (1991). *In the midst of winter: Systemic therapy with families, couples, and individuals with AIDS infection.* New York: W. W. Norton & Company.

Wiens, A. (1993). Autonomy in care: A theoretical framework for nursing. *Professional Nursing, 9,* 95–103.

Worthington, E. (1987). Treatment of families during life transitions: Matching treatment to family response. *Family Process, 26,* 295–308.

Acknowledgments. The qualitative studies underpinning this article were supported in part through a Pace University Scholarly Research Award, two Pace University Summer Research Grants, and a Robert Wood Johnson Foundation Grant. A version of this article was presented at The Lienhard School of Nursing, The Hastings Center, and Dyson Center for Applied Ethics Conference, Family Decision-Making in End-of-Life Decisions, on December 7, 1993, at Pace University.

Response
Kathleen M. Nokes

Six different research studies, spanning the time period between November 1986 and August 1993, were summarized in this article. All of the research involved families in which one person had HIV disease or AIDS. A variety of quantitative and qualitative methodologies were used.

The conceptual framework for this body of research contrasts family cognitive decision-makers with emotional decision-makers. According to this framework, cognitive decision-makers experience less disruption and handle stress more effectively than emotional decision-makers whose decision-making behavior is volatile. A transitional model of HIV illness in the family was developed that consists of three stages: Stage I: Living with HIV; Stage II: The Living-Dying Interval; and Stage III: Bereavement. A number of phases are identified within each of the three stages. Stage I consists of Phase I: Impact; Phase II: Disruption; Phase III: Search for Meaning; Phase IV: Informing Others; and Phase V: Engaging Emotions. Stage II consists of Phase VI: Reorganization; Phase VII: Framing Memories; and Phase VIII: Separation. Stage III consists of Phase IX: Mourning and Phase X: Alignment of the Social Network. The dichotomy between cognitive and emotional decision-making is superimposed upon this transitional model.

All of the research is interpreted through the cognitive/emotional decision-making framework. Stewart believes that nurses need to help families to retain or regain a cognitive decision style. The impact of culture, economics, and education on family behaviors is not addressed in this conceptual framework, which emphasizes cognitive decision-making. The incidence of HIV infection is particularly high in the gay male community and communities of color. The lack of recognition of the impact of factors such as culture and economics may constitute a weakness of the framework, especially when it is applied to families who do not reflect the culture of the American majority.

While Stewart proposes that this transitional model of HIV illness in the family can help to describe end-of-life decisions, it would seem that its purpose could be even broader. The transitional model could be used to address the longitudinal process of living with a person with HIV/AIDS within a family relationship. It is not clear whether phases within each of the stages are dependent upon achieving the components of the prior phase or whether phases can be addressed simultaneously. Because the stages in the transitional model are dependent upon the infected client's stage of HIV disease, they are longitudinal:

Living with HIV comes before the active dying stage, which comes before dying.

This is an impressive body of important research. Some issues, however, either need to be addressed or need clarification. One of the issues is informed consent. Stewart does not address how she obtained Institutional Review Board approval nor does she specify how informed consent was obtained from the families. It is not clear whether the families were given a copy of the audiotapes or how feedback from the rather close relationship that seemed to evolve between Stewart and the families was addressed. Unlike families in which one member has cancer, HIV/AIDS is often diagnosed in more than one member of the family. A typical pattern secondary to heterosexual transmission is a father with AIDS, a mother with HIV disease, and one or more children who are also infected. A common pattern that emerges from male-to-male sexual transmission is that both partners are experiencing a variety of symptoms from HIV disease and one partner may be dying from AIDS. HIV infection of multiple family members is not addressed in this research.

Stewart's initial pilot study was conducted during 1986 to 1987. The term AIDS-related complex (ARC) had been used in the past to describe certain clusters of symptoms; this term is no longer used from either a clinical or public health perspective (Flaskerud, 1992). Rather, the Centers for Disease Control and Prevention in 1993 designated the clinical categories of HIV disease as asymptomatic, acute (primary) HIV, symptomatic, and AIDS.

The finding that three fifths of the sample decided to cope by themselves, never knowing another family with HIV infection and never seeking individual counseling, psychotherapy, or community group services, is striking. Nurses, as direct health care providers, may serve as one of the few persons with whom the family with HIV disease can communicate about their worries, fears, and questions. In the face of overwhelming isolation, this opportunity to comfort and to teach cannot be missed. The nurse working in the ambulatory care setting must recognize the need to provide extra time to these family members; nurses working in the acute care setting must include the needs of the family while intervening for the client; and the nurse working in a home care setting (who probably can best appreciate the extent of this isolation) must be given the extra time and flexibility to address the needs of other family members. It is very likely that these clients will not access the services of the more experienced providers such as the clinical nurse specialist. The nurse who is working as a direct care provider needs to be encouraged and supported to reach out to these families and address their needs. In addition, programs that create support groups may not always be appropriate for these families. While individual interventions are often more costly than group sessions, families may be more willing to use services that are established to meet their individual needs and are delivered in a "safe" environment such as their home.

The transitional model developed by Stewart can be used by health care providers who are working with families and individuals infected/affected by HIV. It is an important contribution to the growing body of knowledge about how to intervene with persons with HIV disease and their families. While it would have been more useful to practicing nurses if Stewart had addressed how the model could be applied to clinical practice, its rich description provides ample background for future work.

REFERENCE

Flaskerud, J. (1992). Overview: HIV disease and nursing. In J. Flaskerud & P. Ungvarski (Eds.), *HIV/AIDS: A guide to nursing care* (pp. 1–29). Philadelphia: W. B. Saunders.

Response
Anselm Strauss

When AIDS and HIV first began to arouse public notice as an incipient epidemic, I was introduced to its complexities by a friend, Pat Biernacki, who was becoming one of the pioneers in outreach work in the streets of San Francisco. At the time, I recollect saying that for a few years we would all be concerned with issues of morality and prevention, but that a major persisting problem, in America at least, would be to manage this new form of chronic illness. It did not take much foresight to predict that, with improved treatment, the people with HIV would be living longer—though eventually dying from AIDS—and would be cared for, like those with other chronic illnesses, both at home and in health facilities. This recollection leads me to the main theme of my commentary on Stewart's article, a commentary stimulated especially by the richness of her quotations from family members and lovers but also by my knowledge both of chronic illness and of behavior around people who are defined as dying.

As with all chronic illnesses, one useful way of thinking about this particular one is to identify some of its major features. Among those are its physiological, social, and psychological ones, but also its political features. Thus, AIDS leads inexorably eventually to death, but when and with what symptomatology are uncertain. Like many other chronic illnesses, it is treated with medications that may bring about many discomforting side effects. Social and psychological responses are also uncertain, both those of the sufferers and their families, friends, and other people. Among the more conspicuous responses are blaming of self and/or victim, rejecting, and stigmatizing, but also forgiving, closing ranks, and so on. The political aspects of HIV/AIDS are startling: the passionate debates, the legislative fights, the assertion of rights. AIDS has certainly contributed to the growing willingness in the media and in common speech to talk openly about death, as compared, say, with the 1960s, when the death and dying movement sought to counter this silence. An integral aspect of this public openness is the public visibility of the AIDS death rate, as knowledge of that rate affects both the immediately involved populations and gets filtered through the media.

But to return to the issue of the "features" of HIV/AIDS: some of these are certainly shared with other chronic illnesses. Yet some of them are, if not unique, at least more rarely characteristic of other illnesses—especially the political and the stigmatic (caused by "gay" activity) aspects. If one scrutinizes the extensive quotations in Stewart's article, in which family members so freely and passionately express themselves, it can be seen that many of their dilemmas, decisions, reactions, and behaviors are not at all unique to families where a member is defined as dying. To mention just a few commonalities: despair follows the dread diagnosis (especially if death is involved)—the many autobiographies of people who have written about this are vivid in their description. Not unusual either is the anger at and acute hopelessness of family members when they find they cannot prevent hospital staffs from keeping their relative or lover alive beyond the point where it is senseless, they believe, to do so. Also, the many closure gestures and rituals that are reflected in Stewart's quotes are well known by anyone who has lived through or studied the last phases of dying and those shortly after death. Also, certain other illnesses precipitate civic action by family members, as they find relief and gratification in working in organizations or groups associated with one or another illness. The quotations suggest many other commonalities.

Yet, what is strikingly different about some of the psychological and behavioral responses associated with dying from AIDS is also reflected in the quotations. These differential responses are connected with the special features of HIV/AIDS. Here are a few examples of those responses. For instance, parents may receive two terrible announcements simultaneously: Your son is dying, and your son is a homosexual! Reactions to this dual announcement—or just the first if you know about the homosexual identity—can be devastating. He brought it on himself. It's my fault, I have failed. What will others, even the other children, think? How do I tell this to others? The quotations reflect reactions such as a wife feeling such as a leper by association; a wife feeling isolated because her husband doesn't want to contaminate her through sexual relations; parents feeling a lack of moral support of the wider family for their dying child; your discovering the very different reactions—supportive and selfish—of your children when you tell them their gay sibling is dying. Among the most striking reactions reported by Stewart are that the bereaving families may experience long-lived alienation from their friends and the wider society but may, to the contrary, also immerse themselves in sustaining efforts on behalf of AIDS organizations.

The moral of my theme-story is that it would be useful, not just theoretically but practically, for all of us, lay people and health professionals alike, to think about HIV/AIDS in terms of similarities and differences of chronicity. Among those chronic illnesses that lead to rapid or eventual death, the phases—physiological, psychological, and social—between the diagnostic announcement and the final relief from bereavement are probably not so very different.

Yet there may be differences concerning those phases, and they are very much worth intense research scrutiny. Whether differences or similarities, I suggest that the *trajectory* model outlined in a previous issue of this journal (Corbin & Strauss, 1991) can be useful for understanding how people live with and through the last phases of life detailed in Stewart's stimulating article. The model guides the researcher or practitioner in discovering and taking into account the diverse viewpoints of all actors in the illness drama, as they intersect and change over the course of the illness. The model insists on that diversity, that interaction of actors, and that temporality. It also ensures that historical movements and social conditions are brought into the inquiry. Reactions and responses to dying are no exception to that kind of encompassing, yet potentially precise conceptualization.

REFERENCE

Corbin, J., & Strauss, A. (1991). A nursing model for chronic illness management based on the trajectory framework. *Scholarly Inquiry for Nursing Practice, 5,* 155–174. Reprinted in Woog, P. (1992). *The chronic illness trajectory framework: The Corbin and Strauss nursing model* (pp. 9–28). New York: Springer Publishing Company.

Chapter 11

Epilogue: A Proactive Model of Health Care

Juliet M. Corbin
Julie Cheitlin Cherry

The chapters in this book are a testimony to what nursing can do and the difference that it can make in the lives of those with chronic conditions. Over and over they remind us why we became nurses and how we view our part in the health care delivery system. Unfortunately, implementing the interventions suggested in these chapters is more a dream than a reality. It isn't that nurses are unwilling. Quite the contrary. They are frustrated by the constraints imposed by a modern health care system that focuses more on profit than on "care." Even in acute care hospitals, long the domain of nurses, there is very little time at the bedside. Nurses are the managers, the overseers of care. All but the most sophisticated tasks are delegated to less educated assistants. They are the ones who care for patients.

It is easy to place all of the blame on the health care system. The profession of nursing, however, also must accept some of the culpability. Rarely, if ever, have nurses pulled together as a total force and used their power to shape change; nor has nursing raised its united voice to stand up to health care providers, insurers, or lawmakers, and others who undermine the delivery of nursing. It is not nurses who have control over their working conditions and the care they deliver. Mostly, it is these other agencies. They have made productivity and reimbursement, rather than patient care, the driving forces behind health care delivery.

The problems in health care are many, there is no doubt. The challenge is to find solutions. Many have been proposed; not much has yet happened. Strangely enough, with all the focus on cost containment, the solutions are still skewed toward crisis-driven illness care. Behind it all lies one very important question: "What drives the present health care system?" The answer is not a simple one, because traditions, cost factors, and special interests are deeply woven into our present health care system. Taking care of sick people is where the financial rewards are. Making sick people well is what health professionals are trained to do and the activity from which they gain much of their work satisfaction. Yet, costs will never be reduced as long as the health care system focuses on caring for sick people. Caring for persons with chronic or any illness requires expert management, costly hospital stays, and sometimes, lengthy regimens. Despite recent efforts to contain health care costs, they are in fact escalating, largely due to the costs of managing chronic conditions ("Chronic Disease Costs," 1997). There are programs aimed at prevention, self-care, and symptom management. For the most part, these programs are few and often operate within an acute care model. Most are poorly funded and have a difficult time being self-sustaining (Federwich, 1997). It is obvious that the present health care delivery system is in need of a major overhaul.

But where do we begin? The time has come to shift the priority away from crisis-driven "acute illness" care, to preventive care, primary, secondary and tertiary, in other words, to go from a "reactive" care model to a "proactive" one. The delivery of acute care is still necessary but should be relegated to a secondary back-up role, with hospitals and other facilities ready to take over when prevention fails. In addition, health promotion and disease management cannot remain the sole domain of providers. Individuals must bear some of the responsibility for their own health and well-being. Health must become a true partnership between providers, recipients, and insurers, thereby increasing the likelihood of receiving quality care at reasonable costs. Finally, access to care must be increased, with the poor having equal access. The time has come to bring health care into the community, rather than keeping it the primary domain of hospitals or other acute care facilities. These thoughts may seem idealistic and perhaps even unobtainable. When considered more thoughtfully, however, they are not radical or even new. Much of the structure for what is proposed is already in place and nurses and others already are implementing many of these ideas (Barrett & Domurat, 1998; Madison, 1997). Patients are increasingly knowledgeable about their medical problems, largely through the Internet and other methods of mass media. They go to their physicians asking for certain tests or medications having already familiarized themselves with what is available. Many supplement their medical regimens with herbal medicines and/or other nontraditional health care forms, sometimes with the awareness and blessing of their providers, more often not.

Nursing is a powerful force! Let it use that power to shape a new health care system. No one else seems to be offering a viable alternative. Nursing has the numbers, educational practices, history of outreach, and philosophical orientation to establish the framework for what could be the standard for health care in the 21st century.

A PROACTIVE MODEL OF CARE

What we are suggesting is a "Proactive Model of Health Care Delivery." In this model, the shift in emphasis is away from acute care to prevention, primary, secondary, and tertiary. Responsibility for health is a shared one, with health professionals and individuals, families and communities equally involved. We are not talking about a halfhearted attempt or sporadic programs aimed at prevention and health maintenance. We are talking about a major philosophic change and orientation toward health care calling for a change in the *focus*, the *setting* and the *directors* of care.

From the time of conception until death persons would take an active role in maintaining their health and, by means of health education, would be empowered to do so. There would be an emphasis on assessment of populations with identification of health risks and interventions instituted to reduce those risks. Services would be geared toward keeping people healthy, with backup facilities available should they become ill. In chronic conditions the focus would be on providing persons with the training and education to maintain stability of their conditions. They would be taught to monitor their health status, to recognize signs of complications, and to act to obtain early intervention.

Rather than physicians, nurses would be the driving force behind the proactive model, as nurses traditionally have been the "teachers" and advocates of health promotion in health care. Physicians would remain in charge of "curing." The settings of care would be "community stations," health care facilities located in community settings where persons live and work. There, nurses would direct an interdisciplinary team that would provide the first line of entry into the health care system. These facilities would:

- Provide education about well childcare, disease prevention, symptom management, and so on;
- Furnish immunizations and other health preventive services;
- Arrange for and coordinate social, economic, and home supportive services;
- Arrange for and coordinate services for the chronically mentally ill;
- Do initial health screening and physicals;
- Render ongoing monitoring and intervention for those with chronic disease;
- Refer persons with medical conditions beyond the scope of outpatient care for "acute" care management as appropriate;
- Be there to promote comeback, provide hands-on care during acute and crisis phases, and arrange for counseling and support during unstable, downward, and dying illness phases;
- Do follow-up care, that is, determine whether persons received appropriate care, were carrying out regimens as directed, needed further intervention, and whether designated patient outcomes were achieved.

Nurses would, of course, still provide acute care in hospitals and through home care agencies, while at the same time being a much more visible force because of their presence in the community. The proposed role for nursing is not far from the public health nursing model of recent times, in which nurses played a significant role in the decrease, and even eradication, of infectious diseases. What is different from the older model is the emphasis on the prevention and management of *chronic* as well as infectious diseases. Education and communication would be the primary tools for implementation of this model. These would not only occur in "community stations" but also through the Internet, reaching out into schools, parks and recreation facilities, clinics, hospitals, and other public places. Monitoring patients' well-being in their homes would occur via the telephone, through e-mail, telemedicine (Nelson, 1997), and other computer-driven devices, such as the Health Buddy.[1] This device monitors patient health status and

---

1. Health Buddy is a product under development by the Health Hero Network, Inc., 2570 West El Camino Real, Suite 222, Mountain View, California 94040.

compliance while at the same time supporting a partnership between providers and recipients. Nurses and other health care professionals would make home visits when necessary. There, they would counsel, monitor, teach, make arrangements and referrals, do hands-on care, coordinate and do follow-up care. There would be more nurse-run special clinics, such as lipid, heart failure, asthma, and diabetes management clinics, either in the community or perhaps connected to a local hospital, where patients could receive intensive monitoring and the education they need to manage their chronic conditions. Nurses would conduct childbirth preparation classes in neighborhoods, then follow with early postpartum and newborn assessment visits. As stated, much of this is already being done through Parish Nursing, in Nurse-Managed Centers, and other nursing outreach programs. Once again, *here* we are talking about a large scale and nation-wide effort that acts on the premise that the only way to reduce health care costs is to promote measures that maintain health and increase access to care, that make full use of nurses, the largest professional body in the health care industry.

There are some potential problems with implementation of such a model. First, Health Maintenance Organizations and other insurers would have to be convinced that the model would cut costs (Greene, Lovely, & Ondrich, 1993). At first, while the "reactive" and "proactive" models coexisted and while the former was phased out, expenditures would be considerable. The new model could be phased in gradually, with small programs implemented in targeted high-risk geographic areas and populations (Clark, 1998). As the newer model takes over, costs should gradually decrease. Second, there may be considerable resistance from physicians and drug companies, who benefit from caring for "illness." In the latter case, they might look to dentistry. Dentists have shifted to a prevention model, but so far they haven't been put out of business! Third, there is the need to convince the general population that it is they, and not health providers, that hold the *key* to wellness. From the time of birth persons must be socialized to take responsibility for their health. Well-being and longevity depend upon health, and health is largely related to lifestyles. There will always be some illness; the effects of heredity, infections, unknown viruses cannot be totally erased. But the incidence of illness, especially of chronic conditions such as those of the cardiovascular system and lung, can be reduced and health care costs kept under control if everyone does his or her part in preventing them.

The Proactive Model of Care presented above is just one suggestion for resolving the present health care crisis. It builds upon what is known about chronic illness and the power of nursing to make a difference in management and, ultimately, in patient outcomes. There must be a way for nurses to deliver the level of care suggested in the foregoing chapters. Though there are many discussions in nursing about its role in health care, it has never united and taken a firm stand. Let it make its voice heard. It can begin by courting those who are most likely to benefit from this approach to care: the general population. Insurers would also be interested if it could be proven that prevention saves money. The year 2000 marks a new millenium. Let it also be the start of a new health care system.

REFERENCES

Barrett, S., & Domurat, E. (November/December, 1998). Taking charge, a new model in chronic disease care. *The Clinical Advisor*, 28–37.

Chronic disease costs could soar. Health report. (1997, April 4), *San Francisco Chronicle*, p. A12.

Clark, C. (1998). Wellness self-care by healthy older adults. *Image, 30 (4)*, 351–355.

Federwisch, A. (1997). Prevention gets attention, but does it get funded? *NURSEweek, 10* (12), 1 & 13.

Greene, V. Lovely, M., & Ondrich, J. (1993). The cost-effectivness of community services in a frail elderly population. *The Gerontologist, 33*, 177–189.

Madison, M. (1997). Stanford saves money by saving lives. (1997, July 11). *San Francisco Chronicle*, p. 3.

Nelson, V. (1997). The bottom line looms large in home care's future. *NURSEweek, 10* (14), 7.

INDEX

Page numbers followed by "t" indicate tables.

Access to care, for women, difficulties in gaining, 47
Acquired immunodeficiency syndrome, 13, 176, 245–293
  blaming, 261
  disclosure, diagnosis, to family, 256–262
  lifestyles, secret from families, 263
  mourning, 280–283
    ritual, 282–283
  Names Project Quilt, 280, 281
  suicide with, 265, 278
Acquired immunodeficiency syndrome-related complex, 246
Affirmation, behavior of another, 26
Affliction. *See* Chronic sorrow
Aggression, pediatric chronic condition, 115
Aging, 51
  chronic illness, 223–244
  grief and, 209
AIDS. *See* Acquired immunodeficiency syndrome
Allergies, 161
Alzheimer's disease, 18, 176
Anger, of sibling, pediatric chronic condition, 115
Angina, relief of, coronary artery bypass surgery, 17
Anti-anginal medications, 17

Anxiety
  gender and, 34
  pediatric chronic condition, 111, 115
  of parent, 120
Approval, moral, in idea of struggle, as burden, 196
ARC. *See* acquired immunodeficiency syndrome-related complex
Arthritis, pediatric chronic condition, 108
Asthma, pediatric chronic condition, 113
Atopic dermatitis, 153
Autism, pediatric chronic condition, 108

Barriers to Health-Promoting Activities for Disabled Persons Scale, multiple sclerosis, 86
Behavioral difficulties, of sibling, pediatric chronic condition, 115
Bereavement process, 247
Biography, 185–190, 227
  defined, 185
Blaming of self, coronary artery bypass surgery, 18–30
Blood test, frequency of, cancer and, 195

Body change, women's experiences with, 54
Body image
  coronary artery bypass surgery, 53
  gender-specific values, 54
Boredom, pediatric chronic condition, 111
Brain injury, pediatric chronic condition, 108
Brief Symptom Index, psychological distress levels, 34
  coronary artery bypass surgery, 34
BSI. *See* Brief Symptom Index
Burn patients, 55

Cancer, 180–201
  activities, modifying, 192
  biography, 185–190
    conceptions of self, 185
    defined, 185
  blood test, frequency of, 195
  conceptions of self, past, giving up, 192
  continuity, 185
  discontinuousness, 185–201
  dread, 193
  frontal lobe, planning for future, 186
  future, expectations of, 186
  grounded theory method, 180–201
  hypochondriac label, avoiding, 189–190, 194
  identity, 190–192
    shifts in, 192
    uncertainty of, 189–190
  illness trajectories, 185–190
  ironical struggle, ethic of, 196
  loss of control, 180–201
  memory, internalizing, 186
  moral approval, in idea of struggle, as burden, 196
  network, supportive, 195
  pacing, 192–193
  pediatric chronic condition, 108
  predictability, loss of, 187
  Problem Centered Family Coping Inventory, 182
  resistance, 188
  resting, 192
  restoration of meaning, as goal of coping, 181
  self-blame, 193
  side effects, weighing benefits against, 195
  stress, defined, 180
  temporal disjunction, 185–201
  temporality, 185–201
  uncertainty abatement work, 192–195
  work processes, 190–192
Cerebral palsy, pediatric chronic condition, 108
Childbirth-related injuries, correction of, 55
Children, chronic conditions of, 106–151, 202–222
  aggression, 115
  anger, of sibling, 115
  anxiety, 111, 115
    of parent, 120
  arthritis, 108
  asthma, 113
  autism, 108
  behavioral difficulties, of sibling, 115
  boredom, 111
  brain injury, 108
  cancer, 108
  cerebral palsy, 108
  chronic grief, of parent, 120
  confidence, parental, 121
  congenital heart defect, 117
  coping, 124
  cystic fibrosis, 108
  depression, 115
    of parent, 120
  diabetes, 108
    insulin-dependent, 112
  divorce, 117
  emotional difficulties, of sibling, 115

entrapment, feelings of, of parent, 120
family, separation from, 111
family-as-unit of analysis studies, 126–129
family environment, 113
family interaction, 124
fatigue, of parent, 120
fear, 111
   of parent, 120
   of sibling, 115
finances, 124
financial pressures, 120
friends, making, keeping, 111
frustration, 111
gender, 113
guilt, 111
hearing disabilities, 108
heart, congenital disorder of, 108
infections, 110
informants, children, parents, teachers as, 112
information seeking, 121
isolation, of parent, 120
jealousy, of sibling, 115
kidney disease, congenital disorder of, 108
leisure, for parents, 118
liver disease, 108, 117
locus of control, maternal, 114
lung, congenital disorder of, 108
maladjustment, of sibling, 115
marital discord, 120
mental health effects, 111
mother
   assessments of, 113
   locus of control, 113
neurological diseases, 108
parents, 116, 123–126
peer relations, 115
Personal Adjustment and Role Skills Scale, 112
physical arduousness, caregiving, 118
poliomyelitis, 127

psychosocial effects, 111
Questionnaire of Resources and Stress, 124
rest, for parents, 118
schizophrenia, 117
school performance, decline in, 115
school teachers, relations with, 145
seizure disorders, 113
self esteem, parental, 121
sense of control, as parental need, 118
separation from home, with chronic condition, 111
siblings, 114–116
   responses, 115
significance of, 108–110
somatization, 115
speech disabilities, 108
spina bifida, 108
stress, parents, 116, 120
ventilator-dependent children, 117
verbal intelligence, 113
visual disabilities, 108
Chronic illness, redefining meaning of, 13
Chronic sorrow, 202–222
   aging, grief and, 209
   antecedents, prior to onset of, 212–213
   bitterness, of parents, 202–222
   chronic, defined, 204
   critical attributes, 206, 207t
   death of child, 211
   defined, 203
   dementia, 202
   depression, 210
      distinguished, 209
      in elderly, 209
   Down's syndrome child, 206
   Duchenne muscular dystropy, 214
   elderly, depression, 209
   empty space phenomenon, 221
   expression of grief, society's expectations for, 205

Chronic sorrow *(continued)*
  grief, visibility of, unresolvable, 206
  guilt, of parents, 202–222
  hiding of grief, society's expectations, 206
  illness trajectory, 213–214
  of later years, 215
  losses, with chronic illness, 202
  mentally retarded children
    developmental milestones, child could not pass, 203, 205
    parents of, 202–222
  of middle years, 214–215
  mood, 209
  multiple sclerosis, 202, 214–215
    chronic emotions of spouse caregiver, 215
  muscular dystrophy, child with, 214
  myelomeningocele child, 206
  parents, 202–222
  premature infants, 205
  progressive nature of, 216
  prolonged grief, chronic sorrow, distinguished, 208
  self-regard, reduced, 209
  time and, 213
  time frame, society's, for expression of grief, 205
  in young family trajectory, 214
Clothes, long-sleeved, with skin disease, 162
Cognitive appraisal model of coping, coronary artery bypass surgery, 19
Cognitive information, to promote self-care, 27
Cognitive strategies, family's, 245–293
Community stations, for health care, 296
Concealment measures, with skin disease, 162
Confidence, parental, pediatric chronic condition, 121

Congenital heart defect, pediatric chronic condition, 117
Consistent Long-Term Retrieval of Selective Reminding Test, Total Recall, multiple sclerosis, 86
Continuity, cancer and, 185
Control, loss of, cancer and, 180–201
Convalescence, defined, 39
Coping
  defined, 17
  as dynamic process, 18
Corbin, Strauss, trajectory model, elderly clients with chronic illness, 223–244
Coronary angioplasty, 37
Coronary artery bypass surgery, 16–35, 36–74
  access to care, women, difficulties in gaining, 47
  active listening, 28
  activity resumption during recovery, 57
  age and, 18
    blamed self, negative relation between, 33
    coping strategies, relationships between, 16–30
    education, coping and, 27t
  Alzheimer's disease, 18
  angina, relief of, 17
  anti-anginal medications, decreased need for, 17
  anxiety, gender and, 34
  avoidance, 18–30
  beauty, women's concern with, 55
  behavior, of another, affirming, 26
  beneficial outcomes of coronary artery bypass surgery, 17
  benefits from surgery, expections, age and, 33
  blamed self, 18–30
  body change, experiences with, 54
  body image, 53
    gender-specific values, 54

Index

Brief Symptom Index, psychological distress levels, 34
changing stressful situation, 18–30
clocks, internal, determining expectations for stages in life cycle, 44
cognitive appraisal model of coping, 19
cognitive information, to promote self-care, 27
convalescence, defined, 39
coping
  defined, 17
  as dynamic process, 18
coronary angioplasty, 37
coronary occlusive disease, timing of development of in women, 44
cosmetic changes in bodies, 55
crisis, midlife, surgical experience triggering, 44
destiny, inability to control, 50
diagnostic procedures, for management of coronary heart disease, gender differences, 46
diet, blaming self for, 28
disturbed mood state, gender and, 34
education, 18
  age, coping and, 27t
  coping strategies, relationships between, 16–30
ego, somatic, 53
emotion-focused coping, 18–30, 20
emotional aid, receiving from another person, 18–30
emotional distress, 17
empathy, capacity of women for, 45
employment status and, 21
entry, into health care system, delayed, women, 47
epiphany quality, of surgery, male, 44
exercise, lack of, blaming self for, 28
exercise tolerance, improved, 17

expectations of surgery, age and, 33
exposure to death, gender differences, 45
extended life expectancy, potential for, 17
family
  disruption, 51
  social support provided by, 26
  turning to, following discharge, 27
fear and, 54
friends
  social support provided by, 26
  turning to, following discharge, 27
function, male concern with, 55
gender, 18, 21
  bias, 37, 46
    in diagnosis, treatment, 70
  coping strategies, relationships between, 16–30
  development, inherent difference in, 44
goals of surgery, expections, age and, 33
graying of America, 51
health professionals
  social support provided by, 26
  turning to, early in experience, 27
highest educational level and, 21
household work, resumption of, 39
incision, meaning of, gender and, 53
independence, relinquishment of, sense of loss, 52
indirect psychological strategies, women, 49
individuation, male gender development and, 44
inevitability of illness, belief in, 47
informational aid, receiving from another person, 18–30
inhibition, women and, 49–50
intergenerational interdependence during illness, 52
internal clocks, determining expectations for stages in life cycle, 44

Coronary artery bypass surgery *(continued)*
  interpretation of clinical events, patient's, understanding of, 37
  interpretive framework, acknowledging individual's, 37
  language
    barrier, between genders, 51
    of women, 50
  learned helplessness, 50
  leisure activities, resumption of, 17
  life expectancy, extended, potential for, 17
  living alone, 39
  male patients, spousal availability, 39
  marital status and, 21
  material aid, giving of, 26
  meanings assigned to surgical experience, gender differ in, 44
  mediastinal incisional discomfort, 57
  medications, anti-anginal, 17
  menses, 54
  mental illness, among women, 50
  midlife crisis, surgical experience triggering, 44
  mother, separation from, gender identity and, 44
  mutilation fears, of female patients, 54
  myocardial infarction, 18
  nature of recovery process, 36–73
  "near death" experience, surgery as, 44
  parameters, to assess progress in recovery, 36–73
  passive psychological strategies, women, 49
  passivity, women and, 49–50
  paternalistic world, medicine, 51
  patient's interpretation of clinical events, understanding of, 37
  perceptions, of another, endorsing, 26
  personal relations, interruption of, 34
  physiologic, psychosocial outcomes, discrepancy between, 17
  positive affect between persons, expression of, 26
  positive aspects of situation, focusing on, 28
  power gradients, between communicants, 50
  powerlessness, expectation of, 50
  problem focused coping, 18–30
  professional careers, interruption of, 34
  Profile of Mood States, 45
  psychological distress levels, Brief Symptom Index, 34
  psychomotor information, to promote self-care, 27
  psychosocial problems, 17
  race and, 21
  reassurance, 28
  relationship orientation, of women, 45
  remapping of relationships, in recovery, 51
  resumption of activities, 39
  role
    negotiation, while healing, 52
    responsibilities, multiple, women, 48
    of women, multiplicity of, 39
  scars
    males and, 56
    meaning of, gender and, 53
  security, sense of, 53
  seeking social support strategies, 33
  seeks social support coping, 20, 22
  self-concept, 53
  self-esteem, 53
  self monitoring, lack of, by women, 48
  sense of wholeness, threat to, 54
  separation from mother

gender identity and, 44
male gender development and, 44
sexual activity, 17
sexual objectification, 54
smoking, blaming self for, 28
social activities, resumption of, 17
social support, seeking, 18–30
sources of social support, change in, 27
stenosis, left main coronary artery, 17
stories of illness, importance of, doubt about, 44
submissiveness, women and, 49–50
support groups, for patients, families, 26
surgical experience, meanings assigned to, gender differ in, 44
surgical incisions, gender responses to, 56
symbolic aid, giving of, 26
symptoms
  awareness of, by women, 48
  reporting in terms of feelings, 51
telephone call-back systems, 26
telephone coaching, 34
timeliness, sense of, for life experiences, 44
treatment procedures, for management of coronary heart disease, gender differences, 46
triple vessel disease, 17
tutor, professional, need for, 33
visiting hours, flexible, 26
Ways of Coping Checklist, 20
  Revised, 20
wishful thinking, 18–30
women
  outliving spouse, 39
  relationship orientation of, 45
work, return to, 17
wound care, 57
Coronary occlusive disease, timing of development of in women, 44

Cost containment, focus on, 295
Covering of skin lesions, with skin disease, 162
Crime, concern about, multiple sclerosis and, 80
Crisis-driven illness care, 295
Cystic fibrosis, pediatric chronic condition, 108

Dementia, 202
Depression
  chronic sorrow, 210
    distinguished, 209
  in elderly, 209
  pediatric chronic condition, 115
  parent, 120
Destiny, inability to control, 50
Developmental life stages, individual, Freud, theory of, 246
Diabetes, 231
  pediatric chronic condition, 108
  insulin-dependent, 112
  Type I, 176t
Diagnosis, receiving, 4
Diagnostic procedures, for management of coronary heart disease, gender differences, 46
Diet, blaming self for, coronary artery bypass surgery, 28
Discontinuousness, cancer and, 185–201
Discovery, diagnosis, cope with implications of, 4
Disturbed mood state, gender and, 34
Divorce, pediatric chronic condition, as cause of, 117
Do Not Resuscitate form, 277
Down's syndrome child, 206
Dread, cancer and, 193
Duchenne muscular dystropy, 214

Educational level, 18
  coping strategies, relationships between, 16–30

Ego, somatic, coronary artery bypass surgery, 53
Elderly
　with chronic illness, 223–244
　depression, 209
Elderly clients with chronic illness, 223–244
Emotion-focused coping, 18–30
Emotional aid, receiving from another person, 18–30
Emotional decision-making, 13
Emotional distress, coronary artery bypass surgery, 17
Emphysema, 176
Employment status, coronary artery bypass surgery, 21
Empty space phenomenon, 221
End-of-life family decision-making, 245–293
Entrapment, feelings of, of parent, pediatric chronic condition, 120
Entry into health care system, delayed, women, 47
Exercise, 81
　lack of, blaming self for, coronary artery bypass surgery, 28
　multiple sclerosis, 80, 91
Exercise tolerance, improved, 17
Expectations of surgery, age and, 33
Exposure to death, gender differences, 45
Expression of grief, society's expectations for, 205
Extended life expectancy, potential for, 17

Family
　decision-making, end-of-life, 245–293
　disruption, coronary artery bypass surgery, 51
　social support provided by, 26
　turning to, following discharge, 27
Fatigue, of parent, pediatric chronic condition, 120
Fear
　coronary artery bypass surgery, 54
　of parent, pediatric chronic condition, 120
　pediatric chronic condition, 111
　of sibling, pediatric chronic condition, 115
Financial pressures, pediatric chronic condition, 120
Flare-ups, skin disease, 157
Freud, Sigmund, individual developmental life stages, theory of, 246
Friends
　making, keeping, pediatric chronic condition, 111
　social support provided by, coronary artery bypass surgery, 26, 27
Frontal lobe, planning for future, 186
Frustration, pediatric chronic condition, 111
Future, expectations of, cancer and, 186

Gender
　anxiety and, 34
　bias, 46
　　coronary artery bypass surgery, 37
　development, inherent difference in, 44
General Self-Efficacy, subscale of Self-Efficacy Scale, multiple sclerosis, 88
Genetic factors, risk for development of chronic condition, 4
Goals of surgery, expectations, age and, 33
Graying of America, 51
Grief. *See* Chronic sorrow
　expression of, society's expectations for, 205
　of parent, pediatric chronic

condition, 120
  prolonged, chronic sorrow, distinguished, 208
  visibility of, unresolvable, 206
Grounded theory, cancer and, 180–201
Guilt, pediatric chronic condition, 111

Health professionals, turning to, early in experience, 27
Health promoting lifestyle, multiple sclerosis, 81–82, 88
  profile, 94
Hearing disabilities, pediatric chronic condition, 108
Heart. See also Coronary artery bypass surgery
  congenital disorder of, pediatric chronic condition, 108
  defect, congenital, pediatric chronic condition, 117
Herbal medicines, 296
Hiding of grief, society's expectations, 206
HIV. See Human immunodeficiency virus
Homemakers, nurturant roles for, 81
Household work, resumption of, after coronary artery bypass surgery, 39
Human immunodeficiency virus, 13, 245–293
  blaming, 261
  disclosure, diagnosis, to family, 256–262
  lifestyles, secret from families, 263
  mourning, 280–283
    ritual, 282–283
  Names Project Quilt, 280, 281
  suicide with, 265, 278
Hypochondriac label, avoiding, 189–190, 194

Identity, cancer and, 190–192
  shifts in, 192
  uncertainty of, 189–190
Incapacity Status Scale, 86
Incision, coronary artery bypass surgery, meaning of, gender and, 53
Income, 79
  quality of life and, 83
Independence, relinquishment of, sense of loss, 52
Individual developmental life stages, Freud, theory of, 246
Individuation, male gender development and, 44
Inevitability of illness, belief in, 47
Infections, pediatric chronic condition, 110
Informants, pediatric chronic condition, children, parents, teachers as, 112
Informational aid, receiving from another person, coronary artery bypass surgery, 18–30
Inhibition, women and, 49–50
Insulin-dependent diabetes, pediatric chronic condition, 112
Intergenerational interdependence during illness, 52
Internal clocks, determining expectations for stages in life cycle, 44
Internet, use of, 296
Interpretation of clinical events, coronary artery bypass surgery, patient's, understanding of, 37
Interpretive framework, coronary artery bypass surgery, acknowledging individual's, 37
Ironical struggle, ethic of, cancer and, 196
Isolation
  of parent, pediatric chronic condition, 120
  from social situations, with skin disease, 162

ISS. *See* Incapacity Status Scale
Itching, with skin disease, 161

Jealousy, of sibling, pediatric chronic condition, 115
Jogging, 82

Kidney disease, pediatric chronic condition, 108
Kubler-Ross, Elizabeth, 247

Lamentation. *See* Chronic sorrow
Language
  barrier, between genders, 51
  of women, 50
Learned helplessness, 50
Leisure
  for parents, pediatric chronic condition, 118
  resumption of, coronary artery bypass surgery, 17
Length of illness, 93
Life expectancy, extended, potential for, 17
  coronary artery bypass surgery, 17
Lifestyle behaviors, risk for development of chronic condition, 4
Liniments, skin disease, 160
Liver disease, pediatric chronic condition, 108, 117
Living alone, 39
Locus of control, maternal, pediatric chronic condition, 114
Long-sleeved clothes, with skin disease, 162
Long-term periodic sadness, experience in reaction to continual losses. *See* Chronic sorrow
Lumbosacral disc disease, 176
Lung, pediatric chronic condition, 108

Maladjustment, of sibling, pediatric chronic condition, 115
Manager, nurse as, 294

Marriage
  discord, pediatric chronic condition, 120
  status, coronary artery bypass surgery, 21
Mass media, use of, 296
Material aid, giving of, coronary artery bypass surgery, 26
Meanings assigned to surgical experience, gender differ in, 44
Mediastinal incisional discomfort, coronary artery bypass surgery, 57
Medications, anti-anginal, 17
Memory, internalizing, cancer and, 186
Mental health effects, pediatric chronic condition, 111
Mental illness, among women, 50
Mentally retarded children
  chronic sorrow, parents of, 202–222
  developmental milestones, child could not pass, 203, 205
  parents of, 202–222
  shock, of parents, 202–222
Midlife crisis, surgical experience triggering, 44
Milestones, child not passing, 203, 205
Moral approval, in idea of struggle, as burden, 196
Mother
  locus of control, pediatric chronic condition, 113
  separation from, gender identity and, 44
Multiple sclerosis, 75–105, 202, 214–215
  age and, 93
  availability of services, 79
  Barriers to Health-Promoting Activities for Disabled Persons Scale, 86
  chronic emotions of spouse caregiver, 215

conflict, 91
Consistent Long-Term Retrieval of Selective Reminding Test, Total Recall, 86
cost, of services, 79
crime, concern about, 80
demands of illness, 93
  perceived, 80
education, 93
everyday life, effect of illness on, 81
exercise, 80, 81, 91
financial resources, 80, 93, 94
functional disability, 93
gender and, 93
General Self-Efficacy subscale of Self-Efficacy Scale, 88
health promoting behaviors, 81–82, 88, 94
homemakers, nurturant roles for, 81
Incapacity Status Scale, 86
income, 79
  quality of life and, 83
interpersonal support, 91
jogging, 82
length of illness, 93
living situations, quality of life and, 83
Neuropsychological Screening Battery for Multiple Sclerosis, 86
number cognitive tests failed, 93
nutrition, 80, 81, 91
perceived health, 80, 93
physical functioning, quality of life and, 83
quality of life, 82–83
Quality of Life Index, 89
reciprocity, 91
recreation, restrictions in, 81
reduced labor-market activity, 81
rest, 80
restrictions in, 81
self-actualization, 91
self-efficacy, 80, 93
self-rated abilities, 93

Self-Rated Abilities for Health Practices Scale, 87
sexual activity and, 81
social support, 79, 81, 91, 93
spinal cord injury, 82
spouse caregiver, chronic emotions of, 215
stress management, 81, 91
stretching exercises, 82
swimming, 82
tennis, 82
time, lack of, 80
tiredness, 80
Muscular dystrophy, child with, 214
Mutilation fears, of female patients, 54
Myelomeningocele child, 206
Myocardial infarction, coronary artery bypass surgery, 18

Near death experience, surgery as, 44
Neurological diseases, pediatric chronic condition, 108
Neuropsychological Screening Battery for Multiple Sclerosis, 86
Nontraditional health care forms, 296
NSBMS. *See* Neuropsychological Screening Battery for Multiple Sclerosis
Nurse, as force behind proactive model, 296
Nutrition, 80, 81, 91

Parents, pediatric chronic condition, 123–126
Parkinson's disease, gradual onset, 176
PARS II. *See* Personal Adjustment and Role Skills Scale
Passive psychological strategies, women, 49
Paternalism in medicine, 51
PCFCI. *See* Problem Centered Family Coping Inventory

Pediatric chronic condition, 106–151, 202–222
  aggression, 115
  anger, of sibling, 115
  anxiety, 111, 115
    of parent, 120
  arthritis, 108
  asthma, 113
  autism, 108
  behavioral difficulties, of sibling, 115
  boredom, 111
  brain injury, 108
  cancer, 108
  cerebral palsy, 108
  chronic grief, of parent, 120
  chronic sorrow, 202–222
  confidence, parental, 121
  congenital heart defect, 117
  coping, 124
  cystic fibrosis, 108
  depression, 115
    of parent, 120
  diabetes, 108
    insulin-dependent, 112
  divorce, 117
  emotional difficulties, of sibling, 115
  entrapment, feelings of, of parent, 120
  family
    environment, 113
    interaction, 124
    separation from, 111
  family-as-unit of analysis studies, 126–129
  fatigue, of parent, 120
  fear, 111
    of parent, 120
    of sibling, 115
  finances and, 120, 124
  friends, making, keeping, 111
  frustration, 111
  gender, 113
  guilt, 111
  hearing disabilities, 108
  heart, congenital disorder of, 108
  infections, 110
  informants, children, parents, teachers as, 112
  information seeking, 121
  isolation, of parent, 120
  jealousy, of sibling, 115
  kidney disease, congenital disorder of, 108
  leisure, for parents, 118
  liver disease, 108, 117
  locus of control, maternal, 114
  lung, congenital disorder of, 108
  maladjustment, of sibling, 115
  marital discord, 120
  mental health effects, 111
  mother
    assessments of, 113
    locus of control, 113
  neurological diseases, 108
  parents, 116, 123–126
  peer relations, 115
  Personal Adjustment and Role Skills Scale, 112
  physical arduousness, caregiving, 118
  poliomyelitis, 127
  psychosocial effects, 111
  Questionnaire of Resources and Stress, 124
  rest, for parents, 118
  schizophrenia, 117
  school performance, decline in, 115
  school teachers, relations with, 145
  seizure disorders, 113
  self-efficacy, parental, 121
  self esteem, parental, 121
  sense of control, as parental need, 118
  separation from home, with chronic condition, 111
  siblings, 114–116
    significance of, 108–110
  somatization, 115
  speech disabilities, 108
  spina bifida, 108

stress, parents, 116, 120
ventilator-dependent children, 117
verbal intelligence, 113
visual disabilities, 108
Peer relations, pediatric chronic condition, 115
Perceptions of another, endorsing, 26
Periodic sadness, long-term, experience in reaction to continual losses. *See* Chronic sorrow
Personal Adjustment and Role Skills Scale, 112
Personal relations, interruption of, coronary artery bypass surgery, 34
Phases of illness, trajectory, 4–5t
Philosophic change, in health care, need for, 296
Physical arduousness, of caregiving, 118
Physical exercise. *See* Exercise
Physical functioning, quality of life and, 83
Physiologic, psychosocial outcomes, discrepancy between, 17
Planning for future, frontal lobe, 186
Poliomyelitis, pediatric chronic condition, 127
Positive affect between persons, expression of, 26
Power gradients, between communicants, 50
Powerlessness, expectation of, 50
Predictability, loss of, cancer and, 187
Premature infants, 205
Pretrajectory phase of illness, 4
Prevention, focus on, 294–299
Proactive model, health care, 294–299
Problem Centered Family Coping Inventory, 182
Problem-focused coping, 18–30
Professional careers, interruption of, coronary artery bypass surgery, 34
Profile of Mood States, 45
Psoriasis, 153
Psychological distress levels, Brief Symptom Index, coronary artery bypass surgery, 34
Psychomotor information, to promote self-care, coronary artery bypass surgery, 27
Psychosocial effects, pediatric chronic condition, 111
Psychosocial reintegration, 6

QLI. *See* Quality of Life Index
Quality of life, 82–83
  living situations, 83
Quality of Life Index, 89
Questionnaire of Resources and Stress, 124

Reactions caused in others, conscious of, with skin disease, 162
Reactive care model, to proactive, 295
Recreation, restrictions in, multiple sclerosis, 81
Regret. *See* Chronic sorrow
Relationship orientation, of women, 45
Remapping of relationships, in recovery, 51
Rest, multiple sclerosis, 80
Restoration of meaning, as goal of coping, 181
Resumption of activities, after coronary artery bypass surgery, 39
Risk for development of chronic condition, genetic, lifestyle factors, 4
Roles
  negotiation, while healing, 52
  responsibilities, multiple, women, 48
  of women, multiplicity of, 39

Sadness. *See* Chronic sorrow
Scars, males and, 56
Schizophrenia, pediatric chronic condition, 117
School performance, decline in, pediatric chronic condition, 115
Seeks social support coping, 20, 22, 33
Seizure disorders, pediatric chronic condition, 113
Self-actualization, 91
Self-blame, cancer and, 193
Self-concept, coronary artery bypass surgery, 53
Self-efficacy, 80, 93
   parental, pediatric chronic condition, 121
Self esteem, chronic illness and, 53, 121
Self monitoring, lack of, by women, 48
Self-rated abilities, 93
Self-Rated Abilities for Health Practices scale, 87
Sense of control, as parental need, pediatric chronic condition, 118
Separation
   from home, with chronic condition, 111
   from mother, gender identity and, 44
Sexual objectification, women and, 54
Siblings, pediatric chronic condition, 114–116
Side effects, weighing benefits against, cancer and, 195
Skin disease, chronic, 152–179
   allergies, 161
   atopic dermatitis, 153
   baths, 160
   boss, problematic relations with, 160
   burdens of living with disease, 157–162
   concealment measures, 162
   covering of skin lesions, 162
   emotional burdens, 157
   flare-ups, 157
   isolation, from social situations, 162
   itching, 161
   liniments, 160
   long-sleeved clothes, 162
   nonacceptance of disease, by family, colleagues, 160
   pain, 161
   preventive measures, 160
   psoriasis, 153
   reactions caused in others, conscious of, 162
   self-control, demand for, 160
   self-monitoring, 160
   self-treatment, 160
   soreness, 161
   spouse, problematic relations with, 160
   stiffness, 161
   stigma, feeling of, 160
   stress, 157, 160
   symptoms, 161
   topical applications, 160
   uncontrollable nature of, 157
   visibility of, 157
   work-role, 161
Smoking, blaming self for, 28
Social activities, resumption of, 17
Soreness, with skin disease, 161
Sorrow, chronic, 202–222
   aging, grief and, 209
   antecedents, prior to onset of, 212–213
   bitterness, of parents, 202–222
   chronic, defined, 204
   critical attributes, 206, 207t
   death of child, 211
   defined, 203
   dementia, 202
   depression
      distinguished, 209
      in elderly, 209
   depression and, 210
   Down's syndrome child, 206

Duchenne muscular dystropy, 214
elderly, depression, 209
empty space phenomenon, 221
expression of grief, society's expectations for, 205
grief, visibility of, unresolvable, 206
guilt, of parents, 202–222
hiding of grief, society's expectations, 206
illness trajectory, 213–214
of later years, 215
losses, with chronic illness, 202
mentally retarded children
    developmental milestones, child could not pass, 203, 205
    parents of, 202–222
of middle years, 214–215
mood, 209
multiple sclerosis, 202, 214–215
    chronic emotions of spouse caregiver, 215
muscular dystrophy, child with, 214
myelomeningocele child, 206
parents, 202–222
premature infants, 205
progressive nature of, 216
prolonged grief, chronic sorrow, distinguished, 208
self-regard, reduced, 209
time and, 213
time frame, society's, for expression of grief, 205
in young family trajectory, 214
Speech disabilities, pediatric chronic condition, 108
Spina bifida, pediatric chronic condition, 108
Spinal cord injury, 82
SRAHP. *See* Self-Rated Abilities for Health Practices scale
Stenosis, left main coronary artery, 17
Stiffness, with skin disease, 161
Stigma, feeling of, with skin disease, 160
Stories of illness, importance of, doubt about, 44
Strauss, Corbin, trajectory model, elderly clients with chronic illness, 223–244
Stress, defined, 180
Stretching exercises, 82
Stroke, acute onset, 176
Support groups, for patients, families, 26
Surgical incisions, gender responses to, 56
Swimming, 82
Symbolic aid, giving of, 26
Symptoms
    appearance of, 4
    awareness of, by women, 48
    reporting in terms of feelings, 51

Telephone call-back systems, 26
Telephone coaching, coronary artery bypass surgery, 34
Temporal disjunction, cancer and, 185–201
Tennis, 82
Time, lack of, 80
Time frame, society's, for expression of grief, 205
Timeliness, sense of, for life experiences, 44
Tiredness, multiple sclerosis, 80
Topical applications, with skin disease, 160
Triple vessel disease, coronary artery bypass surgery, 17
Tutor, professional, need for, 33

Uncertainty abatement work, cancer and, 192–195
Uncontrollable nature, with skin disease, 157

Vaginal-vesicular fistulae, correction of, 55
Ventilator-dependent children, pediatric chronic condition, 117

Visibility, with skin disease, 157
Visiting hours, flexible, 26
Visual disabilities, pediatric chronic condition, 108

Ways of Coping Checklist, Revised, 20
Ways of Coping Scale, 20

WCCL. *See* Ways of Coping Checklist
Wholeness, sense of, coronary artery bypass surgery, threat to, 54
Wishful thinking, coping and, 18–30
Wound care, coronary artery bypass surgery, 57

Springer Publishing Company

Scholarly Inquiry for Nursing Practice

Elizabeth R. Lenz, PhD, RN, FAAN,
Ruth Bernstein Hyman, PhD,
Audrey G. Gift, PhD, RN, FAAN,
and **Pierre Woog,** PhD, Editors

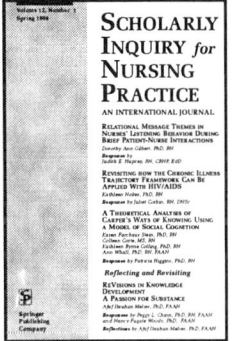

Scholarly Inquiry for Nursing Practice applies the spirit of inquiry to every aspect of nursing practice. What is empathy? How do family caregivers deal with their altered lives? Is nursing an aesthetic experience? Topics are broad ranging, from nursing research (basic and applied), to conceptual model-building and instrument construction, to philosophical perspectives on nursing science.

Articles often cross disciplinary and international borders to bring readers up-to-date, thought-provoking, and penetrating analyses of nursing practice, research and theory. Each article is accompanied by commentary of a noted expert on the topic, so that readers can get an immediate sense of the material's significance in the field.

Sample Contents: Relational Message Themes in Nurses' Listening Behavior During Brief Patient-Nurse Interactions, *Dorothy Ann Gilbert* • Response by *Judith E. Hupcey* • Revisiting How the Chronic Illness Trajectory Framework Can Be Applied with HIV/AIDS, *Kathleen Nokes* • Response by *Juliet Corbin* • The Dark Side of Nursing: Negative Outcomes and Constructive Strategies, *Mary C. Corley* • Response by *Patricia Stevens* • The Theory of Unpleasant Symptoms and Alzheimer's Disease, *Sally A. Hutchinson and Holly Skodol Wilson* • Response by *Elizabeth Lenz and Audrey Gift* • Wives, Husbands, and Daughters of Dementia Patients: Predictors of Caregivers' Health, *Martha B. Sparks* • Response by *Patricia Archbold and Barbara Stewart*

Two issues have been published as books—each winning an AJN Book of the Year Award and one was also selected as Nurse Practitioner Book of the Year.

Abstracted in: Cumulative Index for Nursing and Allied Health Literature, Index Medicus/MEDLINE, International Nursing Index & Nursing Citation Index, Behavioral Medicine Abstracts, Psychological Abstracts, PsychINFO & PsychLIT, Social Services Abstracts, Sociological Abstracts.

Volume 14, 2000 • 4 issues • ISSN 0889-7182

536 Broadway, New York, NY 10012-3955 • (212) 431-4370 • Fax (212) 941-7842

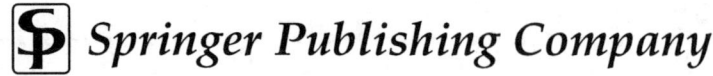**Springer Publishing Company**

CHRONIC ILLNESS TRAJECTORY FRAMEWORKS
The Corbin and Strauss Nursing Model
Pierre Woog, PhD, Editor

"We believe that this book can engender a significant change in how we regard chronic illness disease and the betterment of health."

—**from the Introduction**

A nursing model for chronic illness management, and reactions to it by six nurse experts experienced in the realities of helping people with cancer, cardiac conditions, mental illness, diabetes, multiple sclerosis, and HIV/AIDS. A text for all nurses and nursing students.

Contents:
- Introduction, Pierre Woog
- A Nursing Model for Chronic Illness Management Based upon the Trajectory Framework, *Juliet M. Corbin and Anselm Strauss*
- The Trajectory of Cancer Recovery, *Diane Scott Dorsett*
- Using the Trajectory Framework: Reconceptualizing Cardiac Illness, *Mary H. Hawthorne*
- Applying the Chronic Illness Trajectory Model to HIV/AIDS, *Kathleen M. Nokes*
- Chronic Mental Illness: The Timeless Trajectory, *Marilyn M. Rawnsley*
- Use of the Trajectory Model of Nursing in Multiple Sclerosis, *Suzanne C. Smeltzer*
- Shaping the Course of a Marathon: Using the Trajectory Framework for Diabetes Mellitus, *Elizabeth A. Walker*
- Commentary, *Juliet M. Corbin, & Anselm Strauss*

Named a "Best Book of 1992" by Nurse Practitioner
Translated into Japanese and German • AJN Book of the Year Award
112pp   0-8261-8000-0   hardcover

536 Broadway, New York, NY 10012-3955 • (212) 431-4370 • Fax (212) 941-7842

Chronic illness : research and theory for nursing practice